EDITION 4

ANTIBIOTIC
BASICS FOR
CLINICIANS

The ABCs of Choosing the Right Antibacterial Agent

ALAN R. HAUSER, MD, PhD

Professor, Departments of Microbiology/Immunology and Medicine
Northwestern University
Chicago, Illinois

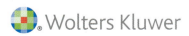

Philadelphia • Baltimore • New York • London
Buenos Aires • Hong Kong • Sydney • Tokyo

Acquisitions Editor: Matt Hauber
Development Editor: Deborah Bordeaux
Editorial Coordinator: Sunmerrilika Baskar
Marketing Manager: Danielle Klahr
Production Project Manager: Frances Gunning
Manager, Graphic Arts & Design: Stephen Druding
Art Director: Jennifer Clements
Manufacturing Coordinator: Margie Orzech
Prepress Vendor: S4Carlisle Publishing Services

Fourth edition

Copyright © 2026 Wolters Kluwer.

Copyright © 2019, 2013, 2007 Lippincott Williams & Wilkins, a Wolters Kluwer business. All rights reserved. This book is protected by copyright. No part of this book may be reproduced or transmitted in any form or by any means, including as photocopies or scanned-in or other electronic copies, or utilized by any information storage and retrieval system without written permission from the copyright owner, except for brief quotations embodied in critical articles and reviews. Materials appearing in this book prepared by individuals as part of their official duties as U.S. government employees are not covered by the above-mentioned copyright. To request permission, please contact Wolters Kluwer at Two Commerce Square, 2001 Market Street, Philadelphia, PA 19103, via email at permissions@lww.com, or via our website at shop.lww.com (products and services).

9 8 7 6 5 4 3 2 1

Printed in Mexico

Library of Congress Cataloging-in-Publication Data

Names: Hauser, Alan R., 1959- author.
Title: Antibiotic basics for clinicians : the ABCs of choosing the right antibacterial agent / Alan R. Hauser.
Description: Fourth edition. | Philadelphia : Wolters Kluwer Health, [2026] | Includes bibliographical references and index. | Summary: "Popular as a classroom text, for review, and as a clinical quick-reference, this time-saving resource helps medical students master the rationale behind antibiotic selection for common bacterial pathogens and infectious diseases. Updated content reflects the latest antibiotic medications available on the market, and new full-color illustrations strengthen users' understanding of the application of antibiotic drug treatment"— Provided by publisher.
Identifiers: LCCN 2024035265 (print) | LCCN 2024035266 (ebook) | ISBN 9781975227579 (paperback) | ISBN 9781975227586 (ebook)
Subjects: MESH: Bacterial Infections—drug therapy | Anti-Bacterial Agents—therapeutic use | Examination Questions | Outline
Classification: LCC RM267 (print) | LCC RM267 (ebook) | NLM WC 18.2 | DDC 615/.329—dc23/eng/20240909
LC record available at https://lccn.loc.gov/2024035265
LC ebook record available at https://lccn.loc.gov/2024035266

This work is provided "as is," and the publisher disclaims any and all warranties, express or implied, including any warranties as to accuracy, comprehensiveness, or currency of the content of this work.

This work is no substitute for individual patient assessment based upon healthcare professionals' examination of each patient and consideration of, among other things, age, weight, gender, current or prior medical conditions, medication history, laboratory data and other factors unique to the patient. The publisher does not provide medical advice or guidance and this work is merely a reference tool. Healthcare professionals, and not the publisher, are solely responsible for the use of this work including all medical judgments and for any resulting diagnosis and treatments.

Given continuous, rapid advances in medical science and health information, independent professional verification of medical diagnoses, indications, appropriate pharmaceutical selections and dosages, and treatment options should be made and healthcare professionals should consult a variety of sources. When prescribing medication, healthcare professionals are advised to consult the product information sheet (the manufacturer's package insert) accompanying each drug to verify, among other things, conditions of use, warnings and side effects and identify any changes in dosage schedule or contraindications, particularly if the medication to be administered is new, infrequently used or has a narrow therapeutic range. To the maximum extent permitted under applicable law, no responsibility is assumed by the publisher for any injury and/or damage to persons or property, as a matter of products liability, negligence law or otherwise, or from any reference to or use by any person of this work.

shop.lww.com

Dedicated to our son, John. Until we see you again.

Preface

Which is more difficult: learning a large body of information or applying the newly learned information? Although the answer is debatable, it is clear that health care professionals must do both. Most health care training programs consist of an initial phase of classroom lectures and small group sessions in which the intricacies of cranial nerves, the Krebs cycle, and renal physiology are mastered. Following this phase, trainees suddenly are immersed in the real world of patients who present with complaints of a cough, a painful lower back, or a fever. As an infectious disease subspecialist, I have often seen this culture shock expressed as the blank look of a medical student when asked, "So, what antibiotic should we start this patient on?" Obviously, a basic understanding of the principles of pharmacology and microbiology is insufficient for most trainees when suddenly faced with the complexities of an infected patient.

This book not only is meant to be a guide to antibiotics for students studying to be physicians, nurses, physician assistants, pharmacologists, or medical technologists but should also prove useful for residents, fellows, and practicing clinicians. It is designed to serve as a bridge between the book knowledge acquired during the initial phases of training and the reflexive prescribing habits of experienced practitioners. Just as the initial bewildering complexities of electrocardiograms and chest radiographs disappear when the first principles underlying these tests are appreciated and understood, so too do the difficulties of antibiotic selection. This book provides the rationale behind antibiotic selection for many common bacterial pathogens and infectious disease presentations so that much of the memorization (and magic and mystery) that usually accompanies proper prescribing of antibiotics is eliminated. Where memorization is unavoidable, learning aids are presented that make the process a little less painful.

This book can be easily read and comprehended in 3 or 4 weeks by a busy student or practitioner. As a result, it is not a comprehensive guide to the antibiotic metropolis but merely an outline of the major thoroughfares of antibiotic therapy so that readers can more easily fill in the residential streets and alleys as they gain experience. In terms of the war analogy used throughout the book, the emphasis is on strategy, not tactics. Thus, only commonly used antibiotics are mentioned, and some oversimplifications and omissions are unavoidable. It is hoped that the reader will be able to master the major concepts and rules so that with subsequent clinical exposure and practice, the nuances and exceptions to these rules may be assimilated.

The fourth edition of this book has been updated and expanded to include newer antibiotics that have become available during the past 5 years. Likewise, sections have been updated to reflect recent changes in treatment guidelines, such as those pertaining to pneumonia and tuberculosis. Where necessary, updated references have been added.

After completing this book, it is hoped that readers will view antibiotics as valuable friends in the fight against infectious diseases and not as incomprehensible foes blocking their progress toward clinical competency. In addition, readers will obtain a foundation that can be built upon throughout their career, as new antibiotics become available.

Acknowledgments

I am indebted to many people who have contributed in large and small ways to this book but would especially like to acknowledge a few individuals. Many thanks to Mike Postelnick, Kristin Darin, and Marc Scheetz for advice and for reviewing portions of this book; Andy Rabin for providing quotes from the medieval literature; and Joe Welch for invaluable advice. Thank you to Kathleen Scogna, Michael Brown, and Steve Boehm at Wolters Kluwer for their assistance, patience, and advice in bringing this project to fruition, and to Matt Hauber, Deborah Bordeaux, and Sunmerrilika Baskar for help throughout the process of putting together the fourth edition of this book. I am grateful to the intelligent and inquisitive medical students at Northwestern University who asked the many questions that inspired this book. And finally, I wish to thank my wife, Anne, and my daughter, Grace, who kept me smiling throughout the whole process.

Contents

Preface   iv
Acknowledgements   v

PART 1 Bacterial Basics

CHAPTER 1   Cell Envelope   3

CHAPTER 2   Protein Production   6

CHAPTER 3   Replication   10

CHAPTER 4   Measuring Susceptibility to Antibiotics   14

PART 2 Antibacterial Agents

CHAPTER 5   Antibiotics That Target the Cell Envelope   21
β-LACTAM ANTIBIOTICS   22
PENICILLINS   27
CEPHALOSPORINS   34
CARBAPENEMS   46
MONOBACTAMS   51
GLYCOPEPTIDES   53
DAPTOMYCIN   58
POLYMYXINS   60

CHAPTER 6   Antibiotics That Block Protein Production   63
RIFAMYCINS   64
AMINOGLYCOSIDES   67
MACROLIDES   71
TETRACYCLINES   74
CLINDAMYCIN   78
OXAZOLIDINONES   80
NITROFURANTOIN   82

CHAPTER 7   Antibiotics That Target DNA and Replication   84
SULFA DRUGS   85
QUINOLONES   90
METRONIDAZOLE   95

CHAPTER 8   Antimycobacterial Agents   97

CHAPTER 9   Summary of Antibacterial Agents   100

PART 3   Definitive Therapy

CHAPTER 10   Gram-Positive Bacteria   107
- STAPHYLOCOCCI   108
- PNEUMOCOCCI   113
- OTHER STREPTOCOCCI   116
- ENTEROCOCCI   119
- LISTERIA MONOCYTOGENES   123

CHAPTER 11   Gram-Negative Bacteria   125
- ENTEROBACTERALES   126
- PSEUDOMONAS AERUGINOSA   132
- NEISSERIA SPP.   136
- CURVED GRAM-NEGATIVE BACTERIA   138
- OTHER GRAM-NEGATIVE BACTERIA   143

CHAPTER 12   Anaerobic Bacteria   149
- CLOSTRIDIUM SPP.   150
- ANAEROBIC GRAM-NEGATIVE BACILLI   153

CHAPTER 13   Atypical Bacteria   155
- CHLAMYDIA   156
- MYCOPLASMA   158
- LEGIONELLA   160
- BRUCELLA   162
- FRANCISELLA TULARENSIS   164
- RICKETTSIA   166

CHAPTER 14   Spirochetes   168
- TREPONEMA PALLIDUM   169
- BORRELIA BURGDORFERI   171
- LEPTOSPIRA INTERROGANS   173

CHAPTER 15   Mycobacteria   175
- MYCOBACTERIUM TUBERCULOSIS   177
- MYCOBACTERIUM AVIUM COMPLEX   180
- MYCOBACTERIUM LEPRAE   182

PART 4 Empiric Therapy

CHAPTER 16 Pneumonia 187

CHAPTER 17 Urinary Tract Infections 194

CHAPTER 18 Pelvic Inflammatory Disease 199

CHAPTER 19 Meningitis 202

CHAPTER 20 Cellulitis 207

CHAPTER 21 Otitis Media 211

CHAPTER 22 Infective Endocarditis 215

CHAPTER 23 Intravascular-Related Catheter Infections 223

CHAPTER 24 Intra-abdominal Infections 226

PART 5 Clinical Cases

PART 6 Review Questions and Answers

APPENDICES 263

1 Dosing of Antibacterial Agents in Adults 263

2 Dosing of Antibacterial Agents in Children 268

3 Dosing of Antibacterial Agents in Adults With Renal Insufficiency 274

4 Antibacterial Agents in Pregnancy 282

5 Generic and Trade Names of Commonly Used Antibacterial Agents 286

6 Medical References 289

7 Literary References 290

Index 291

PART 1

Bacterial Basics

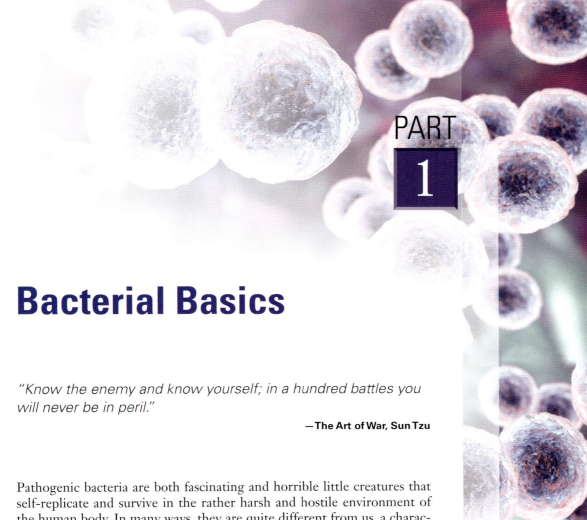

"Know the enemy and know yourself; in a hundred battles you will never be in peril."

—The Art of War, Sun Tzu

Pathogenic bacteria are both fascinating and horrible little creatures that self-replicate and survive in the rather harsh and hostile environment of the human body. In many ways, they are quite different from us, a characteristic that has been exploited by the developers of antimicrobial agents that specifically target these differences. To understand how antibiotics inhibit or kill bacteria, we must first understand the structure and function of these tiny pathogens.

Three aspects of bacteria must be understood to appreciate how antibiotics target and hinder them: the bacterial cell envelope, biosynthetic processes within bacteria, and bacterial replication. Whereas the bacterial cell envelope is a unique structure not present in human cells, bacterial protein production and DNA replication are processes analogous to those used by human cells but which differ from their human counterparts in the components utilized to accomplish them. Each of these three characteristics is discussed in detail in the following chapters.

ADDITIONAL READINGS

Jorgensen JH, Ferraro MJ. Antimicrobial susceptibility testing: a review of general principles and contemporary practices. *Clin Infect Dis.* 2009;49:1749-1755.
Murray PR, Rosenthal KS, Pfaller MA. *Medical Microbiology.* 9th ed. Elsevier; 2020.
Ryan KJ, Ahmad N, Alspaugh JA, et al, eds. *Sherris Medical Microbiology.* 7th ed. McGraw-Hill; 2018.
Wang JC. DNA topoisomerases. *Annu Rev Biochem.* 1985;54:665-697.

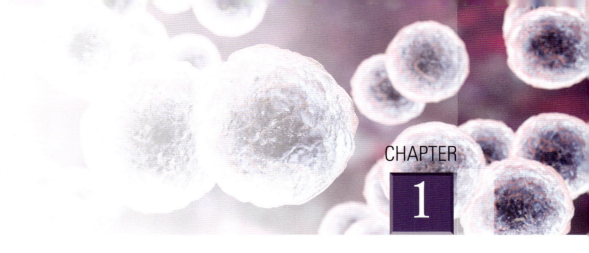

CHAPTER 1

Cell Envelope

"While styles of armor varied and changed from one decade to the next, the basics were a suit of plate armor consisting of a chest piece, a skirt of linked hoops, and arm and leg pieces, all worn over a hauberk or shirt of chain mail and a leather or padded tunic, or a tight-fitting surcoat. . . . Chain mail covered the neck, elbows, and other joints; gauntlets of linked plates protected the hands."

—A Distant Mirror, Barbara W. Tuchman

The **cell envelope** is a protective layer of armor that surrounds the bacterium and allows it to survive in diverse and extreme environments. The cell envelopes of some bacteria consist of a **cytoplasmic membrane** surrounded by a tough and rigid mesh called a cell wall (Figure 1-1); these bacteria are referred to as **gram-positive** bacteria. In contrast, the cell envelope of a **gram-negative** bacterium consists of a cytoplasmic membrane surrounded by a thin cell wall that is itself surrounded by a second lipid membrane called the **outer membrane**. The outer membrane contains large amounts of **lipopolysaccharide (LPS)**, a molecule that is very toxic to humans. The space between the outer membrane and the cytoplasmic membrane, which contains the cell wall, is called the **periplasmic space** or the **periplasm**. Whether a bacterium is gram positive or gram negative can usually be determined by a technique called Gram staining, which colors gram-positive bacteria blue or purple and gram-negative bacteria pink. Gram staining is often the first step used by a hospital microbiology laboratory in identifying an unknown bacterium from a clinical specimen.

As in human cells, the cytoplasmic membrane prevents ions from flowing into or out of the cell itself and maintains the cytoplasm and bacterial components in a

---

Excerpt from *A Distant Mirror: The Calamitous 14th Century* by Barbara W. Tuchman, copyright © 1978 by Barbara W. Tuchman. Used by permission of Alfred A. Knopf, an imprint of the Knopf Doubleday Publishing Group, a division of Penguin Random House LLC. All rights reserved.

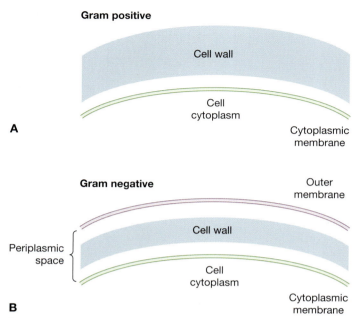

Figure 1-1. Structure of the bacterial cell envelope. A. Gram positive. B. Gram negative.

defined space. The cell wall is a tough layer that gives a bacterium its characteristic shape and protects it from mechanical and osmotic stresses. In gram-negative bacteria, the outer membrane acts as an additional protective barrier and prevents many substances from penetrating into the bacterium. This layer, however, does contain channels called **porins** that allow some compounds such as nutrients to pass through.

Because human cells do not possess a cell wall, this structure is an ideal target for antimicrobial agents. To appreciate how these agents work, we must first understand the structure of the cell wall. This complex assembly is made up of a substance called **peptidoglycan**, which itself consists of long sugar polymers. The polymers are repeats of two sugars: *N*-acetylglucosamine and *N*-acetylmuramic acid (Figure 1-2). If the cell wall were to consist of these polymers alone, it would be quite weak. However, peptide side chains extend from the sugars in the polymers and form cross-links, one peptide to another. These cross-links greatly strengthen the cell wall, just as cross-linking of metal loops strengthened the chain mail armor used by medieval knights.

The cross-linking of peptidoglycan is mediated by bacterial enzymes called **penicillin-binding proteins (PBPs)**. (The reason for this nomenclature will become apparent in later chapters.) These enzymes recognize the terminal two amino acids of the peptide side chains, which are usually D-alanine-D-alanine, and either directly cross-link them to a second peptide side chain or indirectly cross-link them by forming a bridge of glycine residues between the two peptide side chains.

The formation of a tough cross-linked cell wall allows bacteria to maintain their characteristic shapes. For example, some bacteria are rod shaped and referred to as **bacilli**. **Cocci** are spherical in shape. **Coccobacilli** have a morphology that is intermediate between that of bacilli and cocci. Finally, **spirochetes** have a corkscrew shape.

CHAPTER 1 — Cell Envelope

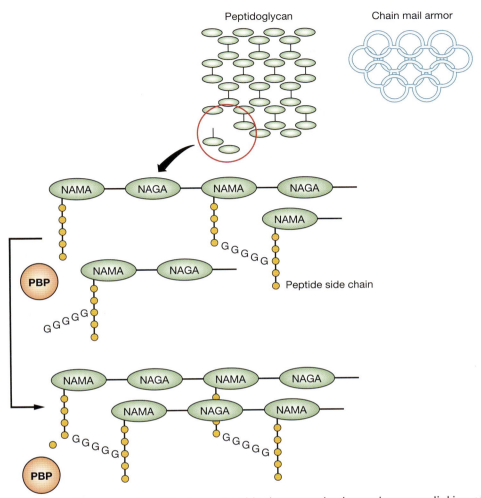

Figure 1-2. Structure of peptidoglycan. Peptidoglycan synthesis requires cross-linking of disaccharide polymers by penicillin-binding proteins (PBPs). GGG, glycine bridge; NAGA, N-acetylglucosamine; NAMA, N-acetylmuramic acid.

QUESTIONS

1. The bacterial cell wall is composed of _____.
2. _____ are enzymes that cross-link peptidoglycan polymers.
3. _____ are rod-shaped bacteria.

ANSWERS

1. peptidoglycan
2. PBPs
3. Bacilli

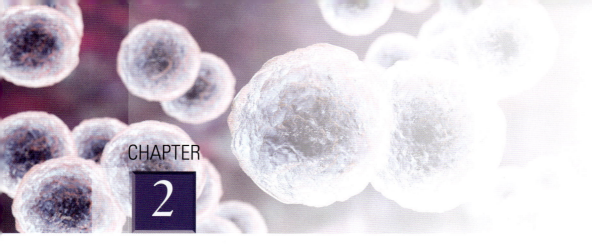

CHAPTER 2

Protein Production

"Plunder fertile country to supply the army with plentiful provisions."

—The Art of War, Sun Tzu

Like all invading armies, bacteria causing an infection need to be resupplied. They require the proper resources to allow for the replacement of old worn-out parts and for building new bacteria. Bacteria acquire these resources from the "country" they are invading, which is the human body. Among the most abundant of the synthesized replacement parts are proteins. The synthesis of these proteins is accomplished using the same general processes that are utilized by human cells (Figure 2-1). First, a number of raw materials or building blocks, such as RNAs, amino acids, and energy-containing nucleoside triphosphates, must be acquired and available within the bacterium. If this condition is met, template bacterial genes are transcribed into RNA by special bacterial enzymes. RNA is then translated into protein. Because some of the bacterial components essential for these processes differ significantly from their human cell counterparts, protein production in bacteria is amenable to inhibition by antibiotics.

RAW MATERIALS

The process of synthesizing new proteins requires abundant amounts of building blocks as well as energy. For example, it is estimated that the energy of three or four nucleoside triphosphates (eg, adenosine triphosphate [ATP] or guanosine triphosphate [GTP]) is required to add a single amino acid to a growing protein. The bacterium generates these raw materials and energy by taking up fuel sources such as glucose from the environment and processing them through metabolic pathways that harness their energy and generate intermediate compounds.

These metabolic pathways are quite complex and differ significantly between bacteria and human cells. They can be used effectively to divide bacteria into two categories: **aerobes** and **anaerobes**. Aerobic bacteria use oxygen from their environment in

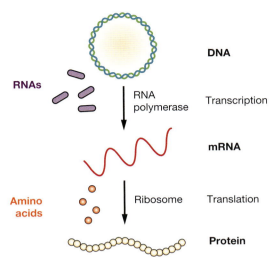

Figure 2-1. An overview of the process by which proteins are produced within bacteria. mRNA, messenger RNA.

the process of metabolism, whereas anaerobic bacteria do not. In fact, strict anaerobes are killed by oxygen because they lack enzymes that detoxify some of the harmful by-products of oxygen, such as hydrogen peroxide and superoxide radicals. *Mycobacterium tuberculosis* is an example of a strict aerobic bacterium; strict anaerobic bacteria include *Clostridium difficile* and *Bacteroides fragilis*. Many bacteria have metabolic pathways that allow them to utilize oxygen when it is present but to function as anaerobes when it is absent. These bacteria are said to be **facultative** with respect to oxygen use and obviously survive fine in the presence or absence of oxygen. Examples of such facultative bacteria include *Escherichia coli* and *Staphylococcus aureus*. Other bacteria grow best in the presence of small amounts of oxygen, less than would be found in air. These bacteria are said to be **microaerophilic**. *Campylobacter jejuni* is an example of a microaerophilic bacterium.

The energy available in the fuel consumed by bacteria is harnessed and stored in the form of nucleoside triphosphates and, in some cases, in the generation of a proton gradient between the interior and exterior of the bacterial cell. The potential energy stored in this gradient is referred to as the **proton motive force**. As protons flow down this gradient (from outside the bacterium to inside the bacterium) and through the cytoplasmic membrane, this energy is utilized to power important processes such as the active transport of nutrients into the cell and the generation of ATP.

TRANSCRIPTION

Transcription is the process by which the information in the DNA of a bacterial gene is used to synthesize an RNA molecule referred to as **messenger RNA (mRNA)**. As in human cells, the enzyme complex **RNA polymerase** is used by bacteria to accomplish this. RNA polymerase binds to DNA and uses it as a template to sequentially add RNAs to a corresponding molecule of mRNA. This process is quite efficient; under ideal conditions, bacterial RNA polymerase can make mRNA at a rate of 55 nucleotides per second.

Although both molecules perform similar functions, bacterial RNA polymerase is structurally and functionally quite distinct from eukaryotic RNA polymerase. (Eukaryotes, unlike bacteria, are organisms that contain nuclei and other membrane-bound organelles within their cells. Examples include animals, plants, fungi, and protozoa.) For example, whereas bacterial RNA polymerase by itself is sufficient to initiate transcription, eukaryotic RNA polymerase requires the help of additional transcription factors. The importance of transcription to the health of the bacterium and the differences between bacterial and eukaryotic RNA polymerases make this enzyme complex an ideal target for antimicrobial compounds.

TRANSLATION

In both eukaryotes and bacteria, macromolecular structures called **ribosomes** do the work of synthesizing proteins from the information present in mRNA, a process called **translation**. These large complexes are composed of both **ribosomal RNA (rRNA)** and proteins. Bacterial ribosomes, however, differ significantly from their eukaryotic counterparts. The **70S bacterial ribosome** is made of a **50S subunit** and a **30S subunit** (Figure 2-2). ("S" stands for Svedberg units, which are a measure of the rate of sedimentation in an ultracentrifuge. Svedberg units, thus, reflect the size of a complex but are not additive.) In contrast, the eukaryotic ribosome is 80S in size and consists of a 60S subunit and a 40S subunit. Each subunit, in turn, is made of multiple rRNA molecules and proteins.

The complete ribosome functions together with another type of RNA, **transfer RNA (tRNA)**, to manufacture new proteins. The ribosome binds to and reads the mRNA template and appropriately incorporates amino acids delivered by the tRNA into the nascent protein based on the information in this template. The importance of translation is indicated by the fact that half of all RNA synthesis in rapidly growing bacteria is devoted to rRNA and tRNA. The essential role played by protein synthesis in bacterial growth and the dissimilarity between the bacterial ribosome and the human ribosome make the former an attractive antibiotic target. Indeed, numerous classes of antimicrobial agents act by binding to and inhibiting the bacterial ribosome.

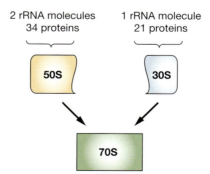

Figure 2-2. Structure of the bacterial ribosome. rRNA, ribosomal RNA.

CHAPTER 2 — Protein Production

QUESTIONS

1. _____ bacteria are those that grow in the absence of oxygen.
2. _____ is an enzyme complex that makes mRNA from a DNA template.
3. The 70S bacterial ribosome consists of _____ and _____ subunits, which themselves consist of _____ and _____.

ANSWERS

1. Anaerobic
2. RNA polymerase
3. 50S, 30S, rRNA, proteins

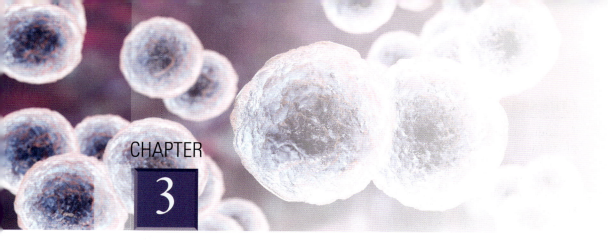

CHAPTER 3

Replication

"We think we have now allotted to the superiority in numbers the importance which belongs to it; it is to be regarded as the fundamental idea, always to be aimed at before all and as far as possible."

—On War, Carl Von Clausewitz

In the battle between bacteria and the human immune response, numbers are key. Bacteria are continuously multiplying in an attempt to overwhelm the host's defensive capabilities, and immune factors are constantly attempting to eradicate the invaders. It is this balance that is often tipped in favor of the human immune response by antibiotics.

An illustrative example of the importance of bacterial multiplication in infection is shigellosis. This form of infectious diarrhea is caused by the bacterium *Shigella* and can occur following ingestion of as few as 200 organisms. Yet, over a short period, these 200 organisms lead to diarrhea in which billions of bacteria are expelled in the feces every day. Obviously, rapid bacterial multiplication is essential for this disease.

Bacterial multiplication occurs by binary fission, the process by which a parent bacterium divides to form two identical daughter cells. This requires the synthesis of numerous biomolecules essential for construction of the daughter cells. Nearly all bacteria have a single circular chromosome, the replication of which is an integral part of cell division. Replication occurs when bacterial enzymes use the existing chromosome as a template for the synthesis of a second identical chromosome. To accomplish this, a ready supply of deoxynucleotides must be available for incorporation into the nascent DNA molecule. This process is more complicated than one might suspect, and other enzymes are also required to regulate the conformation of the DNA to allow for optimal replication of the chromosome. These complex processes afford several opportunities for antimicrobial agents to inhibit bacterial growth.

SYNTHESIS OF DEOXYNUCLEOTIDES

An abundant supply of deoxyadenosine triphosphate (dATP), deoxyguanosine triphosphate (dGTP), deoxycytidine triphosphate (dCTP), and deoxythymidine triphosphate (dTTP) is essential for the production of DNA molecules during DNA replication. Bacteria use several synthetic pathways to manufacture these DNA-building blocks. **Tetrahydrofolate (THF)** is an essential cofactor for several of these pathways and is synthesized as follows (Figure 3-1): The enzyme dihydropteroate synthase uses dihydropterin pyrophosphate and *para*-aminobenzoate (PABA) to generate dihydropteroate, which is subsequently converted to dihydrofolate. Dihydrofolate reductase then converts dihydrofolate into THF. THF is required for the ultimate synthesis of several nucleotides. Although humans readily absorb folate, a precursor of THF, from their diet, most bacteria are unable to do so and must synthesize this cofactor. This synthetic pathway is thus an attractive target for antimicrobial compounds.

DNA SYNTHETIC ENZYMES

The enzyme **DNA polymerase** is responsible for replicating the bacterial chromosome, but other enzymes are also required for this process. One example is the **topoisomerases** that regulate **supercoiling**, or twisting of the DNA. To understand supercoiling, one must appreciate the consequences of having a chromosome composed of helical DNA. The double helix structure of DNA dictates that in a relaxed state, it will contain 10 nucleotide pairs per each helical turn. However, by twisting one end of the DNA while holding the other end fixed, one can increase or decrease the number of nucleotide pairs per helical turn, say to 11 or 9 (Figure 3-2). This results in additional stress on the DNA molecule, which is accommodated by the formation of supercoils. When there is an increase in the number of nucleotide pairs per helical turn, the supercoiling is said to be positive. When there is a decrease, the supercoiling is said to be negative. An analogous process occurs in bacteria. Because parts of the chromosome are "fixed" due to associations with large protein complexes, twists that occur in one portion cannot freely dissipate but accumulate and form supercoils. Where do the twists come from? RNA polymerase is a large molecule that is unable to spin freely while it moves along the bacterial chromosome during transcription. Thus, as RNA polymerase forges its way along the chromosome, separating the DNA strands as it goes, positive supercoiling occurs in front of the enzyme, whereas negative

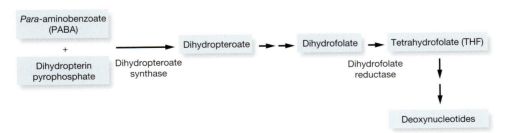

Figure 3-1. Bacterial synthesis of tetrahydrofolate.

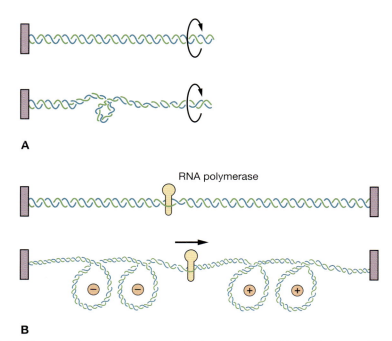

Figure 3-2. Supercoiling of the double helical structure of DNA. A. Twisting of DNA results in the formation of supercoils. B. During transcription, the movement of RNA polymerase along the chromosome results in the accumulation of positive supercoils ahead of the enzyme and negative supercoils behind it. (Adapted from *Molecular Biology of the Cell*, fourth edition by Bruce Alberts, et al. Copyright © 2002 by Bruce Alberts, Alexander Johnson, Julian Lewis, Martin Raff, Keith Roberts, and Peter Walter. Copyright © 1983, 1989, 1994 by Bruce Alberts, Dennis Bray, Julian Lewis, Martin Raff, Keith Roberts, and James D. Watson. Used by permission of W.W. Norton & Company, Inc.)

supercoils accumulate behind it. In theory, excess supercoiling could be a barrier to DNA replication and transcription.

A second consequence of the circular nature of the bacterial chromosome is that, following completion of replication, the two daughter chromosomes will frequently be interlinked (Figure 3-3). This obviously presents an obstacle for the dividing bacterium while it tries to segregate one chromosome to each of the daughter cells.

Bacteria overcome both these problems by producing topoisomerases, enzymes that remove or add supercoiling to DNA. Topoisomerases do this by binding to the DNA, cutting one or both strands of the DNA, passing either a single-strand DNA or a double-stranded DNA through the break, and then religating the DNA. The passage of one or two strands of DNA through the break in essence removes or adds one or two supercoils to the chromosome. It may also unlink two interlocked chromosomes following replication. In this way, bacteria are able to regulate the degree of supercoiling in their chromosomes and allow for separation of chromosomes following DNA replication.

CHAPTER 3 — Replication

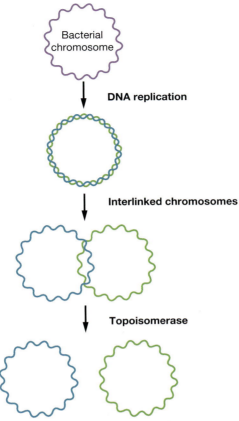

Figure 3-3. Replication of the bacterial chromosome. A consequence of the circular nature of the bacterial chromosome is that replicated chromosomes are interlinked, requiring topoisomerase for appropriate segregation.

QUESTIONS

1. THF is required for several pathways involving the synthesis of _____.
2. The chromosomes of most bacteria are _____.
3. _____ are enzymes that regulate DNA supercoiling.

ANSWERS

1. deoxynucleotides
2. circular
3. Topoisomerases

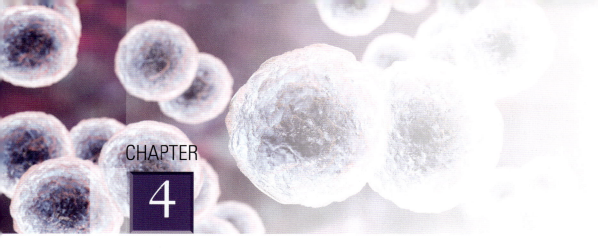

CHAPTER

4

Measuring Susceptibility to Antibiotics

"The best form of defense is attack."

—On War, Carl von Clausewitz

We have discussed three processes of bacteria that are essential for their survival and distinct from corresponding human cell processes: generation of the cell envelope, production of bacterial proteins, and replication of the bacterial chromosome. Each of these processes provides multiple targets for antibiotics that inhibit bacteria. Antibiotics can be divided into two classes: Those antibiotics that kill bacteria are called **bactericidal**, and those that merely suppress bacterial growth are called **bacteriostatic**. Bacteriostatic antibiotics rely on the immune system to eradicate the nonmultiplying bacteria from the patient.

The susceptibility of a bacterial isolate to a given antibiotic is quantified by the **minimum inhibitory concentration (MIC)** and the **minimum bactericidal concentration (MBC)**. As its name implies, the MIC measures the minimum concentration of antibiotic that is still able to suppress the growth of the bacterial isolate under standardized conditions. Likewise, the MBC is the minimum concentration of antibiotic that results in killing of the bacterial isolate under standardized conditions.

In practice, several assays have been developed to measure whether a given bacterial isolate is susceptible or resistant to a particular antibiotic. In the **Kirby-Bauer method**, antibiotic-impregnated wafers are dropped onto agar plates streaked with bacteria. The antibiotics diffuse from the wafers, establishing a gradient with lower concentrations occurring further from the wafer. Bacterial growth will be suppressed in a zone surrounding the wafer, and measurement of the diameter of the zone can be used to determine whether the bacterial strain is susceptible or resistant to the antibiotic. **Etests** operate on a similar principle except that an elongated strip is used instead of a wafer. The strip is impregnated with a decreasing gradient of antibiotic concentrations along its length. When it is dropped onto an agar plate that has been streaked with a lawn of bacteria, the bacteria will grow right up to the end of the strip where little antibiotic is present but will be unable to grow near the end of the strip that contains high concentrations of antibiotics. The spot where the interface of the bacterial lawn and the zone of clearance touches the strip is used to estimate the MIC, a process facilitated by MIC designations marked onto the strip itself. **Broth dilution methods** operate on a similar principle, except that the antibiotic dilutions are created in wells of liquid media rather than in agar. In these assays, the well with the greatest dilution of antibiotic that still does not support the growth of the bacterium identifies the MIC. Today, the microbiology laboratories of most large hospitals rely on machines that utilize these principles to automatically test hundreds of bacterial isolates.

Pearl

The immune system appears to be relatively ineffective in the eradication of bacteria in certain types of infections, such as meningitis and endocarditis. In these infections, bactericidal antibiotics have been used historically instead of bacteriostatic antibiotics.

In the following section, we discuss the individual antibiotics that bind to essential bacterial targets as well as the protective mechanisms that have evolved within bacteria to thwart their action.

Questions

1. _____ antibiotics kill rather than inhibit the growth of bacteria.
2. The _____ method of measuring antibiotic susceptibility utilizes antibiotic-impregnated wafers dropped onto an agar plate streaked with a lawn of bacteria.
3. The _____ method of measuring antibiotic susceptibility utilizes serial dilutions of antibiotics in liquid media.

Answers

1. Bactericidal
2. Kirby-Bauer
3. broth dilution

PART 2

Antibacterial Agents

"The warrior, in accordance with his aims, maintains various weapons and knows their characteristics and uses them well."

— The Book of Five Rings, Miyamoto Musashi

To protect the human body from the onslaught of bacterial pathogens, a large number of antimicrobial compounds have been developed that target points of vulnerability within these invaders. These agents can be grouped into three broad categories based on their mechanism of action: (1) those that target the bacterial cell envelope, (2) those that block the production of new proteins, and (3) those that target DNA or DNA replication.

We now discuss the individual antimicrobial agents. For each, a summary of its antimicrobial spectrum is given in the form of a traffic light. For this purpose, bacteria are broadly grouped into four categories: aerobic gram-positive bacteria, aerobic gram-negative bacteria, anaerobic bacteria, and atypical bacteria. The activity of an antibiotic against a particular category of bacteria is represented by a green light (active), a yellow light (sometimes active), or a red light (not active). Thus, in the example shown in the second figure, one should **go** ahead and use the antibiotic to treat an infection caused by gram-positive bacteria, **stop** if considering using the antibiotic to treat an infection caused by gram-negative bacteria, and proceed with **caution** if treating an infection caused by anaerobic or atypical bacteria. Note that these are only general indications of the antibiotic's activity against these classes of bacteria. There are almost certainly exceptions, and many other factors, such as the antibiotic's ability to achieve high concentrations at the site of the infection, whether it kills or merely inhibits the bacteria, contraindications to the drug, local antibiotic resistance patterns, and the patient's antibiotic history, must be taken into account when actually choosing an appropriate agent. Nonetheless, the traffic light representation is useful as a first step in learning the antimicrobial spectra of individual antibiotics.

HISTORY

Some of the earliest antibacterial agents were antibodies. Serum containing antibodies that bound and inactivated diphtheria toxin was already used to treat individuals with diphtheria in the 1800s. Although most currently used antibiotics are small molecules, antibodies that target toxins made by pathogenic bacteria are experiencing a renaissance. For example, raxibacumab and bezlotoxumab are human monoclonal antibodies that bind a component of *Bacillus anthracis* anthrax toxin and *Clostridioides difficile* toxin B, respectively. It is anticipated that antibodies will again play an important role in the treatment of patients with bacterial infections.

From Markham A. Bezlotoxumab: first global approval. *Drugs*. 2016;76:1793-1798; Migone TS, Subramanian GM, Zhong J, et al. Raxibacumab for the treatment of inhalational anthrax. *N Engl J Med*. 2009;361:135-144.

Groupings of bacteria used in subsequent chapters

Examples

gram-positive bacteria   *Staphylococcus aureus*
Streptococcus pneumoniae
Enterococci
Listeria monocytogenes

gram-negative bacteria   *Haemophilus influenzae*
Neisseria spp.
Enterobacterales
Pseudomonas aeruginosa

anaerobic bacteria   *Bacteroides fragilis*
Clostridium species

atypical bacteria   *Chlamydia* spp.
Mycoplasma spp.
Legionella pneumophila

Traffic light representation of antimicrobial spectrum of activity

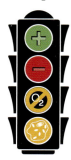

Gram-positive
Gram-negative
Anaerobes
Atypical

ADDITIONAL READINGS

For excellent overviews of antibiotics, please see these references:

Bennett JE, Dolin R, Blaser MJ. *Mandell, Douglas, and Bennett's Principles and Practice of Infectious Diseases*. 9th ed. Elsevier Saunders; 2019.

Mascaretti OA. *Bacteria versus Antibacterial Agents: An Integrated Approach*. ASM Press; 2003.

Walsh C. *Antibiotics: Actions, Origins, Resistance*. ASM Press; 2003.

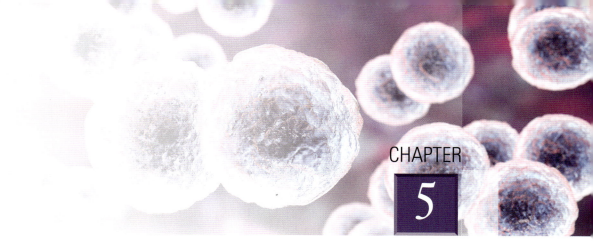

CHAPTER 5

Antibiotics That Target the Cell Envelope

"Though the knights, secure in their heavy armour, had no scruples in riding down and killing the leather-clad foot-soldier, it is entertaining to read of the fierce outcry they made when the foot-soldier retaliated with steel crossbow.... The knights called Heaven to witness that it was not honourable warfare to employ such weapons in battle, the fact being that they realized that armour was no longer the protection to their persons which it was before the days of heavy crossbows...."

—**The Crossbow, Sir Ralph Payne-Gallwey**

If the cell envelope is the bacterium's armor, then β-lactam antibiotics, glycopeptides, daptomycin, and polymyxins are the crossbows capable of piercing it. These antimicrobial agents attack the protective cell envelope, turning it into a liability for bacterium. In the following sections, we discuss how these antibiotics kill bacteria, the types of bacteria they are active against, and their toxicities.

β-Lactam Antibiotics

The exciting story of β-lactam antibiotics began in 1928, when Alexander Fleming noticed that a mold contaminating one of his cultures prevented the growth of bacteria. Because the mold was of the genus *Penicillium*, Fleming named the antibacterial substance "penicillin," the first of a long line of β-lactam agents. Characterization of this compound progressed rapidly, and by 1941, clinical trials were being performed with remarkable success on patients.

The essential core of penicillin is a four-membered ring called a **β-lactam ring** (Figure 5-1). Modifications of this basic structure have led to the development of several useful antibacterial compounds, each with its own characteristic spectrum of activity and pharmacokinetic properties. These include **penicillins**, **cephalosporins**, **carbapenems**, and **monobactams** (Table 5-1). It is important to remember, however, that the antibacterial activity of each β-lactam compound is based on the same basic mechanism (Figure 5-2). Although somewhat of an oversimplification, β-lactam antibiotics can be viewed as inhibitors of penicillin-binding proteins (PBPs) that normally assemble the peptidoglycan layer surrounding most bacteria. It has been hypothesized that the β-lactam ring mimics the D-alanyl-D-alanine portion of the peptide side chain that is normally bound by PBPs when generating cross-links. PBPs thus interact with the β-lactam ring instead of the D-alanyl-D-alanine moiety of the peptide side chain and are not available for the synthesis of new peptidoglycan (Figure 5-3). The disruption of the peptidoglycan layer leads to lysis of the bacterium.

As is the case with all antibiotics, resistance to β-lactams can be divided into two main categories: intrinsic and acquired. **Intrinsic resistance** refers to a resistance mechanism that is intrinsic to the structure or physiology of the bacterial species. For example, the porins in the outer membrane of all *Pseudomonas aeruginosa* strains do not allow passage of ampicillin to the periplasmic space, and all strains of *P. aeruginosa* are, therefore, resistant to this antibiotic. In contrast, **acquired resistance** occurs when a bacterium that was previously sensitive to an antibiotic acquires a mutation or exogenous genetic material that allows it to now resist the activity of that antibiotic. For example, most strains of *P. aeruginosa* are susceptible to the carbapenem imipenem, which gains access to the PBPs of this organism by passing through a specific protein

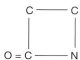

Figure 5-1. The structure of the β-lactam ring.

Table 5-1	β-Lactam Antibiotics
Penicillins	
Cephalosporins	
Carbapenems	
Monobactams	

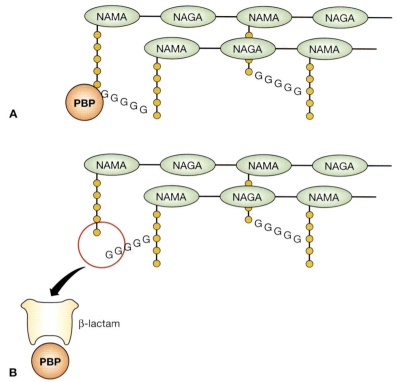

Figure 5-2. Mechanism of action of β-lactam antibiotics. A. Normally, a new subunit of N-acetylmuramic acid (NAMA) and N-acetylglucosamine (NAGA) disaccharide with an attached peptide side chain is linked to an existing peptidoglycan polymer. This may occur by covalent attachment of a glycine (G) bridge from one peptide side chain to another through the enzymatic action of penicillin-binding proteins (PBPs). B. In the presence of a β-lactam antibiotic, this process is disrupted. The β-lactam antibiotic binds the PBPs and prevents them from cross-linking the glycine bridge to the peptide side chain, thus blocking incorporation of the disaccharide subunit into the existing peptidoglycan polymer.

channel found in the outer membrane. However, following exposure to imipenem, spontaneous mutations may occur that result in loss of production of this channel. This, in turn, causes acquired resistance to imipenem. Practically speaking, intrinsic resistance usually implies that all strains of a bacterial species are resistant to a given antibiotic, whereas acquired resistance affects only some strains of a bacterial species.

Resistance usually results from failure of an agent to avoid one of six potential **P**itfalls in the process by which β-lactam antibiotics cause bacterial pathogens to perish rather than persist (Figure 5-4). These are the six **P**s: (1) **P**enetration—β-lactams penetrate poorly into the intracellular compartment of human cells, so bacteria that reside in this compartment are not exposed to them. A β-lactam antibiotic cannot kill a bacterium if it cannot get to it. (2) **P**orins—if a β-lactam antibiotic does reach the bacterium, it must gain access to its targets, the PBPs. In gram-positive bacteria, this is not difficult because the PBPs and the peptidoglycan layer are relatively exposed, but in gram-negative bacteria, they are surrounded by the protective outer membrane.

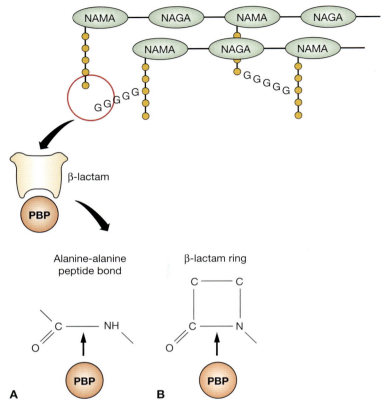

Figure 5-3. Mechanism of penicillin-binding protein (PBP) inhibition by β-lactam antibiotics. A. PBPs recognize and catalyze the peptide bond between two alanine subunits of the peptidoglycan peptide side chain. B. The β-lactam ring mimics this peptide bond. Thus, the PBPs bind to and attempt to catalyze the β-lactam ring, resulting in inactivation of the PBPs.

β-Lactams must breach this membrane by diffusing through porins, which are protein channels in the outer membrane. Many gram-negative bacteria have porins that do not allow passage of certain β-lactams to the periplasmic space. (3) **P**umps—some bacteria produce **efflux pumps**, which are protein complexes that transport antibiotics that have entered the periplasmic space back out to the environment. These pumps prevent antibiotics from accumulating within the periplasm to concentrations sufficient for antibacterial activity. (4) **P**enicillinases (really β-lactamases, but that does not start with P)—many bacteria, both gram positive and gram negative, make **β-lactamases**, enzymes that degrade β-lactams before they reach the PBPs. (5) **P**BPs—some bacteria produce PBPs that do not bind β-lactams with high affinity. In these bacteria, β-lactams reach their targets, the PBPs, but cannot inactivate them. (6) **P**eptidoglycan is absent—there are a few bacteria that do not make peptidoglycan and that, therefore, are not affected by β-lactams. To be effective, β-lactam agents must successfully navigate around each of these potential pitfalls. It is important to note that β-lactam antibiotics are a heterogeneous group of compounds; some may be blocked at certain steps through which others may proceed without difficulty.

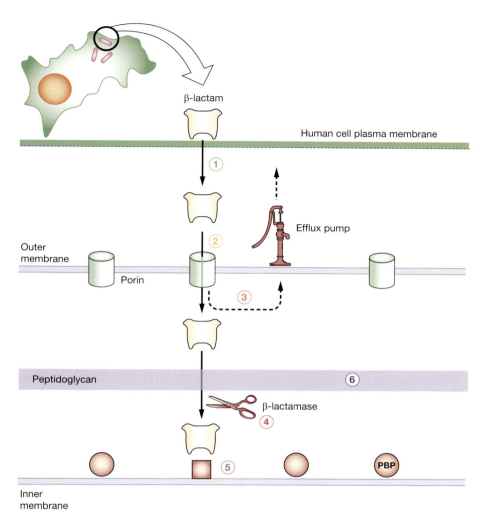

Figure 5-4. Six Ps by which the action of β-lactams may be blocked: **(1)** penetration, **(2)** porins, **(3)** pumps, **(4)** penicillinases (β-lactamases), **(5)** penicillin-binding proteins, and **(6)** peptidoglycan.

Remember

Remember the six **P**s of resistance to β-lactam antibiotics: **P**enetration, **P**orins, **P**umps, **P**enicillinases, **P**BPs, absent **P**eptidoglycan.

History

It was originally thought that antibiotic resistance first occurred as bacteria responded to the therapeutic use of antibiotics in the 20th century. It is now clear that antibiotic resistance genes are thousands of years old and likely evolved along with environmental microbes that naturally produced antimicrobial compounds.

Reprinted by permission from Springer: D'Costa VM, King CE, Kalan L, et al. Antibiotic resistance is ancient. *Nature.* 2011;477:457-461.

One point about β-lactamases: They come in many flavors—that is to say that some are specific for a few β-lactam antibiotics, whereas others have activity against nearly all β-lactam agents. For example, the β-lactamase of *Staphylococcus aureus* is relatively specific for some of the penicillins, whereas the extended-spectrum β-lactamases (ESBLs) made by some strains of *Escherichia coli* and *Klebsiella* spp. ("spp." is the abbreviation for the plural of species) degrade nearly all penicillins, cephalosporins, and monobactams. Different species or strains of bacteria produce different types of β-lactamases that confer upon them unique antibiotic resistance patterns. Thus, generalizations about β-lactamases and their effects on specific antibiotics must be made with caution.

Despite their many limitations, β-lactam antibiotics remain some of the most powerful and broad-spectrum antibiotics available today. They comprise a significant proportion of the total antibiotics prescribed every year.

QUESTIONS

1. All β-lactam antibiotics act by preventing proper construction of the bacterial _____ layer.
2. The four major classes of β-lactam antibiotics are _____, _____, _____, and _____.
3. All β-lactam antibiotics exert their action by binding to _____.
4. _____ are enzymes that cleave β-lactam antibiotics, thus inactivating them.

ANSWERS

1. peptidoglycan
2. penicillins, cephalosporins, carbapenems, monobactams
3. PBPs
4. β-Lactamases

HISTORY

By chance, Alexander Fleming took a 2-week vacation immediately after inoculation of his soon-to-be contaminated agar plates. Because he knew he would not be able to examine the plates for 2 weeks, he incubated them at room temperature instead of 37°C to slow the growth rate of the bacteria. His vacation changed the course of human events. *Penicillium* grows at room temperature but not at 37°C—had Fleming not taken a vacation, he never would have observed the bactericidal effects of the mold. Therefore, vacations truly do make one more productive at work.

From Friedman M, Friedman GW. *Medicine's Ten Greatest Discoveries*. Yale University Press; 1998.

# Penicillins

The penicillins each consist of a thiazolidine ring attached to a β-lactam ring that is itself modified by a variable side chain ("R" in Figure 5-5). Whereas the thiazolidine-β-lactam ring is required for antibacterial activity, the side chain has been manipulated to yield many penicillin derivatives that have altered pharmacologic properties and antibacterial spectra of activity.

As a result of modifications to the R side chain, penicillins come in several classes: the **natural penicillins**, the **antistaphylococcal penicillins**, the **aminopenicillins**, and the **extended-spectrum penicillins** (Table 5-2). In addition, some of the penicillins have been combined with **β-lactamase inhibitors**, which markedly expand the number of bacterial species that are susceptible to these compounds. The members of each class share similar pharmacokinetic properties and spectra of activity but may be quite distinct from members of other classes.

NATURAL PENICILLINS

The natural penicillins, **penicillin G** and **penicillin V**, are the great grandparents of the penicillin antibiotic family but still have much to say about the treatment of antibacterial infections. They are called *natural* penicillins because they can be purified directly from cultures of *Penicillium* mold. The R side chain of penicillin G is shown in Figure 5-6 and consists of a hydrophobic benzene ring.

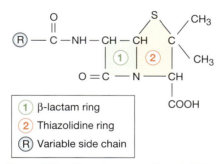

Figure 5-5. The structure of penicillins.

Table 5-2	The Penicillins	
Category	**Parenteral Agents**	**Oral Agents**
Natural penicillins	Penicillin G	Penicillin V
Antistaphylococcal penicillins	Nafcillin, oxacillin	Dicloxacillin
Aminopenicillins	Ampicillin	Amoxicillin, ampicillin
Extended-spectrum penicillins	Piperacillin	
Penicillins plus β-lactamase inhibitors	Ampicillin-sulbactam Piperacillin-tazobactam	Amoxicillin-clavulanate

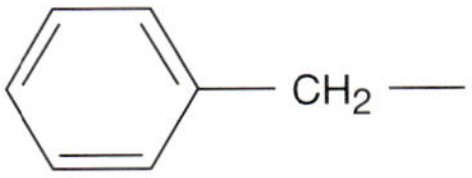

Figure 5-6. R side chain of penicillin G.

Because nearly all bacteria have cell walls composed of peptidoglycan, it is not surprising that the natural penicillins are active against some species of gram-positive, gram-negative, and anaerobic bacteria as well as some spirochetes. Despite this broad range of activity, most bacteria are either intrinsically resistant or have now acquired resistance to the natural penicillins. Understanding the reasons for this can help one remember which species remain susceptible. In turn, the bacterial spectra of the natural penicillins can be used as a foundation for remembering the spectra of the other classes of penicillins. The six **P**s explain resistance to the natural penicillins: (1) **P**enetration—natural penicillins, like most β-lactams, penetrate poorly into the intracellular compartment of human cells, so bacteria that for the most part reside in this compartment, such as *Rickettsia* and *Legionella*, are protected from them. (2) **P**orins—some gram-negative bacteria, such as *E. coli*, *Proteus mirabilis*, *Salmonella enterica*, and *Shigella* spp., have porins in their outer membranes that do not allow passage of the hydrophobic natural penicillins to the periplasmic space. (3) **P**umps—some gram-negative bacteria, such as *P. aeruginosa*, have efflux pumps that prevent the accumulation of penicillins within the periplasm. Although these pumps by themselves may only cause a marginal change in susceptibility, they can work together with penicillinases and porins to have a dramatic effect. (4) **P**enicillinases—many bacteria, both gram positive (staphylococci) and gram negative (some *Neisseria* and *Haemophilus* strains, many enteric species, and some anaerobes, such as *Bacteroides fragilis*), make penicillinases that degrade the natural penicillins. (5) **P**BPs—some bacteria produce PBPs that do not bind natural penicillins with a high affinity (eg, some strains of *Streptococcus pneumoniae*). (6) **P**eptidoglycan—some bacteria, such as *Mycoplasma*, do not make peptidoglycan and, therefore, are not affected by the natural penicillins.

Despite these limitations, natural penicillins are still used to treat infections caused by some gram-positive bacteria, especially streptococci, some anaerobic bacteria, and some spirochetes (Table 5-3). Even a few gram-negative bacteria, such as some strains of *Neisseria meningitidis* and *Haemophilus influenzae*, remain susceptible to penicillin.

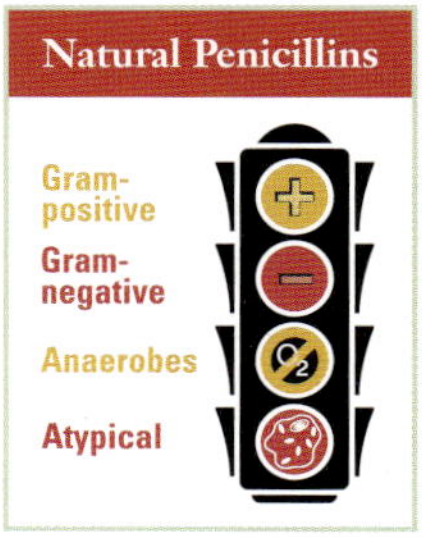

Natural Penicillins

Gram-positive
Gram-negative
Anaerobes
Atypical

Table 5-3	Antimicrobial Activity of Natural Penicillins
Gram-positive bacteria	*Streptococcus pyogenes* Viridans streptococci Some *Streptococcus pneumoniae* Some enterococci *Listeria monocytogenes*
Gram-negative bacteria	Some *Neisseria meningitidis* Some *Haemophilus influenzae*
Anaerobic bacteria	*Clostridia* spp. (except *Clostridioides difficile*) *Actinomyces israelii*
Spirochetes	*Treponema pallidum* *Leptospira* spp.

ANTISTAPHYLOCOCCAL PENICILLINS

The antistaphylococcal penicillins (also called the "penicillinase-resistant penicillins") have bulky residues on their R side chains that prevent binding within the narrow pocket of the staphylococcal β-lactamases (Figure 5-7). As a result, these penicillins are useful in treating infections caused by *S. aureus* and *Staphylococcus epidermidis*. However, they are unable to bind the PBPs of two special groups of staphylococci called methicillin-resistant *S. aureus* (MRSA) and methicillin-resistant *S. epidermidis* (MRSE). Because they cannot bind the PBPs of MRSA and MRSE bacteria, antistaphylococcal penicillins are inactive against them. (Note that methicillin is an antistaphylococcal penicillin that is no longer commercially available but is representative of the entire class of antistaphylococcal penicillins in its spectrum of activity.) Antistaphylococcal penicillins are also less effective than natural penicillins against streptococci and are usually not used to treat them. Nor are these penicillins active against enterococci. Likewise, the bulkiness of the side chains limits the ability of these agents to penetrate most other bacteria, and they are generally only used to treat staphylococcal infections (Table 5-4). This group of antibiotics includes **nafcillin**, **oxacillin**, and **dicloxacillin**.

AMINOPENICILLINS

The aminopenicillins, **ampicillin** and **amoxicillin**, have spectra of activity similar to the natural penicillins with one exception: An additional amino group in their side chain increases their hydrophilicity and allows them to pass through the porins in the outer membranes of some enteric gram-negative rods, such *E. coli*, *P. mirabilis*, *S. enterica*, and *Shigella* spp. (Figure 5-8). This extends the spectra of the aminopenicillins to include these bacteria. Aminopenicillins, however, share the natural penicillins'

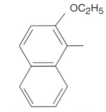

Figure 5-7. R side chain of nafcillin.

Table 5-4	Antimicrobial Activity of the Antistaphylococcal Penicillins
Gram-positive bacteria	Some *Staphylococcus aureus* Some *Staphylococcus epidermidis*

Antistaphylococcal Penicillins
- Gram-positive: +
- Gram-negative: −
- Anaerobes: −
- Atypical: −

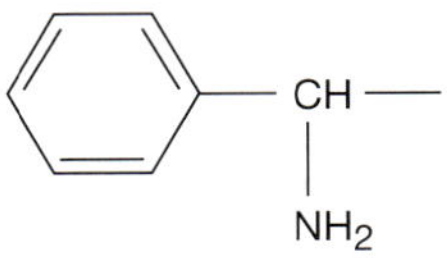

Figure 5-8. R side chain of ampicillin.

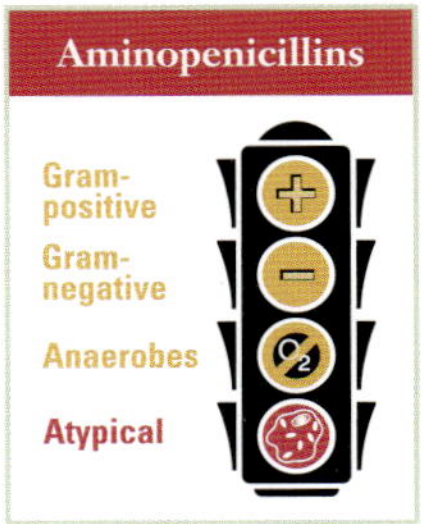

Aminopenicillins

- Gram-positive: +
- Gram-negative: −
- Anaerobes: partial
- Atypical: no

Table 5-5	Antimicrobial Activity of Aminopenicillins
Gram-positive bacteria	*Streptococcus pyogenes* Viridans streptococci Some *Streptococcus pneumoniae* Some enterococci *Listeria monocytogenes*
Gram-negative bacteria	Some *Neisseria meningitidis* Some *Haemophilus influenzae* Some Enterobacterales
Anaerobic bacteria	*Clostridia* spp. (except *Clostridioides difficile*) *Actinomyces israelii*
Spirochetes	*Borrelia burgdorferi*

vulnerability to β-lactamases, and many of the gram-negative bacteria that were initially susceptible to the aminopenicillins are now resistant due to the acquisition of β-lactamase encoding genes (Table 5-5).

EXTENDED-SPECTRUM PENICILLINS

An example of an extended-spectrum penicillin is **piperacillin**. The side chains of this agent allow for even greater penetration into gram-negative bacteria than is seen with the aminopenicillins. Piperacillin's side chain is polar, which increases its ability to pass through the outer membrane porins of some gram-negative bacteria (Figure 5-9).

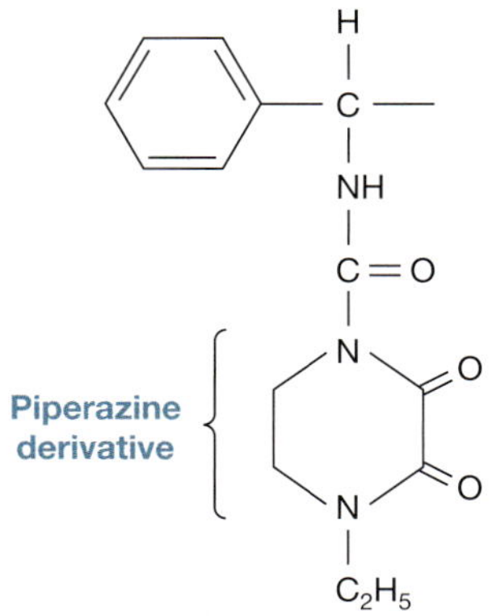

Figure 5-9. R side chain of piperacillin.

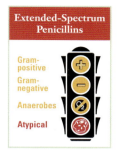

Table 5-6	Antimicrobial Activity of Extended-Spectrum Penicillins
Gram-positive bacteria	*Streptococcus pyogenes* Viridans streptococci Some *Streptococcus pneumoniae* Some enterococci
Gram-negative bacteria	Some *Neisseria meningitidis* Some *Haemophilus influenzae* Some Enterobacterales *Pseudomonas aeruginosa*
Anaerobic bacteria	*Clostridia* spp. (except *Clostridioides difficile*) Some *Bacteroides* spp.

(Incidentally, piperacillin was named for its side chain, which contains a piperazine derivative.) In addition, piperacillin is more resistant to cleavage by gram-negative β-lactamases than are aminopenicillins, although they remain susceptible to some of these enzymes. Thus, compared to the aminopenicillins, piperacillin is more active against gram-negative bacilli, including many strains of *P. aeruginosa*. It maintains some of the gram-positive activity of the natural penicillins but, like the natural penicillins, is susceptible to the β-lactamases of staphylococci. It has modest activity against anaerobes (Table 5-6). In the United States, piperacillin is not available by itself but only in conjunction with the β-lactamase inhibitor tazobactam.

PENICILLIN/β-LACTAMASE INHIBITOR COMBINATIONS

Compounds have been developed to inhibit the β-lactamases of many gram-positive and gram-negative bacteria. These inhibitors are structurally similar to penicillin and, therefore, bind β-lactamases, but instead of being cleaved, they inactivate the β-lactamases. Two of these inhibitors, clavulanate and sulbactam, are used in conjunction with the aminopenicillins to greatly expand their spectra of activity. **Ampicillin-sulbactam** is the parenteral formulation, and **amoxicillin-clavulanate** is the oral formulation of these combinations. Sulbactam and clavulanate inactivate the β-lactamases of many gram-positive, gram-negative, and anaerobic bacteria. As a result, they dramatically broaden the antimicrobial spectrum of the aminopenicillins (Table 5-7). A third inhibitor, tazobactam, is used in conjunction with the extended-spectrum penicillin piperacillin. **Piperacillin-tazobactam** achieves the fullest antimicrobial potential of the penicillins. Tazobactam neutralizes many of the β-lactamases that otherwise inactivate piperacillin, resulting in a marked enhancement of its activity. Thus, piperacillin-tazobactam is the decathlete of the penicillins, with activity against most aerobic gram-positive bacteria, including many β-lactamase–producing staphylococci, most aerobic gram-negative bacteria, and nearly all anaerobic bacteria, except *C. difficile* (Table 5-7). Its excellent activity against gram-positive, gram-negative, and anaerobic bacteria makes piperacillin-tazobactam one of the most widely used antibiotics available today.

Table 5-7	Antimicrobial Activity of Penicillin Plus β-Lactamase Inhibitor Combinations	
Gram-positive bacteria	Some *Staphylococcus aureus* *Streptococcus pyogenes* Viridans streptococci Some *Streptococcus pneumoniae* Some enterococci *Listeria monocytogenes*	
Gram-negative bacteria	*Neisseria* spp. *Haemophilus influenzae* Many Enterobacterales *Pseudomonas aeruginosa* (only piperacillin-tazobactam)	
Anaerobic bacteria	*Clostridia* spp. (except *Clostridioides difficile*) *Bacteroides* spp.	

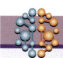

TOXICITY

Adverse reactions to the penicillins are relatively common; an estimated 3% to 10% of people report allergies to these agents, although the actual prevalence is substantially less. Like most antibiotics, penicillins can cause nausea, vomiting, and diarrhea. They also have been associated with drug fever, rash, serum sickness, interstitial nephritis, hepatotoxicity, neurologic toxicity, and hematologic abnormalities. Urticaria, angioedema, and anaphylaxis occur and are referred to as immediate hypersensitivity reactions. Of these, the most feared is anaphylaxis, which is rare but life-threatening. Persons allergic to one penicillin should be considered allergic to all penicillins, and cross-allergenicity may sometimes extend to other β-lactam antibiotics.

The penicillins vary markedly in their activities, especially against gram-negative bacteria. The activities of these agents against gram-negative bacteria can be summarized as follows: (1) The antistaphylococcal penicillins are inactive against gram-negative bacteria. (2) The natural penicillins have activity against some strains of *N. meningitidis* and *H. influenza*, but few other gram-negative bacteria. (3) The spectrum of the aminopenicillins is expanded to include these organisms plus some enteric gram-negative rods, such as certain strains of *E. coli*, *P. mirabilis*, *S. enterica*, and *Shigella* spp. that do not produce β-lactamases. (4) The extended-spectrum penicillins are active against even more enteric gram-negative rods and, importantly, *P. aeruginosa*. (5) Finally, the addition of a β-lactamase inhibitor to an extended-spectrum penicillin extends this list to include most enteric gram-negative bacilli.

REMEMBER

Penicillin G and penicillin V: Which is oral, and which is parenteral?
The letters in penicillin G and penicillin V can be used to remember how these agents are usually administered. Although not actually true, pretend that the "G" in penicillin G means that this drug is destroyed in the stomach ("gastric") and that the "V" in penicillin V means that this drug is destroyed in "veins." Therefore, penicillin G is given intravenously, and penicillin V is given orally.

QUESTIONS

5. Penicillins all share the same basic structure, which consists of a thiazolidine ring linked to a _____ with a modifiable _____.
6. Penicillins act by binding _____, which are bacterial enzymes that function to assemble _____.
7. Natural penicillins have moderate activity against aerobic gram-positive bacteria and anaerobic bacteria but poor activity against aerobic _____ bacteria and most atypical bacteria.
8. Antistaphylococcal penicillins are useful in treating infections caused by _____.
9. Compared to natural penicillins, aminopenicillins have improved activity against _____.
10. Addition of a β-lactamase inhibitor to an aminopenicillin expands the spectra of these agents to include many _____ as well as additional _____ and anaerobes.
11. Compared to aminopenicillins, extended-spectrum penicillins have improved activity against aerobic _____, including _____.
12. When used in combination with β-lactamase inhibitors, extended-spectrum penicillins are active against most aerobic _____, aerobic _____, and _____.

ANSWERS

5. β-lactam ring, side chain
6. PBPs, peptidoglycan
7. gram-negative
8. staphylococci
9. gram-negative bacteria
10. staphylococci, gram-negative bacteria
11. gram-negative bacteria, *P. aeruginosa*
12. gram-positive bacteria, gram-negative bacteria, anaerobic bacteria

ADDITIONAL READINGS

Cho H, Uehara T, Bernhardt TG. Beta-lactam antibiotics induce a lethal malfunctioning of the bacterial cell wall synthesis machinery. *Cell*. 2014;159:1300-1311.
Donowitz GR, Mandell GL. Beta-lactam antibiotics. *N Engl J Med*. 1988;318:419-426.
Donowitz GR, Mandell GL. Drug therapy. Beta-lactam antibiotics. *N Engl J Med*. 1988;318:490-500.
Lax E. *The Mold in Dr. Florey's Coat: The Story of the Penicillin Miracle*. Henry Holt and Company; 2004.
Park MA, Li JT. Diagnosis and management of penicillin allergy. *Mayo Clin Proc*. 2005;80:405-410.
Petri WA Jr. Penicillins, cephalosporins, and other beta-lactam antibiotics. In: Brunton LL, Lazo JS, Parker KL, eds. *Goodman & Gilman's The Pharmacological Basis of Therapeutics*. 10th ed. McGraw-Hill; 2006:1127-1154.
Sanders WE Jr, Sanders CC. Piperacillin/tazobactam: a critical review of the evolving clinical literature. *Clin Infect Dis*. 1996;22:107-123.

Cephalosporins

The cephalosporins received their name from the fungus *Cephalosporium acremonium*, which was the source of the first members of this class. Even more so than penicillins, these agents constitute a large extended family of antibiotics within the β-lactam group. As such, they are appropriately categorized by "generation" (Table 5-8). Because agents in each generation have somewhat similar spectra of activity, this organizational scheme is helpful in remembering the properties of the many cephalosporins.

Each cephalosporin is composed of a nucleus with two side chains (Figure 5-10). The nucleus is 7-aminocephalosporanic acid, which is similar to the nucleus of penicillin, except that the β-lactam ring is fused to a six-membered dihydrothiazine ring instead of a five-membered thiazolidine ring (compare Figures 5-10 to 5-5). The cephalosporin core has two major advantages over the penicillin core: (1) It is intrinsically

Table 5-8 The Cephalosporins

Generation	Parenteral Agents	Oral Agents
First generation	Cefazolin	Cefadroxil, cephalexin
Second generation	Cefotetan,[a] cefoxitin,[a] cefuroxime	Cefaclor, cefprozil, cefuroxime axetil
Third generation	Cefotaxime, ceftazidime, ceftriaxone	Cefdinir, cefpodoxime proxetil, cefixime
Fourth generation	Cefepime	
Fifth generation	Ceftaroline	
Cephalosporin plus β-lactamase inhibitor combinations	Ceftazidime-avibactam, Ceftolozane-tazobactam	
Siderophore cephalosporins	Cefiderocol	

[a]Cephamycins.

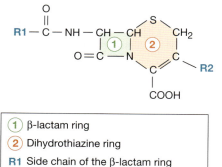

① β-lactam ring
② Dihydrothiazine ring
R1 Side chain of the β-lactam ring
R2 Side chain of the dihydrothiazine ring

Figure 5-10. The structure of cephalosporins.

more resistant to cleavage by β-lactamases and (2) it has two sites, R1 and R2, at which it can be modified. This, in part, explains the large number of cephalosporins commercially available today.

Like other β-lactam antibiotics, the cephalosporins exert their effects by binding and inhibiting PBPs, thereby preventing the appropriate synthesis of peptidoglycan. Although peptidoglycan is a constituent of most bacteria, cephalosporins are not active against certain species and strains of bacteria. As was the case for penicillins, the six **P**s explain resistance to cephalosporins: (1) **P**enetration—cephalosporins, like most β-lactams, penetrate poorly into the intracellular compartment of human cells, so bacteria that for the most part reside in this compartment, such as *Rickettsia* and *Legionella*, are protected from them. (2) **P**orins—some gram-negative bacteria, such as *P. aeruginosa*, have porins in their outer membranes that do not allow passage of many cephalosporins into the periplasmic space. (3) **P**umps—some bacteria, such as *P. aeruginosa*, use efflux pumps to remove antibiotics from the periplasmic space. (4) **P**enicillinases (actually β-lactamases)—many gram-negative bacteria, such as *Enterobacter* and *Citrobacter* spp., make β-lactamases that degrade many cephalosporins. (5) **P**BPs—some bacteria, such as the enterococci and *Listeria monocytogenes*, produce PBPs that do not bind most cephalosporins with a high affinity. (6) **P**eptidoglycan—some bacteria such as *Mycoplasma* do not make peptidoglycan and, therefore, are not affected by the cephalosporins.

Several generalizations about the spectra of activity of cephalosporins can be made. First, with the exception of the fifth-generation agents, each successive generation of agents has broader activity against aerobic gram-negative bacteria. Second, also with several important exceptions, cephalosporins have limited activity against anaerobes. Third, the activities of these agents against aerobic gram-positive bacteria are variable, with the fifth-generation agent ceftaroline having the strongest activity against these bacteria.

FIRST-GENERATION CEPHALOSPORINS

Commonly used first-generation cephalosporins include **cefadroxil** and **cefazolin** (Table 5-8). All agents in this group share similar activities against the different types of bacteria.

The strength of the first-generation cephalosporins is their activity against aerobic gram-positive cocci, such as staphylococci and streptococci (Table 5-9). The R1 side chains of these agents protect their β-lactam rings from cleavage by the staphylococcal β-lactamase (Figure 5-11). As a result, they are useful in the treatment of infections caused by many strains of *S. aureus*. First-generation cephalosporins cannot bind the PBPs of MRSA and MRSE or many highly penicillin-resistant *S. pneumoniae*; these agents are ineffective against these bacteria. Most cephalosporins also lack activity against *L. monocytogenes* and the enterococci.

First-generation cephalosporins have limited activity against aerobic and facultative gram-negative bacteria, primarily because the side chains of these agents, although capable of protecting the β-lactam ring from cleavage by staphylococcal β-lactamases, do not afford protection from the β-lactamases of most gram-negative bacteria. Nonetheless, some strains of *E. coli*, *Klebsiella pneumoniae*, and *P. mirabilis* are susceptible.

First-generation cephalosporins have moderate to poor activity against anaerobes, intracellular bacteria, and spirochetes.

First-Generation Cephalosporins	Table 5-9	Antimicrobial Activity of First-Generation Cephalosporins
Gram-positive: +	Gram-positive bacteria	*Streptococcus pyogenes* Some viridans streptococci Some *Staphylococcus aureus* Some *Streptococcus pneumoniae*
Gram-negative: − Anaerobes: ∅ Atypical: ∅	Gram-negative bacteria	Some *Escherichia coli* Some *Klebsiella pneumoniae* Some *Proteus mirabilis*

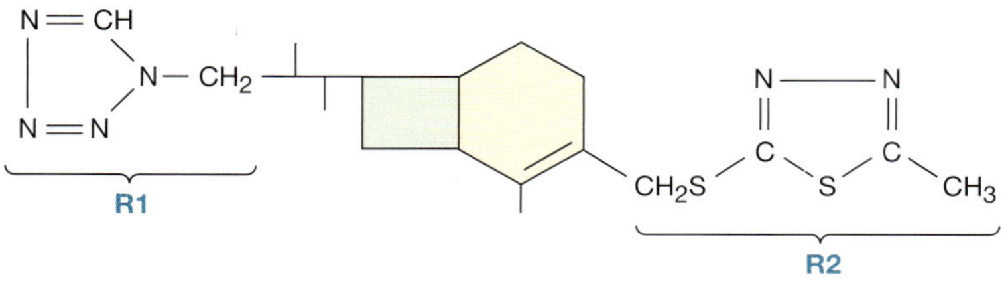

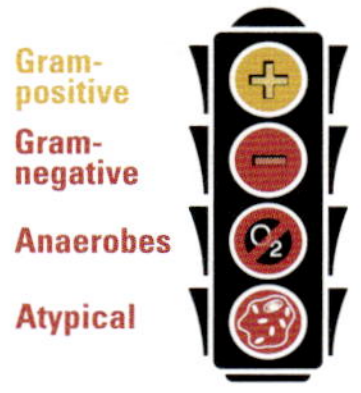

Figure 5-11. Structure of cefazolin.

SECOND-GENERATION CEPHALOSPORINS

Second-generation cephalosporins are divided into two groups: the true cephalosporins, such as **cefuroxime**, and the cephamycins, which include **cefotetan** and **cefoxitin** (see Table 5-8). The cephamycins are derivatives of a parent compound originally isolated from the bacterium *Streptomyces lactamdurans* instead of the fungus *C. acremonium*. They have a methoxy group in place of the hydrogen on the β-lactam ring of the cephalosporin core (Figure 5-12). Thus, these agents are not actually cephalosporins but are included in this group because they are chemically and pharmacologically similar.

Individual second-generation cephalosporins differ in their activity against aerobic gram-positive bacteria (Table 5-10). The true cephalosporins are in general as active against aerobic gram-positive cocci as the first-generation agents. The cephamycins (cefotetan and cefoxitin) have relatively limited activity against this group of bacteria. The strength of the second-generation agents is their increased activity against aerobic and facultative gram-negative bacteria. Second-generation agents are more potent against *E. coli*, *K. pneumoniae*, and *P. mirabilis* than first-generation agents and are also active against *Neisseria* spp. and, in the case of the true cephalosporins, *H. influenzae* (including β-lactamase–producing strains). Because of the additional methoxy group on the β-lactam ring (Figure 5-12), the cephamycins also have enhanced stability to the β-lactamases of some anaerobes, such as *B. fragilis*. However, this added anaerobic activity comes at a cost; it is the methoxy group that results in the diminished activity of the cephamycins against staphylococci and streptococci because of decreased affinity for the PBPs of these bacteria.

CHAPTER 5 — Antibiotics That Target the Cell Envelope

Second-Generation Cephalosporins

Gram-positive
Gram-negative
Anaerobes
Atypical

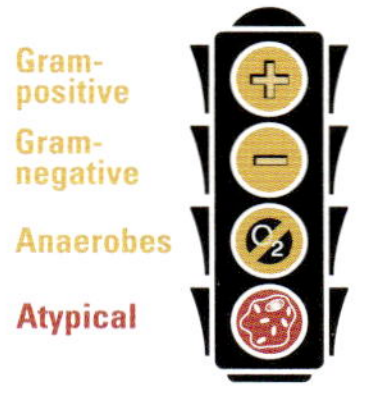

Table 5-10. Antimicrobial Activity of Second-Generation Cephalosporins

Gram-positive bacteria	True cephalosporins have activity equivalent to first-generation agents. Cefoxitin and cefotetan have little activity.
Gram-negative bacteria	Some *Escherichia coli* Some *Klebsiella pneumoniae* *Proteus mirabilis* *Haemophilus influenzae* *Neisseria* spp.
Anaerobic bacteria	Cefoxitin and cefotetan have moderate anaerobic activity.

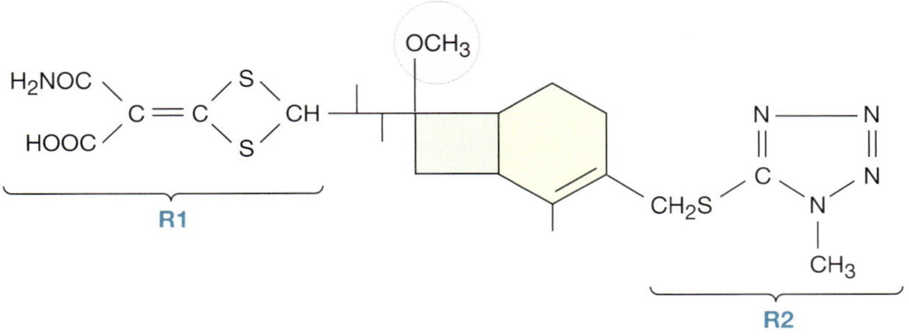

Figure 5-12. Structure of cefotetan. The methoxy group characteristic of the cephamycins is circled.

THIRD-GENERATION CEPHALOSPORINS

Commonly used third-generation cephalosporins include **ceftriaxone**, **cefotaxime**, and **ceftazidime** (see Table 5-8). In general, compounds in this group have moderate activity against aerobic gram-positive bacteria (Table 5-11) and inhibit most strains of penicillin-susceptible *S. pneumoniae*. Third-generation cephalosporins are also active against the spirochete *Borrelia burgdorferi* but have little activity against anaerobic bacteria.

A modification common to many third-generation cephalosporins is the use of an aminothiazolyl group at R1. The presence of this structure at R1 results in increased penetration of these agents through the bacterial outer membrane, increased affinity for PBPs, and increased stability in the presence of some of the plasmid-encoded β-lactamases of aerobic and facultative gram-negative bacteria. Thus, these agents have enhanced activity against *E. coli*, *Klebsiella* spp., *Proteus* spp., *Neisseria* spp., and *H. influenzae* relative to the second-generation cephalosporins, although many strains of *E. coli* and *Klebsiella* have acquired β-lactamases that confer resistance. In addition, some other strains of the Enterobacterales, such as *Enterobacter cloacae*, *Citrobacter freundii*, and *Klebsiella aerogenes*, also initially show susceptibility to third-generation cephalosporins. However, these bacteria harbor chromosomally encoded inducible

Third-Generation Cephalosporins	Table 5-11	Antimicrobial Activity of Third-Generation Cephalosporins
Gram-positive: + Gram-negative: − Anaerobes: O₂ Atypical	Gram-positive bacteria	*Streptococcus pyogenes* Viridans streptococci Many *Streptococcus pneumoniae* Modest activity against *Staphylococcus aureus*
	Gram-negative bacteria	Some *Escherichia coli* Some *Klebsiella pneumoniae* *Proteus* spp. *Haemophilus influenzae* *Neisseria* spp. Some other Enterobacterales
	Spirochetes	*Borrelia burgdorferi*

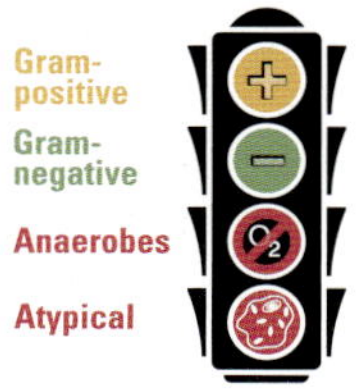

AmpC β-lactamases that may allow the emergence of resistance during treatment. Thus, it is now felt that severe infections caused by these organisms should either not be treated with third-generation cephalosporins or should be treated with these agents in conjunction with a second active agent, even if they appear to be susceptible by in vitro testing.

One shortcoming of most of the third-generation cephalosporins is their lack of activity against *P. aeruginosa*. To address this, the aminothiazolyl R1 side chain of ceftazidime was modified by the addition of an α-hydroxyisobutyric acid group (Figure 5-13), which dramatically increases antipseudomonal activity. Unfortunately, this modification also results in decreased affinity for the PBPs of staphylococci. As a result, ceftazidime has enhanced activity against *P. aeruginosa* but limited activity against *S. aureus*.

Among the third-generation cephalosporins, ceftriaxone is notable for its long half-life. This agent is widely used because of the convenience of its once-per-day dosing.

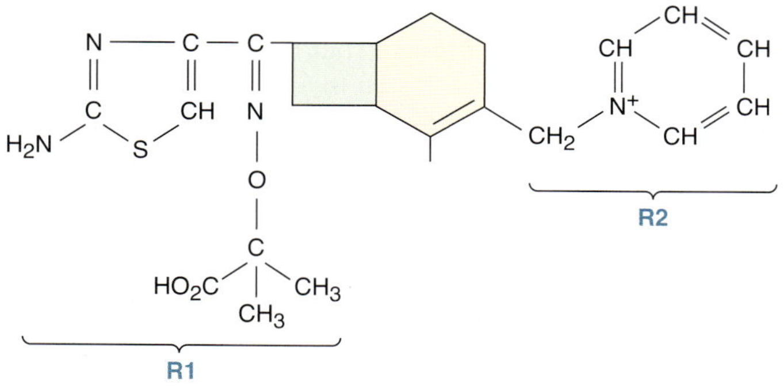

Figure 5-13. Structure of ceftazidime. In ceftazidime, the aminothiazolyl group at R1 typical of third-generation cephalosporins is modified with the addition of a α-hydroxyisobutyric acid group, which enhances activity against *Pseudomonas aeruginosa*.

FOURTH-GENERATION CEPHALOSPORINS

As mentioned earlier, the third-generation cephalosporins are powerful antimicrobial agents but suffer from susceptibility to the chromosomally encoded inducible AmpC β-lactamases of some of the Enterobacterales. In addition, activity against *P. aeruginosa* is gained only at the expense of diminished antistaphylococcal activity. Attempts to address these deficiencies led to modifications of the R2 side chain of the third-generation cephalosporins while leaving the highly successful aminothiazolyl group at R1 unchanged (Figure 5-14). The result of these efforts was the fourth-generation cephalosporin **cefepime** (Table 5-8). The side chains of cefepime allow more rapid penetration through the outer membrane of many gram-negative bacteria, including *P. aeruginosa*. It also binds at a high affinity to many of the PBPs of these bacteria but is relatively resistant to hydrolysis by gram-negative β-lactamases, including the chromosomally encoded inducible AmpC β-lactamases of the Enterobacterales (although the clinical relevance of this is controversial). These properties are attained without the loss of activity against aerobic gram-positive cocci. Thus, this incredibly powerful antibiotic has the best features of the various third-generation cephalosporins (antipseudomonal activity without loss of antistaphylococcal activity) and may also have enhanced activity against many of the Enterobacterales. Cefepime has very limited anaerobic activity (Table 5-12).

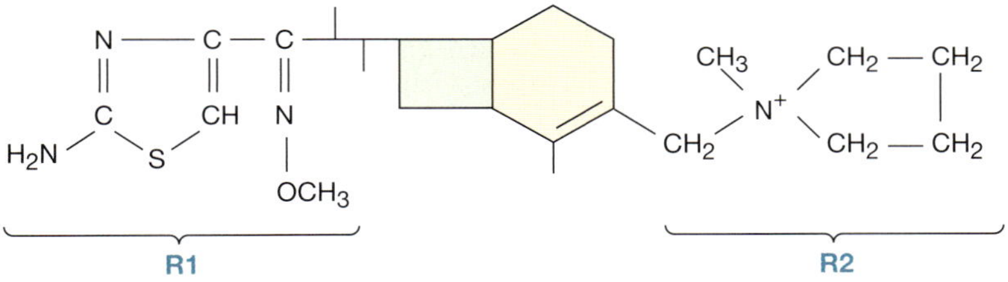

Figure 5-14. Structure of cefepime. The aminothiazolyl group typical of many third-generation cephalosporins is at R1, whereas a polar pyrrolidine group is at R2.

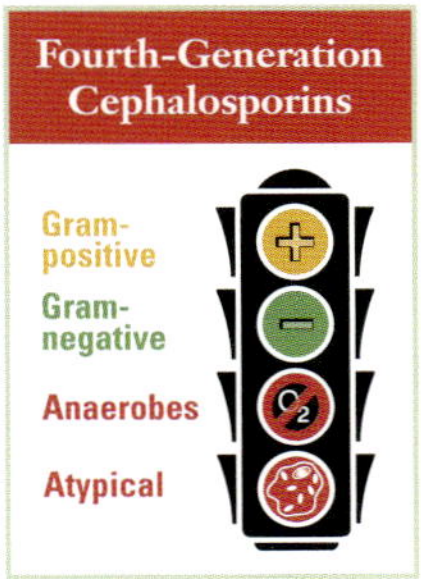

Table 5-12 Antimicrobial Activity of Fourth-Generation Cephalosporins

Gram-positive bacteria	*Streptococcus pyogenes* Viridans streptococci Many *Streptococcus pneumoniae* Modest activity against *Staphylococcus aureus*
Gram-negative bacteria	Some *Escherichia coli* Some *Klebsiella pneumoniae* *Proteus* spp. *Haemophilus influenzae* *Neisseria* spp. Many other Enterobacterales *Pseudomonas aeruginosa*

Fourth-Generation Cephalosporins: Gram-positive +, Gram-negative +, Anaerobes −, Atypical −

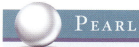

> **PEARL**
>
> The Enterobacterales is a large group of medically important gram-negative bacteria that includes the following genera: *Citrobacter, Enterobacter, Escherichia, Klebsiella, Morganella, Proteus, Providencia, Salmonella, Serratia, Shigella,* and *Yersinia*.

FIFTH-GENERATION CEPHALOSPORINS

Ceftaroline is a new cephalosporin that has expanded activity against aerobic gram-positive cocci, causing some experts to refer to it as a fifth-generation agent (Table 5-8). A 1,3-thiazole ring has been added to the R2 side chain of this cephalosporin, which confers upon it the ability to bind to the PBP of methicillin-resistant staphylococci (Figure 5-15). As a result, ceftaroline has excellent activity against aerobic gram-positive cocci, including MRSA and MRSE and penicillin-resistant *S. pneumoniae* strains (Table 5-13). Its activities against aerobic gram-negative bacteria

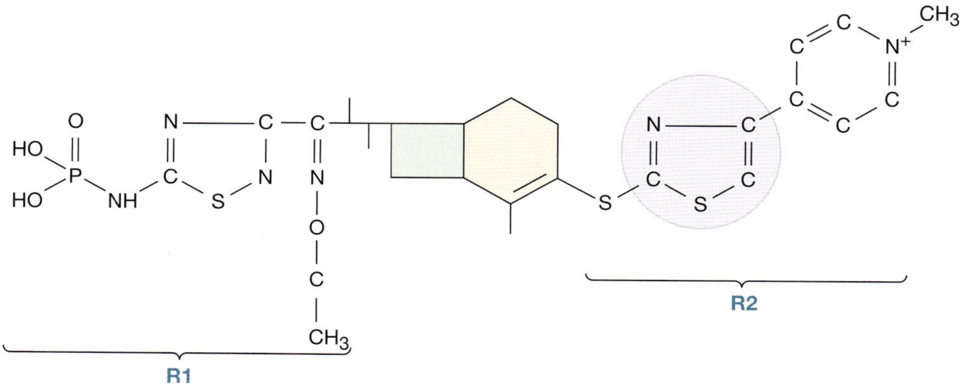

Figure 5-15. Structure of ceftaroline. The circled 1,3-thiazole ring in the R2 side chain confers activity against methicillin-resistant *Staphylococcus aureus* strains.

Fifth-Generation Cephalosporins

- Gram-positive: +
- Gram-negative: −
- Anaerobes: ⊘
- Atypical: ⊘

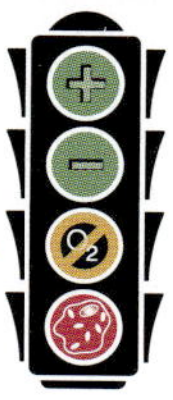

Table 5-13	Antimicrobial Activity of Fifth-Generation Cephalosporins
Gram-positive bacteria	*Streptococcus pyogenes* Viridans streptococci *Streptococcus pneumoniae* Staphylococci
Gram-negative bacteria	Some *Escherichia coli* Some *Klebsiella pneumoniae* *Proteus* spp. *Haemophilus influenzae* *Neisseria* spp. Some other Enterobacterales
Anaerobic bacteria	Some *Clostridium* spp.

are similar to those of cefotaxime and ceftriaxone; it lacks antipseudomonal activity. Ceftaroline also has activity against anaerobic gram-positive bacteria, but not against anaerobic gram-negative bacteria. This agent is administered as the inactive prodrug ceftaroline fosamil, which is rapidly converted to ceftaroline.

CEPHALOSPORIN/β-LACTAMASE INHIBITOR COMBINATIONS

Two recent additions to the cephalosporin family of antibiotics are **ceftazidime-avibactam** and **ceftolozane-tazobactam** (Table 5-8).

Ceftazidime-avibactam broadens the spectrum of ceftazidime by combining it with the β-lactamase inhibitor avibactam. Unlike the β-lactamase inhibitors discussed up to this point, avibactam is not itself a β-lactam but does have structural features of β-lactams, which allows it to be bound by β-lactamases. The addition of avibactam to ceftazidime enhances the latter's activity against Enterobacterales (including ceftazidime-resistant strains) and *P. aeruginosa* (Table 5-14). Arguably, the most useful aspect of this antibiotic is its ability to inhibit the ESBLs, AmpC β-lactamases, and *K. pneumoniae* carbapenemases (KPCs) (see Chapter 11 for a detailed description of these β-lactamases). The net result is enhanced activity against members of the Enterobacterales and good activity against *P. aeruginosa*. This agent may be most useful in the treatment of infections caused by KPC-producing Enterobacterales, for which few alternatives are currently available.

Whereas ceftazidime-avibactam combines an old cephalosporin with a novel β-lactamase inhibitor, ceftolozane-tazobactam combines an old β-lactamase inhibitor with a novel cephalosporin. Ceftolozane has features of ceftazidime, such as the β-hydroxyisobutyric acid group on R1, but has a bulkier R2 side chain, which prevents cleavage by AmpC β-lactamases (compare Figures 5-13 and 5-16). Together, these modifications confer enhanced activity against *P. aeruginosa* (Table 5-15). Tazobactam, which was described in the section on penicillins plus β-lactamase inhibitors, may provide some activity against ESBL-producing Enterobacterales, although this remains controversial.

Table 5-14 Antimicrobial Activity of Cephalosporin Plus β-Lactamase Inhibitor Combinations

Gram-positive bacteria	*Streptococcus pyogenes* Viridans streptococci Many *Streptococcus pneumoniae*
Gram-negative bacteria	*Escherichia coli* (including many carbapenem-resistant strains) *Klebsiella pneumoniae* (including many carbapenem-resistant strains) *Proteus* spp. Other Enterobacterales *Haemophilus influenzae* *Neisseria* spp. *Pseudomonas aeruginosa* (including many highly resistant strains)

Cephalosporin Plus β-Lactase Inhibitor Combinations:
- Gram-positive: +
- Gram-negative: −
- Anaerobes: ○
- Atypical: ○

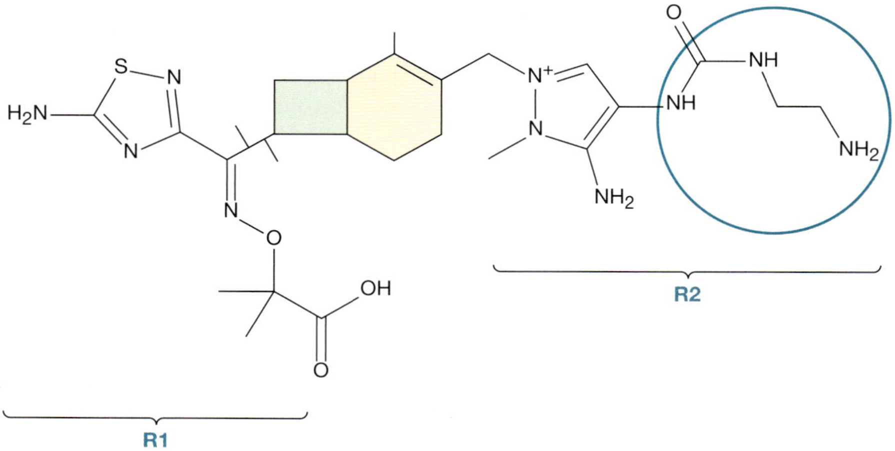

Figure 5-16. Structure of ceftolozane. The R1 side chain is similar to that of ceftazidime, which enhances activity against *Pseudomonas aeruginosa*. However, the R2 group is bulkier than that of ceftazidime or other third-generation cephalosporins (see blue circle), which confers resistance to certain β-lactamases and further enhances antipseudomonal activity.

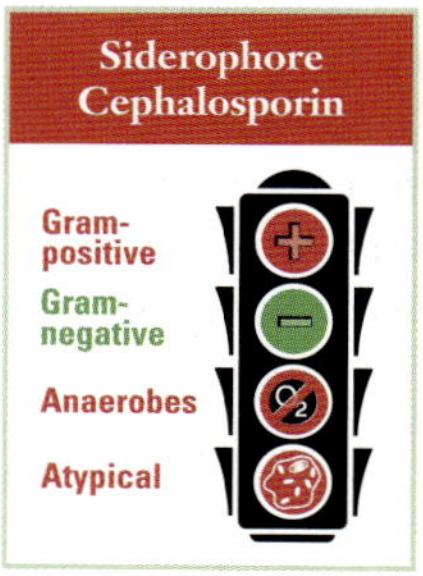

Table 5-15	Antimicrobial Activity of Siderophore Cephalosporins
Gram-negative bacteria	*Escherichia coli* (including many carbapenem-resistant strains) *Klebsiella pneumoniae* (including many carbapenem-resistant strains) *Proteus* spp. Other Enterobacterales *Pseudomonas aeruginosa* (including many highly resistant strains)

SIDEROPHORE CEPHALOSPORINS

A new and exciting class of antibiotics is the siderophore cephalosporins, of which **cefiderocol** is currently approved for use (Table 5-8). In general, cephalosporins gain access to PBPs in the bacterial periplasm by passing through the "front door" porins, outer membrane channels used by bacteria to take up nutrients. In contrast, siderophore cephalosporins use subterfuge and enter "through the back door." How do they do this? Under normal circumstances, siderophores are secreted by bacteria to scavenge iron. The siderophore-iron conjugate is then bound by specific bacterial surface receptors and actively imported into the cell. Cefiderocol, which consists of a siderophore-like structure linked to a cephalosporin antibiotic, tricks bacteria into using their siderophore machinery to actively import it into the periplasm. As a result, siderophore cephalosporins can penetrate the outer membrane barrier of gram-negative bacteria and achieve high concentrations in the periplasm. In addition, the cephalosporin component of cefiderocol, which has side chains similar to

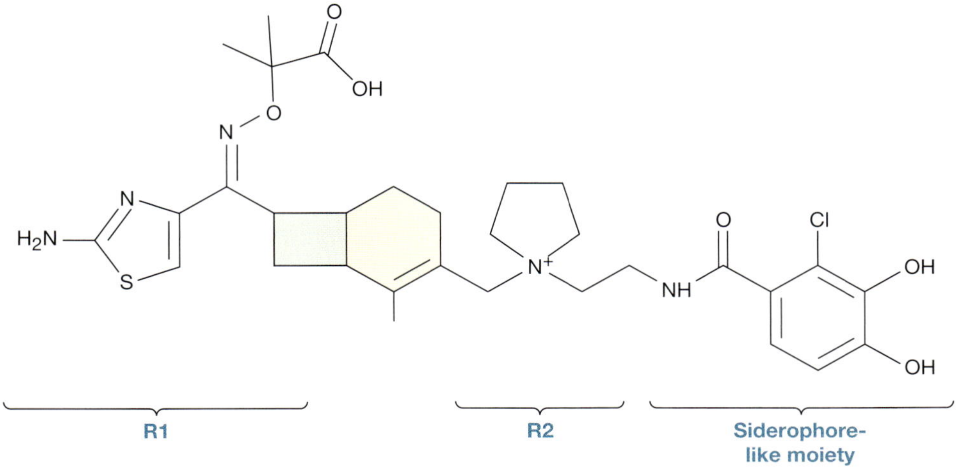

Figure 5-17. Structure of cefiderocol. The R1 group is similar to that of ceftazidime, and the R2 group is similar to that of cefepime. The siderophore-like group is indicated.

those of ceftazidime and cefepime (Figure 5-17), is resistant to degradation by most β-lactamases. The addition of the siderophore moiety adds further stability. The net result is an antibiotic that has in vitro activity against many highly antibiotic-resistant gram-negative bacteria, even those resistant to cephalosporin plus β-lactamase inhibitor combinations and carbapenems. However, some evidence suggests that resistance may emerge during the course of therapy with cefiderocol, and the utility of this antibiotic in patients is still being evaluated. Cefiderocol does not have activity against gram-positive, anaerobic, or atypical bacteria (Table 5-15).

TOXICITY

One of the attractions of the cephalosporins is their relatively favorable safety profile. Rarely, these agents cause immediate hypersensitivity reactions consisting of rash, urticaria, or anaphylaxis. In this regard, approximately 5% to 10% of individuals allergic to penicillin will also have a reaction to cephalosporins. Thus, it is usually recommended that individuals with a history of severe immediate hypersensitivity reactions to penicillin not be treated with cephalosporins. Other rare adverse effects include reversible neutropenia, thrombocytosis, hemolysis, diarrhea, and elevated liver function tests. Cefotetan may cause hypoprothrombinemia and, when used with alcohol, a disulfiram-like reaction. Both of these effects are associated with the methylthiotetrazole moiety at R2 of this agent (see Figure 5-12). Because ceftriaxone is eliminated by biliary excretion, high doses of this agent may result in biliary sludging. Prolonged use of ceftaroline has been linked to neutropenia.

In summary, the cephalosporins vary markedly in their activities, but the following generalizations can be made: (1) With the exception of fifth-generation cephalosporins (ceftaroline), each successive generation has increased activity against aerobic gram-negative rods. (2) Fifth-generation cephalosporins and, to a much lesser degree, first-generation cephalosporins have good activity against aerobic gram-positive bacteria. (3) Some second-generation agents have modest activity against anaerobic bacteria.

History

Cephalosporins were discovered by the Italian scientist Giuseppe Brotzu in the 1940s. He noted that the seawater in the vicinity of a sewage outlet in Cagliari, Italy, periodically cleared, a phenomenon he suspected was due to the production of an inhibitory compound by a microbe growing in the water. He eventually identified the microbe as *C. acremonium* and showed that it did indeed produce a substance that inhibited bacterial growth. This substance became the backbone from which early cephalosporins were synthesized. Interestingly, *Cephalosporium* fungi have been renamed *Acremonium* and occasionally cause infections in people.

Reprinted by permission from Springer: Abraham EP. Cephalosporins 1945-1986. In: Williams JD, ed. *The Cephalosporin Antibiotics*. Adis Press; 1987.

Questions

13. Cephalosporins are grouped into _____ and are all part of the larger class of antibiotics known as _____.
14. Like penicillins, cephalosporins act by binding _____, which are bacterial enzymes that function to assemble peptidoglycan.
15. First-generation cephalosporins are most useful in the treatment of infections caused by aerobic _____ bacteria.
16. Compared to first-generation agents, second-generation cephalosporins have enhanced activity against aerobic _____ bacteria. Some of these agents are also active against _____ bacteria.
17. Third-generation cephalosporins are most useful in the treatment of infections caused by aerobic _____ bacteria.
18. Compared to third-generation agents, fourth-generation cephalosporins have a broader spectrum of activity against aerobic gram-negative bacteria, including _____ and additional members of the _____.
19. Unlike other cephalosporins, fifth-generation cephalosporins have activity against _____ strains.
20. Cephalosporin plus β-lactamase inhibitor combinations are useful for treating multidrug-resistant aerobic _____ bacteria.
21. Use of high doses of _____ has been associated with biliary sludging.
22. Cephalosporins should be used with caution in individuals with severe immediate hypersensitivity reactions to _____.

Answers

13. generations, β-lactams
14. PBPs
15. gram-positive
16. gram-negative, anaerobic

17. gram-negative
18. *P. aeruginosa*, Enterobacterales
19. MRSA
20. gram-negative
21. ceftriaxone
22. penicillins

ADDITIONAL READINGS

Endimiani A, Perez F, Bonomo RA. Cefepime: a reappraisal in an era of increasing antimicrobial resistance. *Expert Rev Anti Infect Ther*. 2008;6:805-824.

Kaye KS, Naas T, Pogue JM, Rossoline GM. Cefiderocol, a siderophore cephalosporin, as a treatment option for infections caused by carbapenem-resistant Enterobacterales. *Infect Dis Ther*. 2023;12(3):777-806. doi:10.1007/s40121-023-00773-6

Petri WA Jr. Penicillins, cephalosporins, and other β-lactam antibiotics. In: Brunton LL, Lazo JS, Parker KL, eds. *Goodman and Gilman's The Pharmacological Basis of Therapeutics*. 11th ed. McGraw-Hill; 2006:1127-1154.

Prober CG. Cephalosporins: an update. *Pediatr Rev*. 1998;19:118-127.

van Duin D, Bonomo RA. Ceftazidime/avibactam and ceftolozane/tazobactam: second-generation β-lactam/β-lactamase inhibitor combinations. *Clin Infect Dis*. 2016;63:234-241.

Zhanel GG, Sniezek G, Schweizer F, et al. Ceftaroline: a novel broad-spectrum cephalosporin with activity against methicillin-resistant *Staphylococcus aureus*. *Drugs*. 2009;69:809-831.

Carbapenems

If β-lactams are viewed as a large extended family of antibiotics, then carbapenems are the arrogant young sons who drive high-powered sports cars and wear flashy clothes. These antibiotics are among the most broadly active antibiotics in use today. As such, they are often the last line of defense against many organisms that are resistant to other antimicrobial agents. Five members of this class, **imipenem, meropenem, ertapenem, meropenem-vaborbactam,** and **imipenem-relebactam**, are commercially available (Table 5-16).

The structures of carbapenems are related to those of penicillins and cephalosporins (Figure 5-18). A β-lactam ring is fused to a five-membered ring with variable side chains. The five-membered ring differs from the thiazolidine ring of penicillin in two ways (see circles in Figure 5-18): A methylene group replaces sulfur, and the ring contains a double bond. In addition, the acylamino root of the penicillin side chain is replaced by a hydroxyethyl group.

This structure results in three properties that account for the carbapenems' incredibly broad spectra of activity. First, these molecules are quite small and have charge characteristics that allow them to utilize special porins in the outer membrane of gram-negative bacteria to gain access to the PBPs. Second, the structures of the carbapenems make them resistant to cleavage by most β-lactamases. Third, the carbapenems have an affinity for a broad range of PBPs from many different kinds of bacteria. As a result of these three properties, the carbapenems are adept at gaining access to the

Table 5-16 The Carbapenems

Parenteral Agents	Oral Agents
Imipenem/cilastatin	None
Meropenem	
Ertapenem	
Meropenem/vaborbactam	
Imipenem/cilastatin/relebactam	

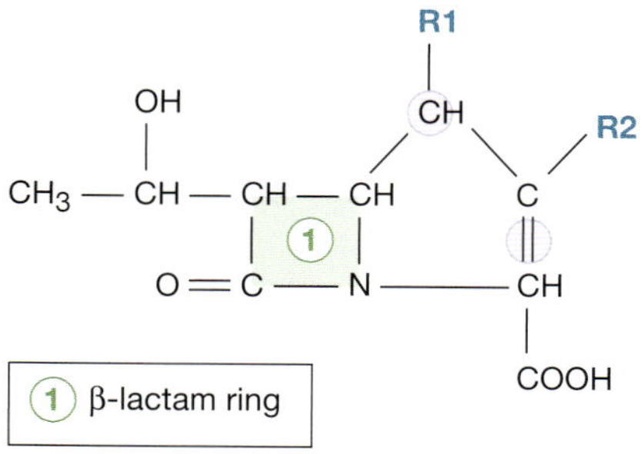

Figure 5-18. The structure of carbapenems. Circles indicate differences from the penicillin core structure.

periplasm, resisting destruction by β-lactamases that reside there, and binding to PBPs to cause bacterial cell death.

Resistance to carbapenems occurs when bacteria overcome the advantageous aspects of these antibiotics. For example, *P. aeruginosa* is prone to develop resistance by acquiring mutations that result in loss of production of the outer membrane porin used by carbapenems to gain access to the periplasm. This often occurs together with overproduction of efflux pumps that limit accumulation of the drugs in the periplasmic space. *Enterococcus faecium* and methicillin-resistant staphylococci are resistant because they produce altered PBPs that do not bind these carbapenems. Finally, some bacteria have acquired the ability to produce extremely powerful β-lactamases that are capable of cleaving carbapenems.

HISTORY

That carbapenems, some of our most powerful antibiotics, are no longer active against some bacteria that were formerly susceptible, underscoring the problem of emerging antimicrobial resistance. In 1946, Alexander Fleming warned against just such an eventuality. ".... the public will demand [the drug and].... then will begin an era.... of abuses. The microbes are educated to resist penicillin and a host of penicillin-fast organisms is bred out which can be passed to other individuals and perhaps from there to others until they reach someone who gets a septicemia or a pneumonia which penicillin cannot save. In such a case the thoughtless person playing with penicillin treatment is morally responsible for the death of the man who finally succumbs to infection with the penicillin-resistant organism. I hope this evil can be averted."

From Penicillin's finder assays its future. *New York Times*. June 26, 1945:21.

IMIPENEM

Imipenem was the first commercially available carbapenem in the United States. Structurally, this compound differs from the other carbapenems in that it lacks an R1 side chain (Figure 5-18). It is rapidly destroyed in the kidney by an enzyme called dehydropeptidase I. As a result, it is administered with cilastatin, an inhibitor of this enzyme.

Imipenem is active against many species of pathogenic bacteria (Table 5-17). Most streptococci, including many penicillin-resistant *S. pneumoniae* strains, are sensitive to this agent, as are many staphylococci (but not the "methicillin-resistant" staphylococci). Imipenem has truly remarkable activity against many different aerobic gram-negative bacteria, including *P. aeruginosa* and many of the highly resistant Enterobacterales, such as *Enterobacter* and *Citrobacter* species. It also has excellent anaerobic coverage and is among the most useful agents in treating infections caused by these organisms. Like most antibiotics, however, it is not active against *C. difficile*.

MEROPENEM

The structure of meropenem differs from that of imipenem at both the R1 and R2 side chains (Figure 5-18). Importantly, whereas imipenem lacks an R1 side chain,

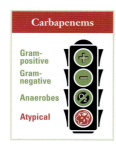

Table 5-17. Antimicrobial Activity of Carbapenems

Gram-positive bacteria	*Streptococcus pyogenes* Viridans streptococci *Streptococcus pneumoniae* Modest activity against *Staphylococcus aureus* Some enterococci *Listeria monocytogenes*
Gram-negative bacteria	*Haemophilus influenzae* *Neisseria* spp. Enterobacterales *Pseudomonas aeruginosa*
Anaerobic bacteria	*Bacteroides fragilis* Most other anaerobes

meropenem has a methyl group at this position, which makes the molecule resistant to cleavage by the renal dehydropeptidase. As a result, meropenem does not need to be administered in conjunction with cilastatin.

Meropenem's spectrum of activity is essentially the same as imipenem. Thus, this agent also has excellent activity against aerobic gram-positive, aerobic gram-negative, and anaerobic bacteria.

ERTAPENEM

Ertapenem also has a methyl group at R1 (see Figure 5-18) and, therefore, is not cleaved by renal dehydropeptidase. It differs from imipenem and meropenem at its R2 side chain, which accounts for its somewhat distinctive antimicrobial and pharmacologic properties. It is less active against aerobic gram-positive bacteria, *P. aeruginosa*, and *Acinetobacter* spp. than the other carbapenems but compensates for this weakness by requiring only once-per-day dosing.

MEROPENEM-VABORBACTAM

Meropenem-vaborbactam is a combination of a carbapenem (meropenem) with a β-lactamase inhibitor (vaborbactam). The addition of vaborbactam addresses one of the holes in meropenem's broad spectrum of activity: members of the Enterobacterales that produce KPCs. KPCs are powerful β-lactamases that can degrade carbapenems, but they are inhibited by vaborbactam. (See Chapter 11 for a detailed description of these β-lactamases.) Vaborbactam does not expand meropenem's already impressive activity against gram-positive or anaerobic bacteria; nor does it enhance its activity against *P. aeruginosa* and *Acinetobacter baumannii*.

IMIPENEM-RELEBACTAM

Imipenem-relebactam is another combination of a carbapenem (imipenem) with a β-lactamase inhibitor (relebactam), and its spectrum of activity is similar to that of meropenem-vaborbactam. As with meropenem-vaborbactam, the addition of relebactam to imipenem expands this carbapenem's activity to include many Enterobacterales that produce KPCs. Unlike meropenem-vaborbactam, however, relebactam restores susceptibility of imipenem to some *P. aeruginosa* strains. In particular, relebactam inhibits the *P. aeruginosa* AmpC β-lactamase, the overproduction of which contributes to imipenem resistance in some strains of *P. aeruginosa*.

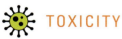
TOXICITY

Carbapenem use is associated with several adverse events, including nausea and vomiting, diarrhea, rash, and drug fever. A more worrisome complication associated with carbapenems is seizures. Patients with preexisting central nervous system disease and renal insufficiency are most at risk for this complication and should be given these drugs with caution. Initially, meropenem was felt to be less likely to cause seizures than imipenem, but this is now controversial.

In summary, carbapenems have excellent activity against a broad spectrum of bacteria, including many aerobic gram-positive bacteria, most aerobic gram-negative bacteria, and most anaerobes. As a result, these compounds are among the most powerful antibacterial agents in use today.

Pearl

Strains of *Enterococcus faecalis* that are susceptible to penicillin are also susceptible to carbapenems (except ertapenem). *E. faecium*, however, is resistant to all carbapenems.

Edwards JR. Meropenem: a microbiological overview. *J Antimicrob Chemother.* 1995;36(suppl A):1-17.

Questions

23. Imipenem is hydrolyzed by dehydropeptidase I in the kidney and, therefore, must be given with _____.
24. Carbapenems have excellent aerobic _____, aerobic _____, and _____ activity.
25. Compared to other carbapenems, ertapenem is less active against aerobic gram-positive bacteria, _____, and _____.

Answers

23. cilastatin
24. gram-positive, gram-negative, anaerobic
25. *P. aeruginosa*, *Acinetobacter* spp.

ADDITIONAL READINGS

Giske CG, Buarø L, Sundsfjord A, et al. Alterations of porin, pumps, and penicillin-binding proteins in carbapenem resistant clinical isolates of *Pseudomonas aeruginosa*. *Microb Drug Resist*. 2008;14:23-30.

Nicolau DP. Carbapenems: a potent class of antibiotics. *Expert Opin Pharmacother*. 2008;9:23-37.

Tiwari A, Tiwari V, Sahoo BM, et al. Carbapenem antibiotics: recent update on synthesis and pharmacological activities. *Curr Drug Res Rev*. 2023;15:35-61.

Yahav D, Giske CG, Gramatniece A, et al. New β-lactam-β-lactamase inhibitor combinations. *Clin Microbiol Rev*. 2021;34:e00115-20. doi:10.1128/CMR.00115-20.

Zhanel GG, Johanson C, Embil JM, et al. Ertapenem: review of a new carbapenem. *Expert Rev Anti Infect Ther*. 2005;3:23-39.

Monobactams

Many of the newer β-lactam antibiotics have extremely broad spectra of activity, but the monobactams go against this trend. **Aztreonam**, the only commercially available monobactam, does only one thing but does it quite well: It kills aerobic gram-negative bacteria. It is available for parenteral use only.

The term *monobactam* has been used to describe several bacterially derived antibiotics that consist of a lone β-lactam ring as opposed to the linked two-ring structures of the penicillins, cephalosporins, and carbapenems (Figure 5-19). Aztreonam is a synthetic monobactam that combines some of the useful features of other β-lactam antibiotics. For example, one of the side chains of aztreonam is identical to that of ceftazidime, which confers activity against *P. aeruginosa* (compare Figures 5-19 with 5-13 in the "Cephalosporins" discussion).

As a result of its designer structural properties, aztreonam gains access to and binds quite well to the PBPs of aerobic gram-negative bacteria and is stable against many of the β-lactamases produced by these organisms (Table 5-18). It has excellent activity against *Neisseria* and *Haemophilus* spp. and intermediate activity against *P. aeruginosa*. Unfortunately, it does not bind the PBPs of gram-positive or anaerobic bacteria and, therefore, is not useful for infections caused by these organisms.

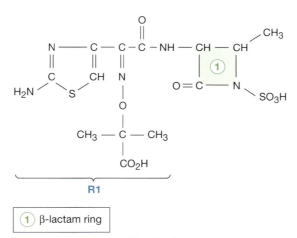

① β-lactam ring

Figure 5-19. The structure of aztreonam. The R1 side chain is similar to that of ceftazidime.

Monobactams	Table 5-18	Antimicrobial Activity of Monobactams
Gram-positive	Gram-negative bacteria	*Haemophilus influenzae*
Gram-negative		*Neisseria* spp.
Anaerobes		Most Enterobacterales
Atypical		Many *Pseudomonas aeruginosa*

Resistance to aztreonam does occur in some members of the Enterobacterales and *P. aeruginosa*, usually as the result of changes in the permeability of the outer membrane of these bacteria or of destruction by β-lactamases.

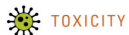

TOXICITY

One of the major advantages of aztreonam is its safety profile. It is not associated with nephrotoxicity and can be viewed as a renal-sparing alternative to the aminoglycosides because both agents have activity against aerobic gram-negative bacteria. Importantly, there are no allergic cross-reactions between aztreonam and other β-lactams, so aztreonam is safe to use in patients with penicillin allergies.

In summary, aztreonam, the only commercially available monobactam, has excellent activity against aerobic gram-negative bacteria but is not useful against gram-positive or anaerobic bacteria. It is a relatively safe drug and can be used in individuals with allergies to other β-lactam agents.

QUESTIONS

26. _____ is the only commercially available monobactam.
27. Aztreonam has excellent activity against aerobic _____ bacteria but lacks activity against aerobic _____ bacteria and _____ bacteria.
28. A particularly useful feature of aztreonam is that it can be used in patients with allergies to other _____ antibiotics.

ANSWERS

26. Aztreonam
27. gram-negative, gram-positive, anaerobic
28. β-lactam

ADDITIONAL READINGS

Asbel LE, Levison ME. Cephalosporins, carbapenems, and monobactams. *Infect Dis Clin North Am.* 2000;14:435-447, xi.
Sykes RB, Bonner DP. Aztreonam: the first monobactam. *Am J Med.* 1985;78:2-10.
Sykes RB, Bonner DP. Discovery and development of the monobactams. *Rev Infect Dis.* 1985;7(suppl 4):S579-S593.

Glycopeptides

Vancomycin is a **glycopeptide** antibiotic, a peptide with a sugar moiety attached to it. **Telavancin, dalbavancin,** and **oritavancin** are a subset of the glycopeptide family called **lipoglycopeptides**—glycopeptides modified to include an additional lipophilic side chain (Table 5-19). Like most peptides, these antibiotics are poorly absorbed in the gastrointestinal tract, so they must be given intravenously to treat systemic infections. Relative to other antibiotics, they are extremely large (Figure 5-20), which

Table 5-19	The Glycopeptides
Parenteral Agents	**Oral Agents**
Vancomycin	None
Dalbavancin	
Telavancin	
Oritavancin	

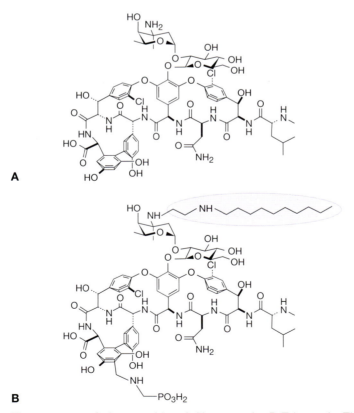

Figure 5-20. The structure of glycopeptides. A. Vancomycin. B. Telavancin. The lipophilic side chain of telavancin is circled.

Table 5-20	Antimicrobial Activity of Glycopeptides
Gram-positive bacteria	*Staphylococcus aureus* *Staphylococcus epidermidis* *Streptococcus pyogenes* Viridans streptococci *Streptococcus pneumoniae* Some enterococci
Anaerobic bacteria	*Clostridium* spp. Other gram-positive anaerobes

prevents them from passing through porins in the outer membranes of gram-negative bacteria. Thus, their activity is restricted to gram-positive organisms (Table 5-20). Within this group, though, their coverage is impressive. They are active against nearly all staphylococci and streptococci, including methicillin-resistant staphylococci and strains of penicillin-resistant *S. pneumoniae*. Susceptibility among enterococci is now variable. Although *L. monocytogenes* usually appears susceptible in vitro, clinical failures have been reported with vancomycin, and glycopeptides should not be used to treat infections caused by this organism. Vancomycin also has good activity against anaerobic gram-positive bacteria, including *C. difficile*.

Like the β-lactams, glycopeptides kill bacteria by preventing the synthesis of the cell wall. They bind to the D-alanyl-D-alanine portion of the peptide side chain of precursor peptidoglycan subunits. Because of the bulk of these compounds, this binding prevents these subunits from being accessed by the PBPs that would normally incorporate them into the growing peptidoglycan polymer (Figure 5-21A).

Some enterococci have developed an ingenious way of resisting glycopeptides. These bacteria encode genes that modify the structure of the peptidoglycan precursor such that the D-alanyl-D-alanine dipeptide is changed, most often to D-alanyl-D-lactate (Figure 5-21B). Glycopeptides are no longer able to recognize and bind to these altered precursors. Unfortunately, the gene clusters that encode this activity in enterococci are transferable and have already been found in *S. aureus*. Thus, it was anticipated that resistance to these agents would occur with increasing frequency in staphylococci as well, although this fear has not been realized to date.

VANCOMYCIN

Vancomycin is the most commonly used member of this class (see Figure 5-20A). It is an old drug initially associated with substantial toxicity. This toxicity, however, is now known to be due to contaminants that resulted from the crude purification process. Newer production techniques have greatly enhanced the safety profile of vancomycin, whereas other agents, such as penicillins, have been progressively limited in their use by increasing resistance. As a result, vancomycin has become a workhorse among antibacterial agents. With increasing use, however, its preeminent position, too, has been threatened by emerging resistance, especially among the enterococci. Although usually given intravenously, it can be given orally to treat bowel infections, such as diarrhea caused by *C. difficile*, but it is not absorbed when administered in this way because it is a modified peptide.

CHAPTER 5 — Antibiotics That Target the Cell Envelope

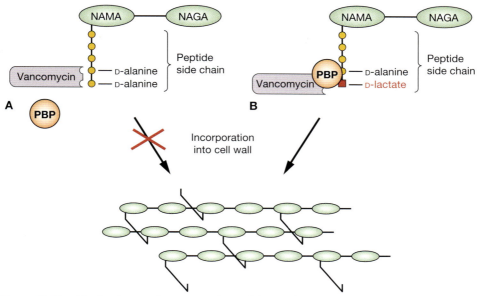

Figure 5-21. Mechanisms of vancomycin activity and resistance. A. Vancomycin binds to the D-alanyl-D-alanine dipeptide on the peptide side chain of newly synthesized peptidoglycan subunits, preventing them from being incorporated into the cell wall by penicillin-binding proteins (PBPs). B. In many vancomycin-resistant strains of enterococci, the D-alanyl-D-alanine dipeptide is replaced with D-alanyl-D-lactate, which is not recognized by vancomycin. Thus, the peptidoglycan subunit is appropriately incorporated into the cell wall. NAGA, *N*-acetylglucosamine; NAMA, *N*-acetylmuramic acid.

HISTORY

Vancomycin was discovered when a missionary from Borneo sent a soil sample to his friend who was an organic chemist at Eli Lilly and Company. The soil sample turned out to harbor a bacterium that made a compound with potent activity against gram-positive bacteria. Eventually, the compound was purified and named vancomycin, which is derived from the word "vanquish."

Griffith RS. Vancomycin use—an historical review. *J Antimicrob Chemother*. 1984;14(suppl D):1-5.

DALBAVANCIN

Structurally, dalbavancin differs from vancomycin in several ways, including the addition of a long lipophilic tail, which classifies it as a lipoglycopeptide. This tail better anchors dalbavancin to the bacterial membrane, which, in turn, keeps it close to the D-alanine-D-alanine–containing peptidoglycan intermediate. This proximity enhances binding of the peptidoglycan intermediate relative to vancomycin and confers upon dalbavancin a greater ability to inhibit peptidoglycan synthesis, allowing this agent to be more potent than vancomycin. The lipophilic tail also dramatically extends the half-life of dalbavancin, allowing once-per-week dosing. Dalbavancin is approved for the treatment of complicated skin and skin structure infections.

TELAVANCIN

Telavancin is a derivative of vancomycin that also has a lipophilic tail (see Figure 5-20B), although its tail is distinct from that of dalbavancin. As with dalbavancin, this modification better anchors telavancin to the bacterial membrane, which, in turn, enhances binding to the D-alanine-D-alanine–containing peptidoglycan intermediate. By binding and intercalating into bacterial cell membranes, the lipophilic side chain of telavancin also promotes loss of membrane potential, pore formation, and leakage of cytosolic contents. Thus, telavancin has two modes of antibacterial activity and may be more potent than vancomycin, although additional studies are necessary to confirm this. Telavancin is approved for the treatment of complicated skin and skin structure infections and hospital-acquired pneumonia caused by susceptible strains of *S. aureus*.

ORITAVANCIN

Oritavancin is also structurally similar to vancomycin but has an additional sugar attached to the peptide core and a distinct lipophilic side chain from dalbavancin and telavancin. These changes confer binding to the bacterial cell membrane and tight affinity of oritavancin to its D-alanine-D-alanine target. Like telavancin, oritavancin also disrupts membrane potential, causes pore formation, and results in leakage of cytosolic contents. The effectiveness of this second mode of bacterial killing is highlighted by the fact that oritavancin is active against vancomycin-resistant enterococci. Similar to dalbavancin, oritavancin can be dosed once per week and is approved for the treatment of complicated skin and skin structure infections.

TOXICITY

Vancomycin may cause nephrotoxicity and hearing loss, especially when administered along with an aminoglycoside. Rarely, neutropenia may occur with the use of this agent. Dalbavancin has been linked to headache. Telavancin has been associated with QT prolongation, dizziness and headache, a metallic/soapy taste in the mouth, and nephrotoxicity. Oritavancin has been linked to headache and dizziness. With all glycopeptides, nausea, vomiting, and diarrhea can occur, and rapid infusion can lead to "red man" syndrome, in which patients develop pruritus and an erythematous rash on the face, neck, and upper torso. Red man syndrome is not a true allergy and can often be avoided by slowing the rate at which the drug is infused.

In summary, glycopeptide antibiotics have excellent activity against most aerobic and anaerobic gram-positive bacteria. Despite increasing resistance, they should continue to be workhorses in the treatment of infections caused by gram-positive bacteria for years to come.

QUESTIONS

29. Glycopeptides have excellent activity against both aerobic and anaerobic _____ bacteria.

30. Recently, resistance to vancomycin has become more common among the _____.

31. Like the β-lactam antibiotics, glycopeptides kill bacteria by preventing proper synthesis of _____.

32. Unlike vancomycin, dalbavancin, telavancin, and oritavancin possess lipophilic side chains, which classify them as _____.

Answers

29. gram-positive
30. enterococci
31. peptidoglycan
32. lipoglycopeptide

ADDITIONAL READINGS

Agarwal R, Bartsch SM, Kelly BJ, et al. Newer glycopeptide antibiotics for treatment of complicated skin and soft tissue infections: systematic review, network meta-analysis and cost analysis. *Clin Microbiol Infect*. 2018;24:361-368.

Courvalin P. Vancomycin resistance in gram-positive cocci. *Clin Infect Dis*. 2006;42(suppl 1):S25-S34.

Kirst HA, Thompson DG, Nicas TI. Historical yearly usage of vancomycin. *Antimicrob Agents Chemother*. 1998;42:1303-1304.

Van Bambeke F. Lipoglycopeptide antibacterial agents in gram-positive infections: a comparative review. *Drugs*. 2015;75:2073-2095.

Walsh C. Deconstructing vancomycin. *Science*. 1999;284:442-443.

Weigel LM, Clewell DB, Gill SR, et al. Genetic analysis of a high-level vancomycin-resistant isolate of *Staphylococcus aureus*. *Science*. 2003;302:1569-1571.

Daptomycin

Daptomycin is a novel cyclic lipopeptide antibiotic that was approved for use in the United States in 2003 (Figure 5-22). The lipid portion of this drug binds to the bacterial cytoplasmic membrane, where it affects overall membrane fluidity. This, in turn, causes membrane depolarization and detachment of enzymes necessary for proper cell wall synthesis. Daptomycin is active against many aerobic gram-positive bacteria, including highly resistant strains such as MRSA, penicillin-resistant *S. pneumoniae*, and some vancomycin-resistant enterococci (Table 5-21). Daptomycin is not active against gram-negative organisms because it cannot penetrate the gram-negative outer membrane to reach the cytoplasmic membrane. Unfortunately, daptomycin has poor activity in the lungs and should not be used to treat pneumonia.

TOXICITY

Daptomycin is relatively well tolerated, but reversible myopathy has been observed at higher doses. Phlebitis, rash, eosinophilic pneumonia, and gastrointestinal adverse effects also occur.

In summary, daptomycin is a potent agent against aerobic gram-positive bacteria and an important drug for the treatment of infections caused by these bacteria.

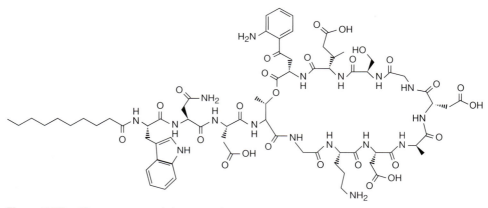

Figure 5-22. The structure of daptomycin.

Table 5-21	Antimicrobial Activity of Daptomycin
Gram-positive bacteria	*Streptococcus pyogenes* Viridans streptococci *Streptococcus pneumoniae* Staphylococci Enterococci
Anaerobic bacteria	Some *Clostridium* spp.

Daptomycin
- Gram-positive: +
- Gram-negative: −
- Anaerobes: ∅
- Atypical: ∅

QUESTIONS

33. The structure of daptomycin is a _____.

34. Daptomycin has excellent activity against aerobic _____ bacteria.

ANSWERS

33. cyclic lipopeptide

34. gram-positive

ADDITIONAL READINGS

Carpenter CF, Chambers HF. Daptomycin: another novel agent for treating infections due to drug-resistant gram-positive pathogens. *Clin Infect Dis.* 2004;38:994-1000.

Humphries RM, Pollett S, Sakoulas G. A current perspective on daptomycin for the clinical microbiologist. *Clin Microbiol Rev.* 2013;26:759-780.

Muller A, Wenzel M, Strahl H, et al. Daptomycin inhibits cell envelope synthesis by interfering with fluid membrane microdomains. *Proc Natl Acad Sci USA.* 2016;113:E7077-E7086.

Rybak MJ. The efficacy and safety of daptomycin: first in a new class of antibiotics for gram-positive bacteria. *Clin Microbiol Infect.* 2006;12(suppl 1):24-32.

Polymyxins

Polymyxins are the prodigal sons of antibiotics. After first being used in the 1950s, they fell into disfavor in the early 1980s because of their perceived toxicities and the availability of safer alternatives. In recent years, however, polymyxins have again become a popular choice of clinicians faced with few options in the treatment of multidrug-resistant gram-negative bacteria.

Two polymyxins are used clinically: polymyxin B and colistin, also known as polymyxin E (Table 5-22). These closely related antibiotics are cationic (positively charged) cyclic peptides with fatty acid side chains (Figure 5-23). The positive charge

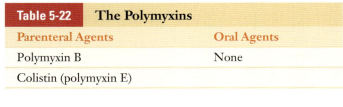

Table 5-22	The Polymyxins
Parenteral Agents	**Oral Agents**
Polymyxin B	None
Colistin (polymyxin E)	

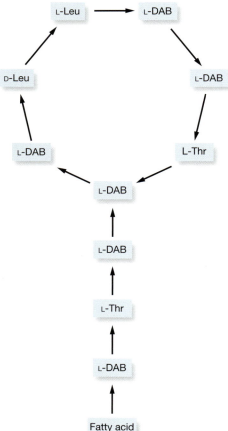

Figure 5-23. The structure of colistin. DAB, diaminobutyric acid; Leu, leucine; Thr, threonine.

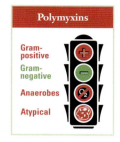

Table 5-23	Antimicrobial Activity of Polymyxins
Gram-negative bacteria	*Pseudomonas aeruginosa* Many Enterobacterales *Haemophilus influenzae*

allows polymyxins to bind to the negatively charged lipopolysaccharide molecules in the bacterial outer membrane, displacing Ca^{++} and Mg^{++} ions that normally stabilize these lipids. The fatty acid tail facilitates further insertion of polymyxins into the outer membrane. The bulkiness of polymyxins disrupts the normally tightly packed lipopolysaccharide molecules, leading to increased permeability and, eventually, lysis of the bacterium. Resistance occurs by several mechanisms, such as alteration of the negative charge associated with lipopolysaccharide, which, in turn, decreases the interaction between polymyxins and lipopolysaccharide. As would be expected, polymyxins have activity against many aerobic gram-negative bacteria, including *P. aeruginosa*, *E. coli*, and *Klebsiella* spp. (Table 5-23). Because polymyxins were infrequently used for several decades, many multidrug-resistant strains of these bacteria remain susceptible to them. However, recent studies have suggested that treatment with these antibiotics is associated with poorer clinical outcomes than comparator antibiotics. As a result, polymyxins tend to be used when alternatives are not available.

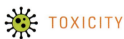 TOXICITY

The toxicity of polymyxins, which earlier led to their disuse, has now been found to be less than previously believed. Nonetheless, they are associated with nephrotoxicity (decreased creatinine clearance) and neurotoxicity (eg, dizziness, weakness, ataxia, paresthesias, vertigo).

In summary, polymyxins have activity against many aerobic gram-negative bacilli and are useful in the treatment of infections caused by these bacteria when resistance precludes the use of other agents.

QUESTIONS

35. Polymyxins bind to and disrupt _____ in the bacterial outer membrane.
36. Polymyxins have activity against aerobic _____ bacteria.

ANSWERS

35. lipopolysaccharide
36. gram-negative

ADDITIONAL READINGS

Biswas S, Brunel JM, Dubus JC, et al. Colistin: an update on the antibiotic of the 21st century. *Expert Rev Anti Infect Ther*. 2012;10:917-934.

Falagas ME, Kasiakou SK. Colistin: the revival of polymyxins for the management of multidrug-resistant gram-negative bacterial infections. *Clin Infect Dis.* 2005;40:1333-1341.

Falagas ME, Rafailidis PI, Matthaiou DK. Resistance to polymyxins: mechanisms, frequency and treatment options. *Drug Resist Updat.* 2010;13:132-138.

Nation RL, Li J. Colistin in the 21st century. *Curr Opin Infect Dis.* 2009;22:535-543.

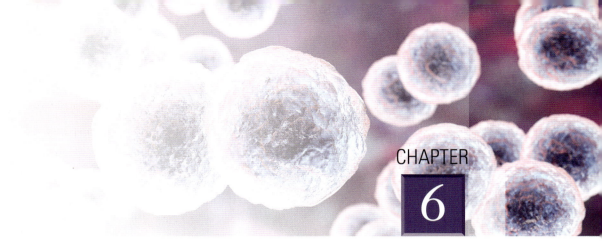

CHAPTER 6

Antibiotics That Block Protein Production

"[Vercingotorix said that] they must direct all their efforts towards cutting the Romans off from forage and supplies.... All villages and isolated buildings must be set on fire in every direction from the Romans' line of march as far as foragers seemed likely to be able to reach."

—Julius Caesar, De Bello Gallico 7.14 (translation by Anne and Peter Wiseman)

Bacteria must constantly use the resources available in their environment to produce new biomolecules that replace old worn-out ones and to build new bacteria. For example, new proteins are continuously being manufactured in a process that involves the synthesis of messenger RNA (mRNA) from DNA genes (transcription) and the subsequent generation of proteins from the mRNA templates (translation). Because these processes are crucial for the growth and multiplication of bacteria, they can be targeted by antibiotics. In the following sections, we discuss the antimicrobial agents that inhibit bacterial transcription and translation.

Rifamycins

The **rifamycins** are "accessory" antibiotics. Just as a stylish purse or sparkling necklace is used to adorn a dress, these antimicrobial agents are added to traditional treatment wardrobes that require a little accentuation for the optimal effect. The rifamycins consist of **rifampin** (also called rifampicin), **rifabutin**, **rifapentine**, and **rifaximin** (Table 6-1). Each has a similar structure that includes an aromatic nucleus linked on both ends by an aliphatic "handle" (Figure 6-1).

Rifamycins act by inhibiting bacterial RNA polymerase. They nestle deep into the DNA/RNA tunnel of this enzyme and, once lodged in this position, sterically block elongation of the nascent mRNA molecule. Resistance develops relatively easily and can result from one of several single mutations in the bacterial gene that encodes RNA polymerase. These mutations each change only a single amino acid at the site where the rifamycins bind to RNA polymerase but are sufficient to prevent this binding. Because single mutations are sufficient to lead to resistance, rifamycins are usually used in combination with other agents to prevent the emergence of resistant strains.

Many of the rifamycins are frequently used in combination regimens for the treatment of mycobacterial infections (Table 6-2). Of the rifamycins, rifampin has been used along with other antibiotics to treat staphylococcal infections. Rifampin is also effective as monotherapy for prophylaxis against *Neisseria meningitidis* and *Haemophilus influenzae*. The use of rifampin alone in prophylaxis is justified by the fact that, usually, very few bacteria are present in the absence of overt disease, thus minimizing the chance that a rifampin resistance mutation will spontaneously occur.

Table 6-1	The Rifamycins
Parenteral Agents	**Oral Agents**
Rifampin	Rifampin
	Rifabutin
	Rifapentine
	Rifaximin

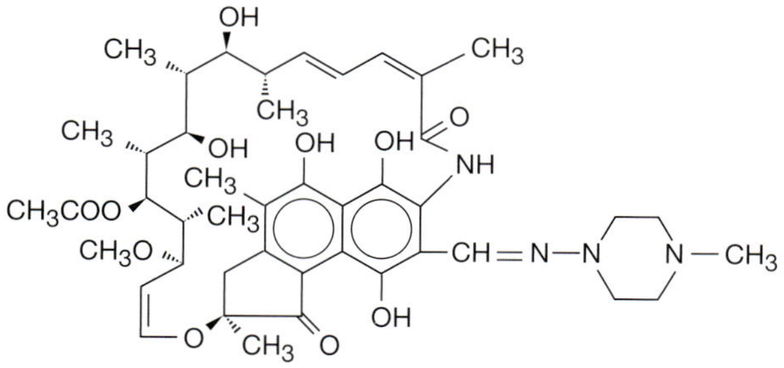

Figure 6-1. The structure of rifampin.

Rifamycins	Table 6-2	Antimicrobial Activity of Rifamycins
Gram-positive	Gram-positive bacteria	Staphylococci
Gram-negative	Gram-negative bacteria	*Haemophilus influenzae* *Neisseria meningitidis*
Anaerobes Atypical	Mycobacteria	*Mycobacterium tuberculosis* *Mycobacterium avium* complex *Mycobacterium leprae*

RIFAMPIN

Rifampin is the oldest and most widely used of the rifamycins. It is also the most potent inducer of the cytochrome P-450 system.

RIFABUTIN

Rifabutin is favored over rifampin in individuals who are simultaneously being treated for tuberculosis and human immunodeficiency virus (HIV) infection because it inhibits the cytochrome P-450 system to a lesser degree than rifampin or rifapentine and thus can be more easily administered along with the many antiretroviral agents that also interact with this system.

RIFAPENTINE

Rifapentine has a long serum half-life, which has led to its use in once-weekly regimens for immunocompetent patients with tuberculosis.

RIFAXIMIN

Rifaximin is a poorly absorbed rifamycin that is used for the treatment of traveler's diarrhea. Because it is not systemically absorbed, it has limited activity against invasive bacteria, such as *Salmonella* and *Campylobacter* spp.

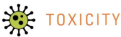

TOXICITY

The rifamycins are potent inducers of the cytochrome P-450 system. Thus, they may dramatically affect the levels of other drugs metabolized by this system. Rifamycins also commonly cause gastrointestinal complaints such as nausea, vomiting, and diarrhea and have been associated with hepatitis. Skin rashes and hematologic abnormalities may occur. Of note, rifampin causes an orange-red discoloration of tears, urine, and other body fluids, which can lead to patient anxiety and the staining of contact lenses. Rifabutin has been associated with uveitis.

The rifamycins are used primarily as components of multidrug regimens for mycobacterial infections and some staphylococcal infections. The ease with which bacteria develop resistance to these agents precludes their use as monotherapy in active disease.

History

The name *rifamycin* was derived from the French movie *Rififi*, which was popular at the time these agents were discovered.

From Sensi P. History of the development of rifampin. *Rev Infect Dis.* 1983;5(suppl 3):S402-S406 by permission of Oxford University Press.

Questions

1. Rifampin binds bacterial _____ and inhibits synthesis of _____.
2. Rifampin is used primarily in the treatment of diseases caused by _____ and _____.
3. The rifamycins are usually used in conjunction with other antimicrobial agents because _____ to rifamycins develops during monotherapy.

Answers

1. RNA polymerase, mRNA
2. mycobacteria, staphylococci
3. resistance

Additional Readings

Burman WJ, Gallicano K, Peloquin C. Comparative pharmacokinetics and pharmacodynamics of the rifamycin antibacterials. *Clin Pharmacokinet.* 2001;40:327-341.

Campbell EA, Korzheva N, Mustaev A, et al. Structural mechanism for rifampicin inhibition of bacterial RNA polymerase. *Cell.* 2001;104:901-912.

Huang DB, DuPont HL. Rifaximin—a novel antimicrobial for enteric infections. *J Infect.* 2005;50:97-106.

Munsiff SS, Kambili C, Ahuja SD. Rifapentine for the treatment of pulmonary tuberculosis. *Clin Infect Dis.* 2006;43:1468-1475.

Aminoglycosides

The **aminoglycosides** are among the oldest antibiotics, dating back to the purification of **streptomycin** from the bacterium *Streptomyces griseus* in 1944. **Neomycin** became available in 1949, followed by **gentamicin** in 1963, **tobramycin** in 1967, **amikacin** in 1972, and **plazomicin** in 2018 (Table 6-3). (Although streptomycin is still occasionally used, it has been largely supplanted by the newer aminoglycosides and will not be discussed further here.) Like penicillin, these agents initially were active against both gram-negative and gram-positive bacteria. Unlike penicillin, though, the aminoglycosides have maintained their effectiveness against many of these bacteria despite over 70 years of use and today are commonly administered antibiotics.

Aminoglycosides are positively charged molecules that are quite large (Figure 6-2), although still only one-third the size of vancomycin. Each aminoglycoside molecule consists of two or more sugars bound by a glycosidic linkage to a central six-membered ring that contains amino group substituents. The name *aminoglycoside* is derived from the *amino* groups and the *glycosidic* linkage. Unlike vancomycin, the aminoglycosides have excellent activity against aerobic gram-negative bacteria because their size does not prevent their passage through the bacterial outer membrane. Rather, the positively charged nature of aminoglycosides allows them to bind to the negatively charged outer membrane and results in the formation of transient holes through which the antibiotic molecules move. Access to the bacterial ribosomes, which are the targets of aminoglycosides, still requires penetration of the bacterial cytoplasmic membrane. This is accomplished by an energy-dependent active bacterial transport mechanism that requires oxygen and an active proton motive force. For these reasons, aminoglycosides work poorly

Table 6-3	The Aminoglycosides
Parenteral Agents	**Oral Agents**
Gentamicin	Neomycin[a]
Tobramycin	
Amikacin	
Plazomicin	

[a]Not absorbed when given orally. Used for bowel decontamination.

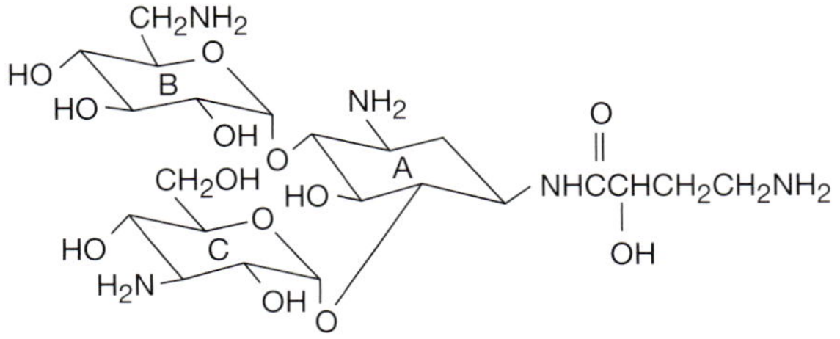

Figure 6-2. The structure of the aminoglycoside amikacin. Features of aminoglycosides include amino sugars (**B**, **C**) bound by glycosidic linkages to a relatively conserved six-membered ring (**A**) that itself contains amino group substituents.

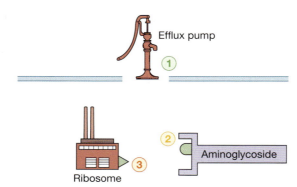

Figure 6-3. Bacterial resistance to aminoglycosides occurs via one of three mechanisms that prevent the normal binding of the antibiotic to its ribosomal target: (1) Efflux pumps prevent accumulation of the aminoglycoside in the cytosol of the bacterium. (2) Modification of the aminoglycoside prevents binding to the ribosome. (3) Mutations within the ribosome prevent aminoglycoside binding.

in anaerobic and acidic environments such as abscesses and have no activity against anaerobic bacteria. Each aminoglycoside acts by binding to the 30S subunit of the bacterial ribosome, which causes mismatching between the mRNA codon and the charged aminoacyl-transfer RNA (tRNA). This, in turn, promotes protein mistranslation.

For reasons that are unclear, resistance to aminoglycoside antibiotics remains relatively rare. When it does occur, it is usually the result of one of three mechanisms (Figure 6-3): (1) decreased accumulation within the bacterium, which most likely reflects the presence of efflux pumps; (2) bacterial "aminoglycoside-modifying enzymes" (AMEs) such as acetyltransferases, nucleotidyltransferases, and phosphotransferases, which modify the drug and prevent it from binding ribosomes; and (3) mutation of the bacterial ribosome in such a way that the aminoglycoside can no longer bind to it. (This last mechanism appears to be relatively rare.) Resistance is not always class wide. For example, because of its unique side chains, amikacin is resistant to modification by some AMEs that are active against gentamicin and tobramycin, and plazomicin is active against many bacteria resistant to the other aminoglycosides.

Aminoglycosides have excellent activity against aerobic gram-negative bacteria (Table 6-4). These agents are commonly used to treat infections caused by members

Table 6-4	Antimicrobial Activity of Aminoglycosides
Gram-positive bacteria	Used synergistically against some: Staphylococci Streptococci Enterococci *Listeria monocytogenes*
Gram-negative bacteria	*Haemophilus influenzae* Enterobacterales
Mycobacteria	*Mycobacterium tuberculosis* *Mycobacterium avium* complex

of the Enterobacterales. Because of disappointing results in animal studies, aminoglycosides are usually used in combination with another active agent in severe infections, even against bacterial strains that are highly sensitive. These agents are active to a much lesser degree against aerobic gram-positive bacteria. The uptake of aminoglycosides is enhanced by antibiotics that inhibit bacterial cell wall synthesis, such as β-lactams and vancomycin. Thus, in some aerobic gram-positive bacteria such as enterococci, aminoglycosides have synergistic efficacy when used with these agents even when the bacterium is moderately resistant to aminoglycosides. Lower amounts of aminoglycosides, referred to as *synergistic dosing*, are given when they are used with cell wall–active agents to treat aerobic gram-positive bacteria. Some of the aminoglycosides are also active against certain mycobacteria species such as *Mycobacterium tuberculosis* and *Mycobacterium avium* complex.

GENTAMICIN

Gentamicin is the most commonly used of the aminoglycosides. It is active against both aerobic gram-negative and aerobic gram-positive bacteria.

TOBRAMYCIN

For practical purposes, tobramycin has the same spectrum of activity as gentamicin and is used similarly. In general, most gentamicin-resistant strains also lack susceptibility to tobramycin. Unlike gentamicin, however, tobramycin lacks activity against enterococci and should not be used for infections caused by this bacterium.

AMIKACIN

Strains of aerobic gram-negative bacteria that are resistant to gentamicin and tobramycin may remain susceptible to amikacin. Thus, this agent has better overall activity against these bacteria. Like tobramycin, however, amikacin lacks clinically significant activity against enterococci.

PLAZOMICIN

Plazomicin is the most recent addition to the family of aminoglycosides. The addition of a unique group to the aminoglycoside core allows this antibiotic to resist modification by AMEs. This in turn allows plazomicin to retain activity against many members of the Enterobacterales (especially multidrug-resistant *Escherichia coli* and *Klebsiella pneumoniae* strains) that are resistant to other aminoglycosides.

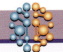

Remember

Unlike tobramycin, neomycin, and streptomycin, the aminoglycosides gentamicin and plazomicin are spelled without a "y." This has led to the commonly prescribed antibiotic gentamicin being one of the most frequently misspelled medical words. Other contenders include "pruritic" and "guaiac."

TOXICITY

The major factor limiting the use of aminoglycosides is their toxicity. These agents are associated with relatively high frequencies of nephrotoxicity and ototoxicity. Aminoglycosides penetrate human cells poorly except for proximal renal tubule cells, where they are concentrated. As a result, approximately 5% to 10% of patients who receive aminoglycosides will develop nephrotoxicity or decreased renal function. This incidence can be as high as 50% in patients who have specific risk factors for toxicity, such as increased age and concomitant exposure to other renal toxins. Fortunately, the damage to the kidneys is usually reversible, and renal function often returns to normal after discontinuation of the drug. Note that renal toxicity is usually only observed after 3 to 4 days of therapy, so aminoglycosides can be safely given for a short period without placing the patient at significant risk for this adverse effect. Ototoxicity consists of two types: auditory impairment, which may lead to irreversible hearing loss, and vestibular toxicity, which results in disturbances in balance.

The aminoglycosides remain potent agents for the treatment of many infections caused by aerobic gram-negative bacteria. They also possess synergistic activity with cell wall–active agents and are useful as adjunctive therapy against some aerobic gram-positive bacteria. Toxicity continues to be a concern with their use.

QUESTIONS

4. The aminoglycosides have excellent activity against aerobic _____ bacteria.
5. The aminoglycosides are used at synergistic doses along with cell wall–active agents to treat some aerobic _____ bacteria.
6. The two major toxicities associated with the aminoglycosides are _____ and _____.

ANSWERS

4. gram-negative
5. gram-positive
6. nephrotoxicity, ototoxicity

ADDITIONAL READINGS

Chambers HF. Aminoglycosides. In: Burunton LL, Lazo JS, Parker KL, eds. *Goodman and Gilman's the Pharmacological Basis of Therapeutics*. 11th ed. McGraw-Hill; 2006:1155-1172.
Gonzalez LS III, Spencer JP. Aminoglycosides: a practical review. *Am Fam Physician*. 1998;58:1811-1820.
Mingeot-Leclercq MP, Glupczynski Y, Tulkens PM. Aminoglycosides: activity and resistance. *Antimicrob Agents Chemother*. 1999;43:727-737.
Saravolatz LD, Stein GE. Plazomicin: a new aminoglycoside. *Clin Infect Dis*. 2020;70:704-709.

Macrolides

Macrolide antibiotics follow the old adage "jack of all trades, master of none." These agents are active against some gram-positive bacteria, some gram-negative bacteria, some atypical bacteria, some mycobacteria, and even some spirochetes. However, they are not reliably effective against most bacteria in any one group. Nonetheless, they remain very useful agents for the treatment of specific types of infections, such as respiratory infections, and for treatment directed toward specific organisms. The macrolide group of antibiotics consists of **erythromycin**, **clarithromycin**, and **azithromycin** (Table 6-5).

All macrolides consist of a large cyclic core called a macrocyclic lactone ring (Figure 6-4) (hence the name *macrolide*). This ring is decorated with sugar residues. Macrolides bind tightly to the 50S subunit of the bacterial ribosome at a location that blocks the exit of the newly synthesized peptide. Thus, macrolides function in a manner similar to the aminoglycosides in that they target ribosomes and prevent protein production. Resistance is becoming increasingly common and occurs by one of several mechanisms: (1) inhibition of drug entry and accumulation—macrolides have difficulty penetrating the outer membrane of most aerobic gram-negative bacilli and are actively pumped out of some resistant bacteria. For example, some gram-positive bacteria, such as *Streptococcus pneumoniae*, contain a *mef* gene that encodes an efflux pump that impairs accumulation of macrolides within the bacterium. (2) Enzyme-mediated ribosome binding site alteration—some bacteria acquire resistance to macrolides by

Table 6-5	The Macrolides	
Parenteral Agents	**Oral Agents**
Erythromycin	Erythromycin
	Clarithromycin
Azithromycin	Azithromycin

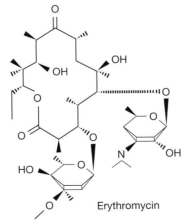

Figure 6-4. The structure of erythromycin.

methylating the portion of the 50S ribosome normally bound by these drugs, preventing this interaction. For example, this type of resistance is encoded by the *erm* gene in *S. pneumoniae*. Methylation of the ribosome in this way also results in resistance to clindamycin and streptogramins, which act by binding the bacterial ribosome and inhibiting protein translation as well. (3) Mutation of the ribosome binding site—rarely, mutations occur that affect the portion of the bacterial ribosome bound by macrolides. Regardless of the mechanism, resistance to one member of the macrolide group usually implies resistance to all members.

As a group, the macrolides are active against various bacteria (Table 6-6). They are effective against some staphylococci and streptococci, although not usually methicillin-resistant staphylococci and penicillin-resistant streptococci. A large hole in the spectrum of macrolides is that most aerobic gram-negative bacilli are resistant, but some *Neisseria*, *Bordetella*, and *Haemophilus* strains are susceptible. Macrolides are not useful in the treatment of most anaerobic infections. On the other hand, they are active against many atypical bacteria and some mycobacteria and spirochetes.

ERYTHROMYCIN

Erythromycin, the oldest of the macrolides, was discovered in 1952 and contains a 14-member macrocyclic lactone ring (Figure 6-4). It is less useful than the other macrolides in the treatment of respiratory infections because it lacks significant activity against *H. influenzae*. Because it has a spectrum of activity similar to clarithromycin and azithromycin but is less well tolerated, it has been replaced by these newer agents.

CLARITHROMYCIN

Clarithromycin is a semisynthetic derivative of erythromycin and also consists of a 14-member macrocyclic lactone ring. It has somewhat greater activity against aerobic gram-positive bacteria and *H. influenzae* than erythromycin.

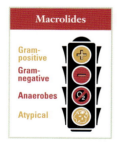

Table 6-6	Antimicrobial Activity of Macrolides
Gram-positive bacteria	Some *Streptococcus pyogenes* Some viridans streptococci Some *Streptococcus pneumoniae* Some *Staphylococcus aureus*
Gram-negative bacteria	*Neisseria* spp. Some *Haemophilus influenzae* *Bordetella pertussis*
Atypical bacteria	*Chlamydia* spp. *Mycoplasma* spp. *Legionella pneumophila* Some *Rickettsia* spp.
Mycobacteria	*Mycobacterium avium* complex *Mycobacterium leprae*
Spirochetes	*Treponema pallidum* *Borrelia burgdorferi*

AZITHROMYCIN

Azithromycin has a modified 15-member macrocyclic lactone ring that allows it to better penetrate the outer membrane of some aerobic gram-negative bacteria. Hence, it has somewhat better activity against these bacteria and is useful in the treatment of *H. influenzae*. One of its main advantages is that it is taken up in high amounts by tissues and then slowly released over subsequent days. Thus, a 5-day course of oral therapy results in therapeutic drug levels in the blood for 10 days.

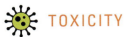

TOXICITY

The macrolides are relatively safe drugs, causing mostly mild adverse reactions. Erythromycin is associated with gastrointestinal symptoms such as nausea, vomiting, and diarrhea and with thrombophlebitis following intravenous administration, but clarithromycin and azithromycin are usually tolerated quite well. However, QT prolongation leading to polymorphic ventricular tachycardia does occur with use of these agents, and azithromycin has been linked to a small increase in cardiovascular deaths. Erythromycin and clarithromycin, but not azithromycin, are also capable of inhibiting the cytochrome P-450 system and thereby affecting levels of other drugs.

The macrolides have some activity against aerobic gram-positive bacteria, aerobic gram-negative bacteria, atypical bacteria, mycobacteria, and spirochetes. Within each of these groups, however, several species are resistant to these agents, and macrolides, therefore, must be used with caution as empiric agents.

QUESTIONS

7. Among the macrolides, _____ has the best aerobic gram-negative coverage and is, therefore, useful against _____.
8. _____ and _____ are macrolides that are better tolerated than erythromycin.
9. Macrolides have relatively poor activity against _____ bacteria.
10. The structures of all macrolides contain a _____ lactone ring.
11. _____ may cause thrombophlebitis following intravenous administration.

ANSWERS

7. azithromycin, *H. influenzae*
8. Azithromycin, clarithromycin
9. anaerobic
10. macrocyclic
11. Erythromycin

ADDITIONAL READINGS

Leclercq R. Mechanisms of resistance to macrolides and lincosamides: nature of the resistance elements and their clinical implications. *Clin Infect Dis*. 2002;34:482-492.
Neu HC. New macrolide antibiotics: azithromycin and clarithromycin. *Ann Intern Med*. 1992;116:517-519.
Zuckerman JM. The newer macrolides: azithromycin and clarithromycin. *Infect Dis Clin North Am*. 2000;14:449-462.

Tetracyclines

The **tetracyclines** are a class of antibiotics that date back to the 1950s. Today, six members of this group are commonly used: **tetracycline**, **doxycycline**, **minocycline**, **tigecycline**, **eravacycline**, and **omadacycline** (Table 6-7).

The core structure of the tetracyclines consists of four fused six-membered rings (Figure 6-5). This structure allows the tetracyclines to interact with the 30S subunit of the bacterial ribosome and prevent binding by tRNA molecules loaded with amino acids. In this way, protein synthesis is blocked. Resistance to tetracyclines most commonly occurs by one of two mechanisms. Exogenous genes are acquired that encode efflux pumps, which prevent intracellular accumulation of these drugs. Alternatively, genes may be acquired that encode ribosomal protection proteins. These factors alter the conformation of the bacterial ribosome such that tetracyclines no longer bind them but protein translation remains unaffected.

Tetracyclines are active against some aerobic gram-positive bacteria, such as *S. pneumoniae*, and some aerobic gram-negative bacteria, such as *H. influenzae* and *N. meningitidis* (Table 6-8). These agents also have some anaerobic activity and can be used to treat infections caused by some spirochetes, such as *Borrelia burgdorferi* and *Treponema pallidum*. The strength of this class of drugs, however, is its activity against atypical bacteria, including rickettsiae, chlamydiae, and mycoplasmas.

TETRACYCLINE

Tetracycline was discovered in 1953 but is still used today. It is available in an oral formulation.

Table 6-7	The Tetracyclines
Parenteral Agents	**Oral Agents**
Doxycycline	Tetracycline
Tigecycline	Doxycycline
Eravacycline	Minocycline
Omadacycline	Omadacycline

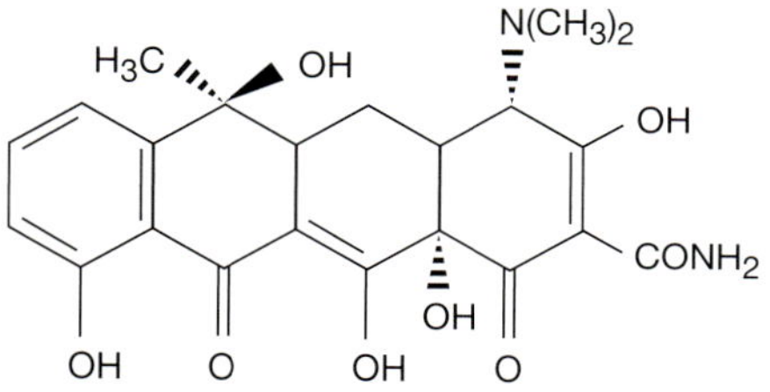

Figure 6-5. The structure of tetracycline.

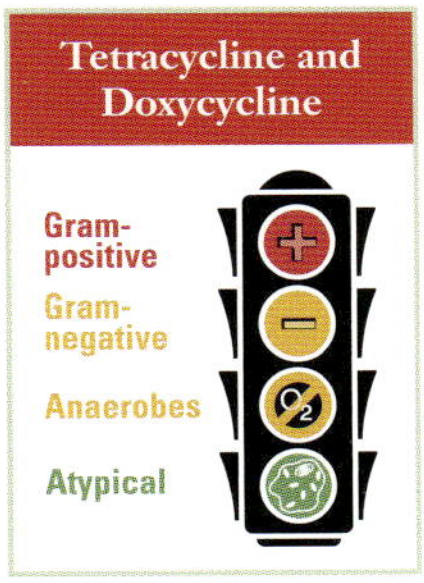

Table 6-8. Antimicrobial Activity of Tetracycline and Doxycycline

Tetracycline and Doxycycline	
Gram-positive bacteria	Some *Streptococcus pneumoniae*
Gram-negative bacteria	*Haemophilus influenzae* *Neisseria meningitidis*
Anaerobic bacteria	Some *Clostridia* spp.
Spirochetes	*Borrelia burgdorferi* *Treponema pallidum*
Atypical bacteria	*Rickettsia* spp. *Chlamydia* spp. *Mycoplasma* spp.

Gram-positive: +
Gram-negative: ±
Anaerobes: ±
Atypical: +

DOXYCYCLINE

The spectrum of activity of doxycycline is essentially the same as tetracycline. It is more commonly used because of its longer half-life, which allows for twice per day dosing.

MINOCYCLINE

The spectrum of activity of minocycline is similar to that of the other tetracyclines except that this agent is preferable for the treatment of methicillin-resistant staphylococcal infections. Minocycline is also occasionally used for infections caused by *Mycobacterium leprae*.

TIGECYCLINE, ERAVACYCLINE, OMADACYCLINE

Tigecycline, eravacycline, and omadacycline are the newest tetracyclines. Each contains modifications to the core tetracycline structure. For example, tigecycline contains a glycyl amide group on the terminal six-membered ring of the core tetracycline structure (Figure 6-6). For each of these agents, the core structure modifications prevent recognition by many bacterial efflux pumps and make them insensitive to modifications of the 30S ribosomal subunit that confer resistance to other tetracyclines.

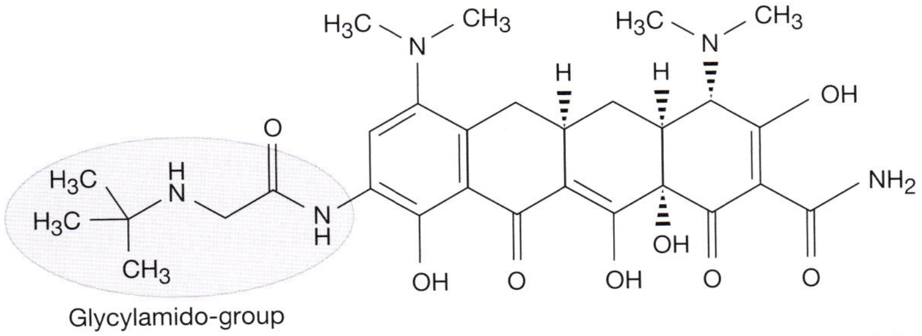

Figure 6-6. The structure of tigecycline. The glycylamido group that distinguishes tigecycline from the other tetracyclines is circled.

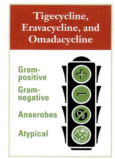

Table 6-9	Antimicrobial Activity of Tigecycline, Eravacycline, and Omadacycline
Gram-positive bacteria	*Streptococcus pyogenes* Viridans group streptococci *Streptococcus pneumoniae* Staphylococci Enterococci *Listeria monocytogenes*
Gram-negative bacteria	*Haemophilus influenzae* *Neisseria* spp. Enterobacterales
Anaerobic bacteria	*Bacteroides fragilis* Many other anaerobes
Atypical bacteria	*Mycoplasma* spp.

Because these mechanisms account for the bulk of the resistance to tetracyclines, tigecycline, eravacycline, and omadacycline have impressively broad in vitro antimicrobial spectra (Table 6-9). They are active against most aerobic gram-negative bacteria. However, *Pseudomonas aeruginosa* and *Proteus* spp., which produce efflux pumps that do recognize this agent, are usually resistant. Most aerobic gram-positive bacteria, including methicillin-resistant staphylococci, vancomycin-resistant enterococci, and penicillin-resistant *S. pneumoniae*, are susceptible to these agents, as are anaerobic and atypical bacteria. Despite their impressively broad spectra of activity, these agents should not be used indiscriminately. Tigecycline has been associated with worse overall outcomes in severe infections compared to comparator agents, perhaps because it is rapidly cleared from serum and urine. As a result, the US Food and Drug Administration recommends that it only be used when alternative treatments are not suitable. Similarly, experts recommend that eravacycline not be used as monotherapy in bloodstream or complicated urinary tract infections. Omadacycline is not recommended for infections caused by Enterobacterales producing extended-spectrum β-lactamases or carbapenemases because of decreased potency and an unfavorable pharmacokinetic-pharmacodynamic profile.

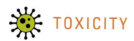 TOXICITY

The tetracyclines are relatively safe drugs, but several contraindications must be kept in mind. One of the core rings of these agents is a potent chelator of metal ions such as calcium. This may result in the gray to yellow discoloration of actively forming teeth and deposition in growing bone. For these reasons, the tetracyclines should not be given to pregnant women and given cautiously to children younger than 8 years. Hypersensitivity reactions such as rashes and anaphylaxis occur but are not common. An exception is the blue-black hyperpigmentation of skin and mucous membranes observed relatively frequently with minocycline use. The tetracyclines are also associated with phototoxicity. Gastrointestinal side effects such as nausea, vomiting, and esophageal ulceration are also seen, as is hepatotoxicity.

The tetracyclines are an old class of antibiotics that are still used for treating infections caused by certain organisms, particularly atypical pathogens. Tigecycline, eravacycline, and omadacycline are newer variants of these agents with broad in vitro activity against aerobic and anaerobic bacteria, including some species resistant to many other antibiotics, but their clinical effectiveness remains controversial. Toxicity precludes their use in pregnant women and requires that they be used cautiously in young children.

QUESTIONS

12. Tetracyclines inhibit bacterial growth by binding to bacterial _____.
13. Tetracyclines have excellent activity against _____ bacteria.
14. Because of problems with discoloration of teeth and deposition in bones, tetracyclines should not be used in _____ and should be used with caution in _____.
15. The newer tetracyclines are _____, _____, and _____.
16. The newer tetracyclines have in vitro activity against many highly resistant aerobic _____ and _____ bacteria, as well as anaerobic and _____ bacteria.

ANSWERS

12. ribosomes
13. atypical
14. pregnant women, children
15. tigecycline, eravacycline, omadacycline
16. gram-positive, gram-negative, atypical

ADDITIONAL READINGS

Chopra I, Roberts M. Tetracycline antibiotics: mode of action, applications, molecular biology, and epidemiology of bacterial resistance. *Microbiol Mol Biol Rev*. 2001;65:232-260.
Chukwudi CU. rRNA binding sites and the molecular mechanism of action of the tetracyclines. *Antimicrob Agents Chemother*. 2016;60:4433-4441.
Grossman TH. Tetracycline antibiotics and resistance. *Cold Spring Harb Perspect Med*. 2016;6:a025387.
Karlowsky JA, Steenbergen J, Zhanel GG. Microbiology and preclinical review of omadacycline. *Clin Infect Dis*. 2019;69:S6-S15.
Lee YR, Burton CE. Eravacycline, a newly approved fluorocycline. *Eur J Clin Microbiol Infect Dis*. 2019;38:1787-1794.
Stein GE, Babinchak T. Tigecycline: an update. *Diag Microbiol Infect Dis*. 2013;75:331-336.

Clindamycin

Clindamycin, which was introduced in 1966, is a synthetic derivative of the antibiotic lincomycin. Together, these agents comprise the lincosamide antibiotic group and are characterized by the common structure of an amino acid linked to an amino sugar (Figure 6-7). Only clindamycin, which is available in both oral and intravenous forms, is commonly used today. There has been a resurgence of interest in clindamycin because of its activity against many strains of community-acquired methicillin-resistant *S. aureus* and because of its potential efficacy in the treatment of toxin-mediated diseases caused by staphylococci and streptococci.

The lincosamide antibiotics bind to the 50S subunit of the bacterial ribosome and inhibit protein synthesis. Theoretically, then, these agents should prevent the production of bacterial toxins, and they are often used for this reason as adjunctive therapy in toxic shock syndrome caused by streptococci or staphylococci. Clindamycin's mechanism of action is very similar to that of the macrolides. In fact, their binding sites overlap. Thus, some strains of bacteria that are resistant to macrolides because of ribosomal modification are also resistant to clindamycin. Most gram-negative bacteria are intrinsically resistant to clindamycin because their outer membranes resist penetration by this drug.

Clindamycin's utility lies in its activity against two groups of bacteria: aerobic gram-positive bacteria and anaerobic bacteria (Table 6-10). In particular, it is active against many staphylococci and streptococci, including some strains of community-acquired methicillin-resistant *S. aureus*. Likewise, it has relatively broad activity against anaerobic bacteria, although some *Bacteroides fragilis* and clostridial strains are resistant. As mentioned previously, it is not useful against aerobic gram-negative bacteria or atypical bacteria.

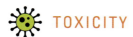

TOXICITY

The major toxicity of clindamycin, which has limited its use, is the occurrence of *Clostridioides difficile* colitis in 0.01% to 10% of individuals who receive it. Clindamycin kills many components of the normal bacterial flora in the bowel, allowing for overgrowth by *C. difficile*, which is resistant to this drug. In the most serious form of *C. difficile*

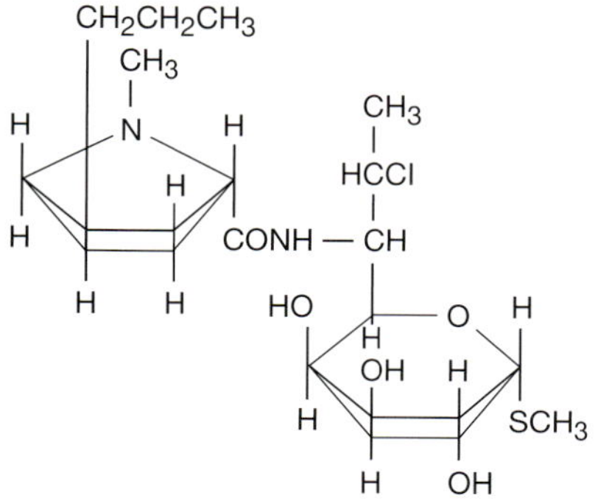

Figure 6-7. The structure of clindamycin.

Clindamycin	Table 6-10	**Antimicrobial Activity of Clindamycin**
Gram-positive / Gram-negative / Anaerobes / Atypical	Gram-positive bacteria	Some *Streptococcus pyogenes* Some viridans group streptococci Some *Streptococcus pneumoniae* Some *Staphylococcus aureus*
	Anaerobic bacteria	Some *Bacteroides fragilis* Some *Clostridium* spp. Most other anaerobes

colitis, plaques of necrotic debris are seen lining the colon, which is referred to as *pseudomembranous colitis*. Clindamycin has also been associated with diarrhea not caused by *C. difficile* and with rash.

Clindamycin remains a useful drug for the treatment of some infections caused by aerobic gram-positive and anaerobic bacteria. It is not active against aerobic gram-negative or atypical bacteria. Caution must be exercised regarding the relatively frequent occurrence of *C. difficile* colitis associated with its use.

QUESTIONS

17. Clindamycin is active against many aerobic _____ bacteria and _____ bacteria.
18. Resistance to _____ may also lead to resistance to clindamycin in some bacteria.
19. Use of clindamycin may lead to life-threatening _____.

ANSWERS

17. gram-positive, anaerobic
18. macrolides or erythromycin
19. pseudomembranous colitis

ADDITIONAL READINGS

Falagas ME, Gorbach SL. Clindamycin and metronidazole. *Med Clin North Am*. 1995;79:845-867.
Fass RJ, Scholand JF, Hodges GR, et al. Clindamycin in the treatment of serious anaerobic infections. *Ann Intern Med*. 1973;78:853-859.
Mason KJ, Dietz A, Deboer C. Lincomycin, a new antibiotic. I. Discovery and biological properties. *Antimicrob Agents Chemother*. 1962;2:554-559.
Russell NE, Pachorek RE. Clindamycin in the treatment of streptococcal and staphylococcal toxic shock syndromes. *Ann Pharmacother*. 2000;34:936-939.
Sutter VL. In vitro susceptibility of anaerobes: comparison of clindamycin and other antimicrobial agents. *J Infect Dis*. 1977;135(suppl):S7-S12.

HISTORY

The class of lincosamide antibiotics received its name from the site where the bacterium that produced lincomycin was isolated: Lincoln, Nebraska.

Oxazolidinones

The **oxazolidinones** consist of two currently approved antibiotics: **linezolid** and **tedizolid**. Unlike many of the drugs discussed up to this point, which were isolated from bacteria or fungi, oxazolidinones are completely synthetic compounds.

Linezolid and tedizolid have excellent activity against most aerobic gram-positive bacteria, including methicillin-resistant staphylococci, penicillin-resistant *S. pneumoniae*, and vancomycin-resistant enterococci (Table 6-11). They also have in vitro activity against some aerobic gram-negative, anaerobic, and atypical bacteria, but they currently are not used to treat infections caused by these organisms. Linezolid and tedizolid are available in both oral and intravenous formulations and achieve similarly high serum levels when given by either route. Tedizolid has the advantage of once-daily dosing.

LINEZOLID

Linezolid's structure consists of an oxazolidinone core that has been modified at several sites (Figure 6-8). By binding the 50S subunit of the bacterial ribosome, it prevents association of this subunit with the 30S subunit, thus blocking ribosome assembly. It also inhibits protein synthesis by preventing the formation of the first peptide bond of the nascent peptide. Although linezolid is a new agent not found in nature and its structure unique among antimicrobial agents, resistance has already been detected. It is the consequence of a single amino acid mutation within the gene encoding a portion

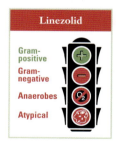

Table 6-11 Antimicrobial Activity of Linezolid

Gram-positive bacteria	*Streptococcus pyogenes*
	Viridans group streptococci
	Streptococcus pneumoniae
	Staphylococci
	Enterococci

Figure 6-8. The structure of linezolid.

of the bacterial ribosome. Interestingly, some aerobic gram-negative bacilli such as *Escherichia coli* are intrinsically resistant to linezolid because they produce efflux pumps active against this compound.

TEDIZOLID

Tedizolid's structure is similar to that of linezolid except for the addition of a D-ring on the left-hand side and a hydroxymethyl group in place of the acetamide group on the right-hand side (Figure 6-8). The additional D-ring allows for tighter binding to the bacterial ribosome, and the hydroxymethyl group avoids steric hindrance by some ribosome modifications that prevent linezolid binding. The net result is that tedizolid is more potent and slightly more active against resistant strains than linezolid.

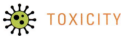

TOXICITY

The oxazolidinones are in general well tolerated. Like most antibiotics, they cause gastrointestinal symptoms such as nausea, vomiting, and diarrhea. Thrombocytopenia, anemia, and leukopenia occur relatively frequently but are reversible. Neuropathy and lactic acidosis have also been reported. Tedizolid may be associated with somewhat fewer of these toxicities than linezolid. These agents should not be given with monoamine oxidase (MAO) inhibitors and should be used with caution with serotonin receptor inhibitors because this combination can lead to the serotonin syndrome, which consists of fever, agitation, mental status changes, and tremors.

Oxazolidinones are an important addition to our antimicrobial armamentarium. These drugs have excellent activity against aerobic gram-positive bacteria, including many of those resistant to other antibiotics.

QUESTIONS

20. Linezolid has excellent activity against resistant gram-positive bacteria such as _____-resistant staphylococci and _____-resistant enterococci.
21. This agent binds to bacterial _____ and inhibits protein synthesis.
22. Compared to linezolid, tedizolid has the advantage of _____-daily dosing.

ANSWERS

20. methicillin, vancomycin
21. ribosome
22. once

ADDITIONAL READINGS

Burdette SD, Trotman R. Tedizolid: the first once-daily oxazolidinone class antibiotic. *Clin Infect Dis*. 2015;61:1315-1321.
Hamel JC, Stapert D, Moerman JK, et al. Linezolid, critical characteristics. *Infection*. 2000;28:60-64.
Moellering RC. Linezolid: the first oxazolidinone antimicrobial. *Ann Intern Med*. 2003;138:135-142.
Swaney SM, Aoki H, Ganoza MC, et al. The oxazolidinone linezolid inhibits initiation of protein synthesis in bacteria. *Antimicrob Agents Chemother*. 1998;42:3251-3255.

Nitrofurantoin

Nitrofurantoin is an old drug, having been first marketed in 1953. It belongs to a group of compounds called the *nitrofurans* (Figure 6-9). Because nitrofurantoin achieves only low levels in the blood but is concentrated in the urine, it has been used almost exclusively for the treatment of acute cystitis. It is not recommended for pyelonephritis because these infections are often associated with bacteremia. The mechanism of action of nitrofurantoin remains poorly characterized but it may bind ribosomes and inhibit translation. This, in turn, may adversely affect carbohydrate metabolism within bacteria. Nitrofurantoin has activity against many of the organisms that commonly cause community-acquired urinary tract infections, including aerobic gram-negative bacteria (except *Proteus* spp. and *P. aeruginosa*) and aerobic gram-positive bacteria, such as enterococci and *Staphylococcus saprophyticus* (Table 6-12). Contributing to its longevity is that emergence of resistance has been rare. Nitrofurantoin is only available in an oral formulation.

TOXICITY

Nitrofurantoin use has been associated with several adverse reactions, including nausea, vomiting, rash, pulmonary hypersensitivity reactions and interstitial pneumonitis, hepatitis, hemolytic anemia, and peripheral neuropathy.

Nitrofurantoin is a "niche" antibiotic with excellent activity against many of the bacteria that commonly cause community-acquired acute cystitis. It does not achieve therapeutically active levels in body tissues outside the urinary tract and should not be used to treat other types of infections.

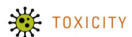

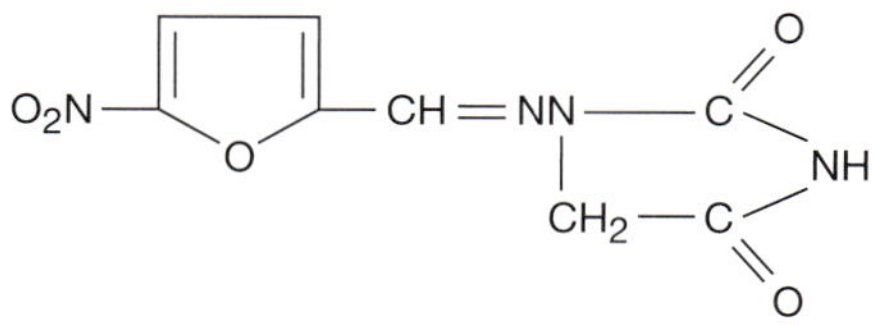

Figure 6-9. The structure of nitrofurantoin.

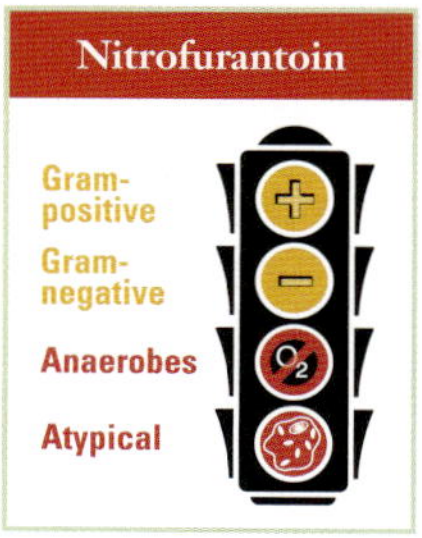

Nitrofurantoin	Table 6-12	Antimicrobial Activity of Nitrofurantoin
Gram-positive: +	Gram-positive bacteria	*Staphylococcus saprophyticus* Enterococci
Gram-negative: − Anaerobes: O₂ Atypical: ⊗	Gram-negative bacteria	Most Enterobacterales

Only in the context of acute cystitis.

QUESTIONS

23. Nitrofurantoin has excellent activity against many of the aerobic _____ and _____ bacteria that commonly cause community-acquired acute cystitis.

24. Nitrofurantoin does not achieve high _____ levels and, therefore, should not be used to treat systemic infections or pyelonephritis.

25. Despite decades of use, very little _____ to nitrofurantoin has emerged.

ANSWERS

23. gram-negative, gram-positive

24. blood

25. resistance

ADDITIONAL READINGS

Cunha BA. New uses for older antibiotics: nitrofurantoin, amikacin, colistin, polymyxin B, doxycycline, and minocycline revisited. *Med Clin North Am*. 2006;90:1089-1107.

Cunha BA. Nitrofurantoin: an update. *Obstet Gynecol Surv*. 1989;44:399-406.

Mandell GL, Bennett JE, Dolin R. *Mandell, Douglas, and Bennett's Principles and Practice of Infectious Disease*. 7th ed. Churchill Livingstone/Elsevier; 2010:515-520.

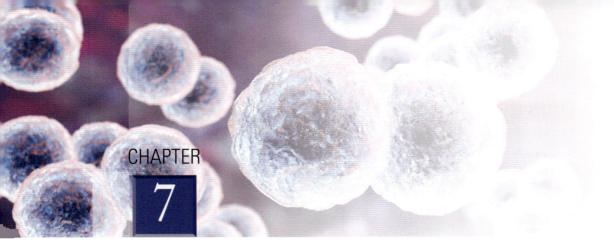

CHAPTER 7

Antibiotics That Target DNA and Replication

"What made the French naval effort so formidable was their excellent Admiral, Jean de Vienne, whose aim was to control the Channel and prevent English reinforcements reaching Guyenne and Brittany."

—The Hundred Years War, Desmond Seward

In the battle between bacterial invaders and the human immune response, superiority in numbers is often crucial. Bacteria have an advantage in this regard because they are capable of rapidly dividing; in a sense, they continuously reinforce themselves through rapid replication. Several antibiotics block the arrival of these reinforcements by inhibiting bacterial DNA replication and thus bacterial multiplication. In the following sections, we discuss these antimicrobial agents in detail.

Sulfa Drugs

Sulfa drugs are very old and date back to the early part of the 20th century. Thus, this class of antibiotics predates even the penicillins. In this section, we discuss two members of this group that are still widely used: **trimethoprim-sulfamethoxazole** and **dapsone** (Table 7-1). A third member, sulfisoxazole, is used in conjunction with erythromycin to treat otitis media in children.

As its name suggests, trimethoprim-sulfamethoxazole is actually a combination of two antimicrobial agents: trimethoprim and sulfamethoxazole. Trimethoprim is not a sulfa drug but acts on the same general pathway as these drugs. It is not as old as the sulfa drugs but nonetheless traces its roots back to the 1950s and 1960s. The breakthrough in the development of trimethoprim-sulfamethoxazole, however, came when it was discovered in 1968 that these two agents had potent activity when used in combination. Over the past 30 years, trimethoprim-sulfamethoxazole has been used to treat various bacterial infections.

Trimethoprim-sulfamethoxazole inhibits bacterial growth by preventing the synthesis of *tetrahydrofolate* (THF), the active form of folic acid. THF is an essential cofactor for metabolic pathways that generate deoxynucleotides, which are the building blocks of DNA (Figure 7-1). Sulfamethoxazole does this by mimicking *para*-aminobenzoate (PABA) and thereby competitively inhibiting the enzyme dihydropteroate synthase that normally incorporates PABA into the synthesis pathway of THF (Figures 7-1 and 7-2). Trimethoprim, on the other hand, is a structural analog of dihydrofolate and, therefore, inhibits dihydrofolate reductase, which is required for the conversion of dihydrofolate to THF (Figures 7-1 and 7-3). Thus, these two antibiotics inhibit

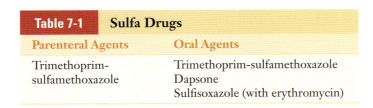

Table 7-1	Sulfa Drugs
Parenteral Agents	**Oral Agents**
Trimethoprim-sulfamethoxazole	Trimethoprim-sulfamethoxazole Dapsone Sulfisoxazole (with erythromycin)

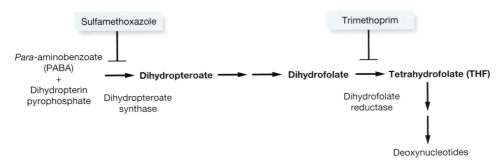

Figure 7-1. Inhibition of tetrahydrofolate synthesis by trimethoprim-sulfamethoxazole.

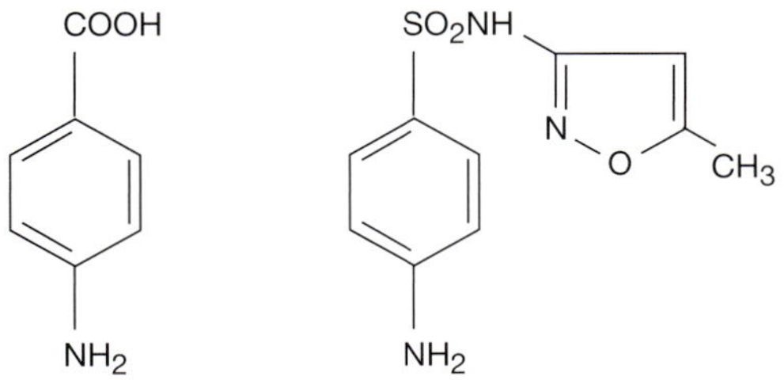

Para-aminobenzoic acid Sulfamethoxazole

Figure 7-2. The structure of sulfamethoxazole is similar to that of *para*-aminobenzoic acid.

distinct steps in the same pathway and in that way block the production of compounds essential for bacterial growth while decreasing the probability that bacterial resistance will develop. Nonetheless, the emergence of resistant strains has limited the use of trimethoprim-sulfamethoxazole. Bacteria become resistant to both of these agents by producing altered forms of their target enzymes that are not inhibited by the antibiotics or by changes in permeability that prevent the accumulation of the antibiotics within bacteria. Some strains overproduce PABA, which, at high concentrations, is capable of successfully competing with sulfamethoxazole for dihydropteroate synthase, resulting in sulfamethoxazole resistance.

Trimethoprim-sulfamethoxazole has activity against a broad range of aerobic gram-positive and aerobic gram-negative bacteria (Table 7-2). However, as might be expected with an agent that has been widely used for such an extended period, many strains that were intrinsically susceptible have now acquired resistance. Still, many streptococci and staphylococci remain susceptible to this drug combination, as does *Listeria monocytogenes*. Some strains of Enterobacterales such as *Escherichia coli*, *Salmonella* spp., and *Shigella* spp. are also susceptible, as are some strains of *Haemophilus influenzae*. Anaerobes and atypical bacteria tend to be resistant to trimethoprim-sulfamethoxazole.

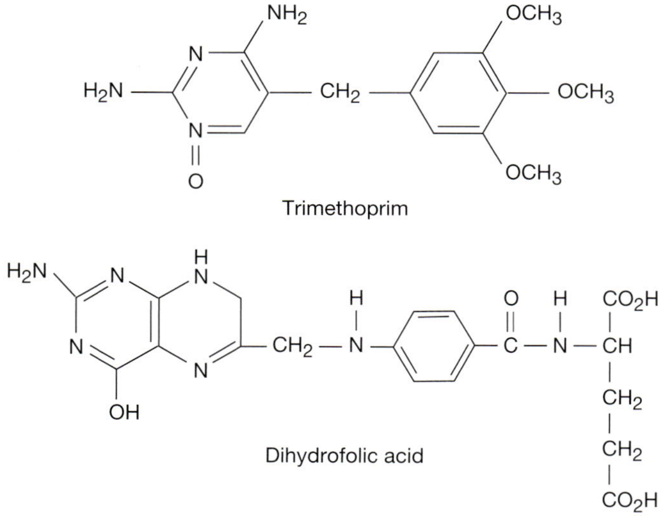

Figure 7-3. The structure of trimethoprim is similar to that of dihydrofolic acid.

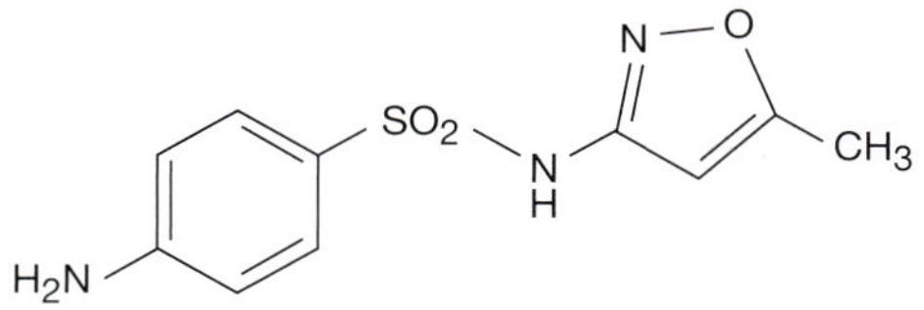

CHAPTER 7 — Antibiotics That Target DNA and Replication

Sulfamethoxazole

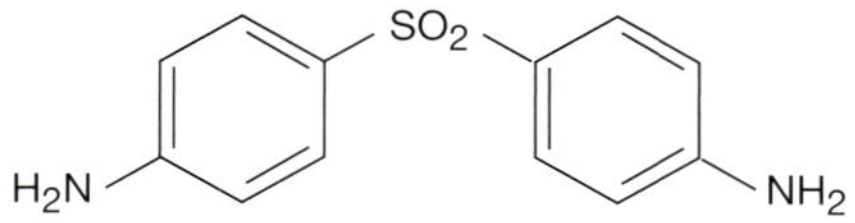

Dapsone

Figure 7-4. Comparison of the structures of sulfamethoxazole and dapsone.

This agent is available in both oral and parenteral formulations. When given orally, both drugs are well absorbed, and serum levels approach those achieved with intravenous (IV) administration.

Dapsone is a second sulfa drug that is used today. Its structure is related to that of sulfamethoxazole (Figure 7-4), and it acts by the same mechanism. Its spectrum of activity, however, is quite distinct. Dapsone's use as an antibacterial agent is limited to the treatment of leprosy, which is caused by *Mycobacterium leprae* (Table 7-2).

HISTORY

Sulfa drugs were the first antibacterial agents used in the United States. In 1935, sulfachrysoidine was used to treat a 10-year-old girl with meningitis caused by *H. influenzae*. The patient's father, who was a physician, had heard about the use of this sulfa drug in Germany to successfully treat bacterial infections. He, therefore, asked whether some sulfachrysoidine could be obtained for the treatment of his daughter. This was done, but the therapy unfortunately failed and the girl died.

From Carithers HA. The first use of an antibiotic in America. *Am J Dis Child.* 1974;128:207-211.

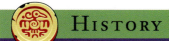

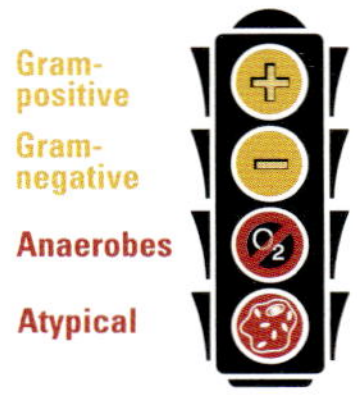

Table 7-2	Antimicrobial Activity of Sulfa Drugs	
Trimethoprim-sulfamethoxazole		
Gram-positive bacteria		Some *Streptococcus pneumoniae* Some staphylococci *Listeria monocytogenes*
Gram-negative bacteria		Some *Haemophilus influenzae* Some Enterobacterales
Dapsone		
		Mycobacterium leprae

TOXICITY

Because human cells do not synthesize folic acid, they lack dihydropteroate synthase, the target of sulfamethoxazole. Human cells do contain dihydrofolate reductase, which they use to recycle THF to dihydrofolate, but trimethoprim is 50,000 to 100,000 times more active against the bacterial enzyme than the human enzyme. Thus, one might expect that trimethoprim-sulfamethoxazole would be associated with relatively little toxicity, but this turns out not to be the case. It is associated with gastrointestinal effects as well as fever, rash (including Stevens-Johnson syndrome), leukopenia, thrombocytopenia, hepatitis, and hyperkalemia. For reasons that are unclear, human immunodeficiency virus (HIV)-infected individuals are particularly prone to trimethoprim-sulfamethoxazole toxicity. Dapsone causes similar adverse effects and, in addition, has been associated with hemolysis and methemoglobinemia.

Sulfa drugs are very old antibiotics that are still frequently used today. Trimethoprim-sulfamethoxazole is used for the treatment of some infections caused by aerobic gram-positive and aerobic gram-negative bacteria. Dapsone is an agent of choice for leprosy.

Pearl

Some bacteria, like human cells, are capable of taking up folic acid from their environment and thus do not need to synthesize this factor. For example, enterococci are inhibited by trimethoprim-sulfamethoxazole when grown on a laboratory medium, which does not contain folic acid. Trimethoprim-sulfamethoxazole, however, is not useful in treating enterococcal infections because these bacteria are capable of using folic acid present in the human body.

From Wisell KT, Kahlmeter G, Giske CG. Trimethoprim and enterococci in urinary tract infections: new perspectives on an old issue. *J Antimicrob Chemother.* 2008;62:35-40 by permission of Oxford University Press.

QUESTIONS

1. Trimethoprim and sulfamethoxazole are structurally unrelated antibiotics that both inhibit the synthesis of _____.
2. This combination of antibiotics has activity against some aerobic _____ and aerobic _____ bacteria.
3. Individuals infected with _____ are particularly prone to the toxicity of trimethoprim-sulfamethoxazole.
4. Dapsone's primary antibacterial use is for the treatment of _____.

ANSWERS

1. THF
2. gram-positive, gram-negative
3. HIV
4. leprosy

ADDITIONAL READINGS

Burchall JJ. Mechanism of action of trimethoprim-sulfamethoxazole. II. *J Infect Dis*. 1973;128(suppl):437-441.

Huovinen P. Increases in rates of resistance to trimethoprim. *Clin Infect Dis*. 1997;24(suppl 1):S63-S66.

Masters PA, O'Bryan TA, Zurlo J, et al. Trimethoprim-sulfamethoxazole revisited. *Arch Intern Med*. 2003;163:402-410.

Meyers WM. Leprosy. *Dermatol Clin*. 1992;10:73-96.

Quinolones

The **quinolones**, like the penicillins, are a group of antibiotics that resulted from serendipity flavored with a healthy dose of rational drug design. The discovery of this class of antimicrobial agents can be traced to the observation that a byproduct generated during the synthesis of chloroquine, an antimalarial compound, possessed modest activity against gram-negative bacteria. The subsequent modification of this compound led to agents with potent activity against aerobic gram-negative, aerobic gram-positive, and even some anaerobic bacteria. Of the quinolones, **ciprofloxacin**, **levofloxacin**, **ofloxacin**, **moxifloxacin**, **delafloxacin**, and **gemifloxacin** are the most frequently prescribed (Table 7-3). Gemifloxacin is no longer available in the United States.

All commercially available quinolones possess a core dual-ring structure (Figure 7-5). During modification of this core, it was discovered that addition of a fluorine atom enhanced potency, and as a result, this alteration has been incorporated into all the quinolones commonly used today. For this reason, these drugs are called *fluoroquinolones* to distinguish them from older agents such as nalidixic acid that lack this fluorine.

Quinolones work by inhibiting two topoisomerases, bacterial enzymes that regulate DNA supercoiling. These topoisomerases are named DNA gyrase and topoisomerase IV. Quinolones stabilize the complex that forms between topoisomerases and DNA at the stage of DNA strand breakage but before religation, resulting in the accumulation of double-stranded breaks in the chromosome. These breaks cause arrest of the DNA replication machinery, leading to inhibition of DNA synthesis and, eventually, bacterial death.

Resistance to quinolones results from spontaneous mutations that occur in specific regions of the genes encoding DNA gyrase and topoisomerase IV. Unfortunately,

Table 7-3	The Quinolones
Parenteral Agents	**Oral Agents**
Ciprofloxacin	Ciprofloxacin
Levofloxacin	Levofloxacin
Moxifloxacin	Moxifloxacin
Delafloxacin	Delafloxacin
	Gemifloxacin
	Ofloxacin

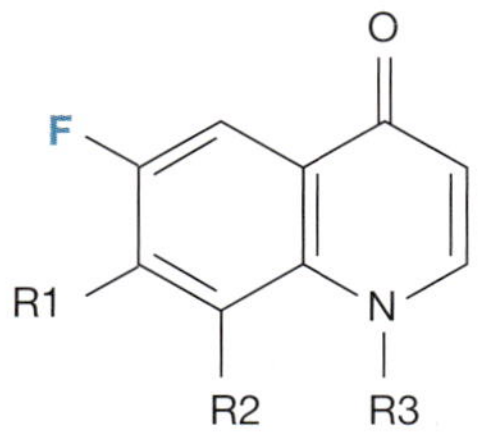

Figure 7-5. The core structure of the quinolones.

a single mutation in one of these genes is often sufficient to significantly reduce sensitivity to the quinolones. Bacteria with such a mutation are better able to survive in the presence of quinolones, thus allowing for the occurrence of secondary mutations over time that further increase the resistance to the quinolones. Eventually, bacteria with specific mutations in both the DNA gyrase and topoisomerase genes emerge; such bacteria are highly resistant to quinolones. Because a single mutation is capable of starting this process, it is not surprising that quinolone resistance is a major factor limiting the use of these agents. A second mechanism of resistance is the overexpression of efflux pumps in some bacteria. Because these efflux pumps tend to export several different antibiotics in addition to the quinolones, this can lead to cross-resistance between quinolones and other classes of antibiotics. A third mechanism is the production of factors that protect DNA gyrase and topoisomerase IV from binding by quinolones.

The quinolones have broad activity against various bacteria (Table 7-4). Their strength is their activity against aerobic gram-negative bacteria. In general, they are highly active against most members of the Enterobacterales, *Haemophilus* spp., and *Neisseria* spp. They are also effective against some staphylococci and streptococci, many atypical bacteria, and even some mycobacteria.

CIPROFLOXACIN

Ciprofloxacin is one of the oldest fluoroquinolones still in common use. Like many of the fluoroquinolones, it contains a piperazine derivative at the R1 side chain, which greatly enhances its activity against aerobic gram-negative bacteria (Figure 7-6). (Note that addition of a piperazine derivative to the penicillin core structure results in piperacillin, which also has enhanced activity against gram-negative bacteria.) It is the most potent of the quinolones against aerobic gram-negative bacteria and is effective against *Pseudomonas aeruginosa*. This is balanced by rather weak aerobic gram-positive activity. Ciprofloxacin is also active against many atypical bacteria and some mycobacteria.

Table 7-4	Antimicrobial Activity of the Quinolones
Gram-positive bacteria	Some *Staphylococcus aureus* *Streptococcus pyogenes* Viridans group streptococci *Streptococcus pneumoniae*
Gram-negative bacteria	*Neisseria* spp. *Haemophilus influenzae* Many Enterobacterales Some *Pseudomonas aeruginosa*
Anaerobic bacteria	Some *Clostridia* spp. Some *Bacteroides* spp.
Atypical bacteria	*Chlamydia* *Mycoplasma pneumoniae* *Legionella* spp.
Mycobacteria	*Mycobacterium tuberculosis* *Mycobacterium avium* complex *Mycobacterium leprae*

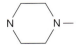

Figure 7-6. The R1 side chain of ciprofloxacin is a piperazine derivative, which enhances activity against aerobic gram-negative bacteria.

LEVOFLOXACIN AND OFLOXACIN

Structurally, levofloxacin and ofloxacin are very closely related. *Ofloxacin* is a racemic mixture of an active and inactive stereoisomer, whereas *levofloxacin* is composed solely of the active stereoisomer. Thus, these two agents have the same spectra of activity, but levofloxacin is generally 2-fold more potent and, as a result, more commonly used. Levofloxacin is not quite as active as ciprofloxacin against aerobic gram-negative bacteria but is still effective against infections caused by most of these bacteria, including *P. aeruginosa*. Relative to ciprofloxacin, levofloxacin has enhanced activity against aerobic gram-positive bacteria and is effective in the treatment of severe infections caused by *Streptococcus pneumoniae*, including those strains that are penicillin resistant.

MOXIFLOXACIN AND GEMIFLOXACIN

These agents, especially gemifloxacin, have enhanced activity against *S. pneumoniae* (including penicillin-resistant strains) and atypical bacteria. This comes at the expense of aerobic gram-negative activity, especially against *P. aeruginosa*. Moxifloxacin contains a methoxy group at R2, which increases potency against anaerobic bacteria (Figure 7-7).

DELAFLOXACIN

Delafloxacin is the newest of the quinolones and has the most modifications to the quinolone core structure (Figure 7-8). Unlike the other quinolones, it lacks a basic group at R1, giving the agent an overall weak acid character that is thought to enhance bacterial uptake in acidic environments, such as the phagolysosome and abscesses. A chlorine residue at R2 increases the stability of delafloxacin, enhancing activity against aerobic gram-positive and anaerobic bacteria. The large aromatic ring at R3 further enhances interactions with DNA gyrase and topoisomerase IV, which allows delafloxacin to maintain activity in the presence of mutations that confer resistance to other quinolones. Together, these modifications confer strong activity against aerobic gram-positive bacteria, such as staphylococci and streptococci. In fact, unlike the other quinolones, delafloxacin is active against many strains of methicillin-resistant *Staphylococcus aureus* and is approved for the treatment of acute skin and soft tissue infections. Delafloxacin is also active against aerobic gram-negative bacteria such as *P. aeruginosa* and many members of the Enterobacterales and has in vitro activity against some anaerobic and atypical bacteria.

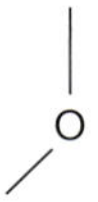

Figure 7-7. The R2 side chain of moxifloxacin is a methoxy group, which enhances activity against anaerobic bacteria.

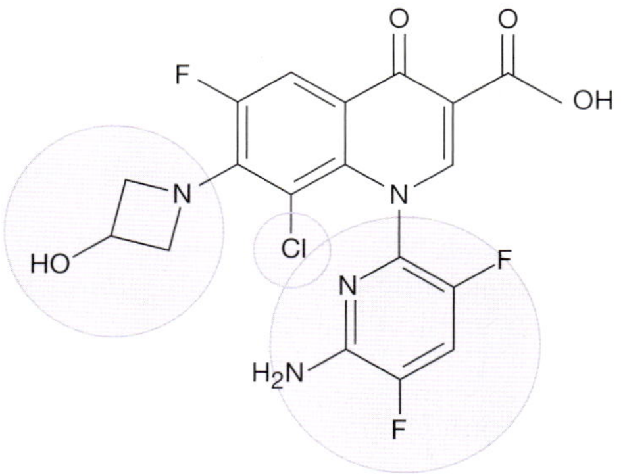

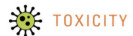

Figure 7-8. The structure of delafloxacin, which highlights changes to the R1, R2, and R3 side chains that confer on this quinolone its unique spectrum of activity.

 TOXICITY

Quinolones were initially thought to be well tolerated, but several problematic adverse reactions have become apparent during the years in which these antibiotics have been widely used. Gastrointestinal symptoms are the most common side effect, seen in 5% to 10% of individuals taking these agents. Adverse effects involving the nervous system such as headache, dizziness, or peripheral neuropathy occur in approximately 5% of patients, whereas rashes occur in approximately 1% to 2%. Quinolones cause cartilage abnormalities in juvenile animals, so they should be avoided when possible in children younger than 18 years of age and not used at all in pregnant women. Achilles tendon rupture has been reported in the elderly. Quinolone use has been associated with prolongation of the QT interval on electrocardiograms. Thus, these agents may predispose to ventricular arrhythmias such as torsades de pointes, especially when they are used in conjunction with other agents that also prolong the QT interval. Some reports suggest that quinolone use results in the development of *Clostridioides difficile*-associated diarrhea more frequently than most antibiotics. Because of the risk of serious adverse reactions, the U.S. Food and Drug Administration has recommended that fluoroquinolones not be used to treat certain uncomplicated infections.

PEARL

In general, the quinolones have good activity against *S. pneumoniae* and are especially useful for infections caused by penicillin-resistant strains of this bacterium. However, ciprofloxacin should be used with caution in the treatment of serious infections caused by *S. pneumoniae* because treatment failures have been reported.

From Mandell LA, Wunderink RG, Anzueto A, et al. Infectious Diseases Society of America/American Thoracic Society consensus guidelines on the management of community-acquired pneumonia in adults. *Clin Infect Dis.* 2007; 44(suppl 2):S27-S72 by permission of Oxford University Press.

Quinolones are useful in treating infections caused by aerobic gram-negative bacteria, atypical bacteria, and some aerobic gram-positive bacteria and mycobacteria. Some members also have activity against *P. aeruginosa* or anaerobic bacteria.

QUESTIONS

5. As a group, the fluoroquinolones are most useful in the treatment of aerobic _____ infections, although they also have activity against aerobic _____ bacteria, atypical bacteria, and mycobacteria.

6. Of the fluoroquinolones, _____ is most active against *P. aeruginosa*.

7. _____ is the only approved fluoroquinolone with activity against methicillin-resistant *S. aureus*.

8. The quinolones target bacterial _____ and _____, which leads to breaks in the bacterial chromosome.

9. Fluoroquinolones should be given to children with caution because of concerns about possible damage to _____.

ANSWERS

5. gram-negative, gram-positive

6. ciprofloxacin

7. delafloxacin

8. DNA gyrase, topoisomerase IV

9. cartilage

ADDITIONAL READINGS

Bolon MK. The newer fluoroquinolones. *Med Clin N Am*. 2011;95:793-817.

Drlica K, Malik M, Kerns RJ, et al. Quinolone-mediated bacterial death. *Antimicrob Agents Chemother*. 2008;52:385-392.

O'Donnell JA, Gelone SP. Fluoroquinolones. *Infect Dis Clin North Am*. 2000;14:489-513.

Redgrave LS, Sutton SB, Webber MA, et al. Fluoroquinolone resistance: mechanisms, impact on bacteria, and role in evolutionary success. *Trends Microbiol*. 2014;22:438-445.

Saravolatz LD, Leggett J. Gatifloxacin, gemifloxacin, and moxifloxacin: the role of 3 newer fluoroquinolones. *Clin Infect Dis*. 2003;37:1210-1215.

Stein GE, Goldstein EJ. Fluoroquinolones and anaerobes. *Clin Infect Dis*. 2006;42:1598-1607.

Turban A, Guerin F, Din A, Cattoir V. Updated review on clinically-relevant properties of delafloxacin. *Antibiotics*. 2023;12:1241. doi:10.3390/antibiotics12081241

Metronidazole

Metronidazole, a 5-nitroimidazole, was discovered in the 1950s. It continues to be an important and frequently used antibiotic for the treatment of infections caused by anaerobic bacteria.

Metronidazole is a small molecule that can passively diffuse into bacteria. An important component of its structure is a nitro group that extends from the core five-membered ring (Figure 7-9). This group must be reduced (ie, accept electrons) for metronidazole to be active. As part of their metabolic machinery, anaerobic bacteria possess low redox potential electron transport proteins, which are capable of donating electrons to this nitro group. Aerobic bacteria, however, lack these proteins, perhaps because they are incompatible with the presence of oxygen, which itself is an extremely potent electron acceptor. For this reason, metronidazole's spectrum of activity is limited to obligate anaerobic bacteria and some microaerophilic bacteria that normally thrive in the presence of low concentrations of oxygen. Once reduced, the nitro group is thought to form free radicals that lead to breaks in DNA molecules and subsequent bacterial death.

Resistance to metronidazole is rare among obligate anaerobic bacteria. When it does occur, it is thought to result from a decrease in the capacity of the electron transport proteins to reduce the nitro group of metronidazole. The development of resistance in the microaerophilic bacterium *Helicobacter pylori* is more common, although the mechanism remains unclear.

Metronidazole is effective against nearly all anaerobic gram-negative bacteria, including *Bacteroides fragilis*, and most anaerobic gram-positive bacteria, including *Clostridium* spp. (Table 7-5). It is one of the few antibiotics that has activity against *C. difficile*. The microaerophilic (ie, optimal growth in low levels of oxygen) bacterium *H. pylori* is also frequently susceptible.

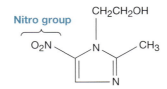

Figure 7-9. The structure of metronidazole.

Metronidazole	Table 7-5	Antimicrobial Activity of Metronidazole
Gram-positive ⊖ Gram-negative ⊖ Anaerobes ⊕ Atypical ⊖	Anaerobic bacteria	*Bacteroides fragilis* *Clostridium* spp. Most other anaerobes

Both oral and IV formulations of metronidazole are available. Oral metronidazole is extremely well absorbed and results in serum levels comparable to those following IV administration.

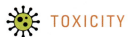
TOXICITY

Metronidazole is relatively well tolerated but is associated with some minor toxicities, such as nausea and epigastric discomfort. It can also cause an unpleasant metallic taste and "furring" of the tongue. Occasionally, metronidazole is associated with neurologic complaints, including headache, dizziness, and peripheral neuropathy. Metronidazole can lead to a disulfiram-like reaction; ingestion of alcohol should be avoided while taking this drug.

Metronidazole retains excellent activity against obligate anaerobic bacteria and is useful in the treatment of some microaerophilic bacteria, such as *H. pylori*.

QUESTIONS

10. Metronidazole has excellent activity against most _____ bacteria.
11. Metronidazole also has activity against some _____ bacteria, such as *H. pylori*.
12. Aerobic bacteria are not killed by metronidazole because they do not _____ its nitro group.

ANSWERS

10. anaerobic
11. microaerophilic
12. reduce

ADDITIONAL READINGS

Bartlett JG. Metronidazole. *Johns Hopkins Med J*. 1981;149:89-92.
Edwards DI. Nitroimidazole drugs—action and resistance mechanisms. I. Mechanisms of action. *J Antimicrob Chemother*. 1993;31:9-20.
Finegold SM. Metronidazole. *Ann Intern Med*. 1980;93:585-587.

HISTORY

Metronidazole was discovered because of its activity against protozoans. However, a patient being treated with metronidazole for *Trichomonas vaginalis* vaginitis, a protozoan infection, was noted to have marked improvement in her gingivitis, which was caused by anaerobic bacteria. This led to investigations of metronidazole's activity against anaerobic bacteria.

From Mascaretti OA. *Bacteria Versus Antibacterial Agents: An Integrated Approach*. ASM Press; 2003.

CHAPTER 8

Antimycobacterial Agents

They robbed and burned all the villages, so that you could well go a whole day's journey and never find anyone occupying a village or land tilled. Then corn was dear, and flesh and cheese and butter, because there was none in the land. Wretched men starved with hunger....

—**The Anglo-Saxon Chronicles, translated and edited by Michael Swanton**

Like residents of regions devastated by prolonged wars, patients afflicted with mycobacterial infections tend to become weakened and emaciated and may even die due to the chronicity of the disease process. These slowly progressing infections are caused by bacteria that are themselves slow growing. Because many antimicrobial agents have poor activity against slowly dividing bacteria, mycobacteria are prone to develop resistance to antibiotics. As a result, treatment of infections caused by mycobacteria requires multiple antimicrobial agents for extended periods. Different species of mycobacteria cause different diseases, each of which requires its own unique therapeutic regimen. In this chapter, we focus on several agents used for the treatment of common mycobacterial infections.

Tuberculosis is caused by *Mycobacterium tuberculosis*. The disfiguring disease leprosy is caused by *Mycobacterium leprae*. A long list of other mycobacteria, often referred to as "nontuberculous mycobacteria," also cause various diseases in humans. For example, *Mycobacterium avium* complex is a group of mycobacteria that frequently cause disease in immunocompromised hosts, particularly those infected with human immunodeficiency virus (HIV). Agents commonly used to treat mycobacterial infections include **isoniazid**, **rifamycin**, **pyrazinamide**, **ethambutol**, **clarithromycin**, and **azithromycin**. Other agents occasionally used in the treatment of mycobacterial infections include amikacin, bedaquiline, pretomanid, linezolid, delamanid, streptomycin, cycloserine, ethionamide, capreomycin, *p*-aminosalicylic acid, clofazimine, dapsone, and the quinolones.

ISONIAZID

Isoniazid has little activity against most bacteria but is capable of killing both intracellular and extracellular *M. tuberculosis*. It is thought to inhibit an enzyme essential for the synthesis of mycolic acid, an important constituent of the *M. tuberculosis* cell envelope. This may explain the specificity of isoniazid for mycobacteria because other bacteria do not make mycolic acid. Resistance occurs with mutations in the gene that encodes catalase-peroxidase, which is required to convert isoniazid to its active form. Likewise, mutations in the gene encoding the target enzyme essential for mycolic acid synthesis also result in resistance. Isoniazid is associated with rash, fever, hepatotoxicity, and peripheral neuropathy. The prophylactic administration of pyridoxine prevents neuropathy.

RIFAMPIN, RIFABUTIN, AND RIFAPENTINE

Unlike isoniazid, the rifamycins are active against a broad spectrum of bacteria. These agents, which inhibit bacterial RNA polymerase, are discussed in more detail in the "Rifamycins" section of Chapter 6. Mycobacteria readily become resistant to rifamycins when they are used as monotherapy for active disease. Resistance is the result of mutations in the gene that encodes RNA polymerase.

PYRAZINAMIDE

Pyrazinamide targets a protein essential for restarting stalled ribosomes. This agent kills mycobacteria only at acidic pH. Fortunately, intracellular *M. tuberculosis* resides within an acidic phagosome, and this drug is active against intracellular organisms. Resistance results from mutations in the gene encoding pyrazinamidase, an enzyme essential for converting pyrazinamide into its active form. Adverse effects include hepatotoxicity and elevated serum levels of uric acid, which may lead to gout.

ETHAMBUTOL

Ethambutol targets an enzyme involved in the synthesis of the mycobacterial cell wall. Mutations in the gene encoding this enzyme result in resistance. The major toxicity is optic neuritis, which may lead to decreased visual acuity and loss of red-green discrimination.

CLARITHROMYCIN AND AZITHROMYCIN

Clarithromycin and azithromycin prevent protein translation by targeting the ribosomes of many different bacteria, including some mycobacteria. These agents are discussed in more detail in the "Macrolides" section of Chapter 6.

In summary, several antibiotics are active against mycobacteria. Some of these agents, such as isoniazid, are used specifically to treat mycobacterial infections, whereas other agents, such as rifampin, show activity against a broad range of bacterial genera. Because mycobacteria are prone to develop resistance to antimicrobial compounds and are difficult to eradicate, treatment regimens usually contain multiple agents and continue for months. Toxicity is problematic and must be carefully monitored over the extended periods that these agents are given.

QUESTIONS

1. Mycobacterial infections are usually treated with _____ drugs for extended periods.
2. _____, _____, _____, and _____ are first-line agents for the treatment of *M. tuberculosis*.
3. Isoniazid, rifampin, and pyrazinamide all may cause _____.

ANSWERS

1. multiple
2. Isoniazid, rifamycin, pyrazinamide, ethambutol
3. hepatotoxicity

ADDITIONAL READINGS

Miotto P, Cirillo DM, Migliori GB. Drug resistance in *Mycobacterium tuberculosis*: molecular mechanisms challenging fluoroquinolones and pyrazinamide effectiveness. *Chest.* 2015;147:1135-1143.

Nahid P, Dorman SE, Alipanah N, et al. Official American Thoracic Society/Centers for Disease Control and Prevention/Infectious Diseases Society of America Clinical Practice Guidelines: treatment of drug-susceptible tuberculosis. *Clin Infect Dis.* 2016;63:e147-e195

Nahid P, Mase SR, Migliori GB, et al. Treatment of drug-resistant tuberculosis: an official ATS/CDC/ERS/IDSA clinical practice guideline. *Am J Respir Crit Care Med.* 2019;200:e93-e142.

Shi W, Zhang X, Jiang X, et al. Pyrazinamide inhibits trans-translation in *Mycobacterium tuberculosis*. *Science.* 2011;333:1630-1632.

Vilchèze C, Wang F, Arai M, et al. Transfer of a point mutation in *Mycobacterium tuberculosis* inhA resolves the target of isoniazid. *Nat Med.* 2006;12:1027-1029.

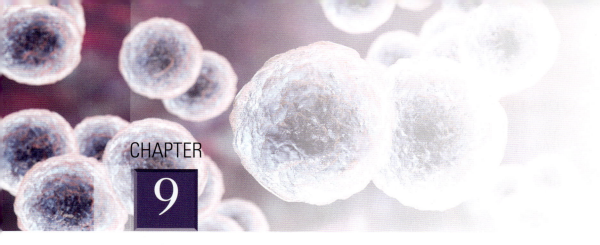

CHAPTER 9

Summary of Antibacterial Agents

Now let us take a deep breath and review what we have learned. Probably, the most apparent fact is that there are a lot of antibiotics used to treat bacterial infections! Certainly, it has gotten progressively more difficult to master this topic over the years as more and more antimicrobial agents have been developed. Yet, by grouping these agents based on their spectra of activity, the subject becomes manageable.

Let us start with aerobic gram-positive bacteria. A quick review of the antibiotics in the preceding sections indicates that certain agents have robust activity against gram-positive organisms, whereas other agents have modest activity and still others have very limited or no activity (Figure 9-1). Those agents with activity against most gram-positive bacteria are β-lactam/β-lactamase inhibitor combinations, carbapenems (including carbapenem/β-lactamase inhibitor combinations), glycopeptides, oxazolidinones, and daptomycin. When empirically treating probable gram-positive infections, the use of one of these agents in the correct setting will likely be effective. Remember this group of high-power agents! However, even these antibiotics are not perfect—each has its weaknesses. For example, carbapenems and β-lactam/β-lactamase inhibitor combinations are not active against methicillin-resistant *Staphylococcus aureus*. Obviously, vancomycin will not kill vancomycin-resistant enterococci. Resistance to the oxazolidinones and daptomycin has already been reported among gram-positive bacteria. So do not forget to check susceptibilities and modify treatment accordingly. Many agents have modest activity against gram-positive bacteria (Figure 9-1). These antibiotics are active against some gram-positive bacteria, but not others. Some, such as aminoglycosides and rifampins, should only be used in combination with other agents active against this class of bacteria.

Aerobic gram-negative bacteria are particularly troublesome causes of infection, and a large number of antimicrobial agents have been developed to target these bacteria (Figure 9-2). Those with the broadest activity include some penicillin/β-lactamase inhibitor combinations, third- and fourth-generation cephalosporins, cephalosporin/β-lactamase inhibitor combinations, siderophore cephalosporins, carbapenems

CHAPTER 9 — Summary of Antibacterial Agents

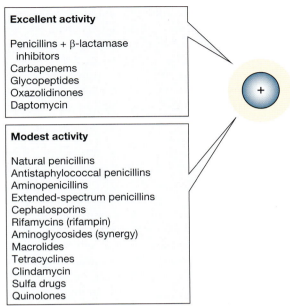

Figure 9-1. Antibiotics for the treatment of infections caused by aerobic gram-positive bacteria.

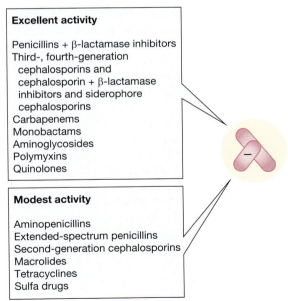

Figure 9-2. Antibiotics for the treatment of infections caused by aerobic gram-negative bacteria.

(including carbapenem/β-lactamase inhibitor combinations), monobactams, aminoglycosides, polymyxins, and quinolones. These agents share the ability to penetrate the outer membrane barrier of most gram-negative pathogens and avoid inactivation by common resistance mechanisms. Nonetheless, a significant number of gram-negative bacteria will be resistant to agents in one or more of these classes, and susceptibilities of individual bacterial strains must still be checked to ensure optimal therapy. A second group of antibiotics has modest activity against gram-negative bacteria; these agents are useful in the treatment of infections caused by some gram-negative bacteria (Figure 9-2).

Anaerobic bacteria have a propensity to cause mixed infections and are difficult to culture. As a result, these infections are often treated empirically, which requires a thorough understanding of the spectra of activity of individual antibiotics. Three groups of agents are active against an especially broad range of anaerobic bacteria: the penicillin/β-lactamase inhibitor combinations, the carbapenems (including carbapenem/β-lactamase inhibitor combinations), and metronidazole (Figure 9-3). These agents will effectively treat most anaerobic bacteria encountered in clinical practice. One important exception is *Clostridioides difficile*, a cause of antibiotic-associated diarrhea, which is often treated with oral vancomycin. Although lacking the near-universal spectra of activity of the first group of agents, a large number of antibiotics are still useful in the treatment of anaerobic infections and make up a second tier of anaerobic drugs (Figure 9-3). These agents are used to treat infections caused by one or a subset of anaerobic bacteria with known susceptibilities.

Atypical bacteria are hard to visualize by routine methods such as Gram staining or are difficult to grow on laboratory media. Although this classification is not perfect, it does allow for a way of thinking about this diverse group of bacteria with regard to antimicrobial therapy. Some of the bacteria included in this group are *Chlamydia* spp., *Mycoplasma* spp., *Legionella pneumophila*, *Brucella* spp., *Francisella tularensis*,

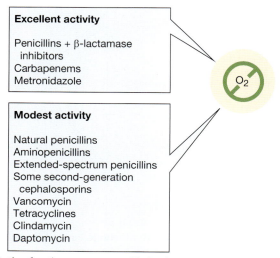

Figure 9-3. Antibiotics for the treatment of infections caused by anaerobic bacteria.

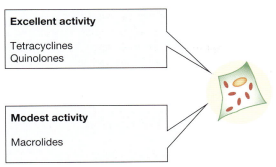

Figure 9-4. Antibiotics for the treatment of infections caused by atypical bacteria.

and *Rickettsia* spp. Many of these bacteria reside within macrophages or other host cell types. As a result, antibiotics that penetrate well into host cells have the best activity against these organisms. These include the tetracyclines and the quinolones (Figure 9-4). The macrolides are also effective against infections caused by many of these bacteria.

Knowing which antibiotic classes have activity against the different groups of bacteria is a useful way to learn how to choose appropriate antimicrobial agents. However, one must remember that the antimicrobial activity of agents within some classes differs significantly. For example, the quinolones are not listed as having anaerobic activity, yet moxifloxacin is effective against infections caused by some of these bacteria. Likewise, tigecycline, eravacycline, and omadacycline have much broader activity than the other members of the tetracycline antibiotics. Thus, the activities summarized in this chapter should be thought of as general guidelines with many exceptions.

PART 3

Definitive Therapy

"You can attain proficiency in this path by seeing through the opponent's strategy, and by knowing the strengths and weaknesses of the opponent's tactics."

—The Book of Five Rings, Miyamoto Musashi

The choice of which antibiotic to prescribe for the treatment of a bacterial infection usually must be made in one of three types of situations. First, a patient may be suspected or known to have a bacterial infection, but the bacterial species responsible for the illness has not yet been identified. Treatment in such cases is referred to as **empiric therapy** and consists of an antimicrobial agent or agents that are active against the bacteria most associated with the disease syndrome afflicting the patient (eg, community-acquired pneumonia). Often in such cases, clinical samples will be obtained prior to starting antimicrobial therapy, and these samples will be cultured or otherwise tested in an attempt to identify the causative bacterium. If the bacterial species responsible for the illness is identified, therapy is narrowed to specifically target this particular organism. For example, a sputum sample obtained from a patient with community-acquired pneumonia may grow *Streptococcus pneumoniae*, and it is then the clinician's job to choose the best antibiotic regimen to treat the pneumonia. The prescribed regimen would be referred to as **definitive therapy** because the causative organism is known. A final decision regarding antimicrobial therapy is often made several days later, when the antibiotic susceptibilities of the cultured bacterium are reported. At that time, activity, cost, convenience of dosing, penetration, and other factors are used to choose the most appropriate antibiotic from the list of agents to which the bacterium is susceptible.

In this section, we focus on definitive therapy. Essential to choosing the best antimicrobial regimens for definitive therapy is knowing which antibiotics have activity against the individual bacterial pathogens, so we discuss the preferred antimicrobial agents for the bacteria most commonly encountered in clinical practice. The emphasis is on parenteral agents used to treat severe infections. As with the traffic lights in the preceding sections, we somewhat arbitrarily divide the common bacterial pathogens into the following groups: gram-positive bacteria, gram-negative bacteria, anaerobic bacteria, and atypical bacteria. In this way, the information presented in this section reviews and solidifies the knowledge you have gained in the preceding section. Two additional groups of bacteria are also discussed: spirochetes and mycobacteria.

Note that in clinical practice, a large variety of factors enter into the decision of which antimicrobial agent is prescribed for a particular patient. Consideration is given to the allergy profile of the patient, the penetration of different agents to the site of infection, cost, ease of administration, and recent antibiotic exposure history, which may suggest a risk of resistance to certain agents. It is often preferred to use an agent with a narrow spectrum of activity over one with a broad spectrum of activity. Here, however, we focus only on the susceptibility of specific kinds of bacteria to antibiotics, because this is the point from which most prescribing decisions begin.

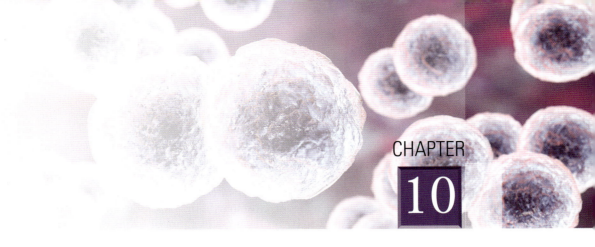

CHAPTER 10

Gram-Positive Bacteria

"'A terrible worm in an iron cocoon,' as he was called in an anonymous poem, the knight rode on a saddle rising in a higher ridge above the horse's backbone with his feet resting in very long stirrups so that he was virtually standing up and able to deliver tremendous swinging blows from side to side with any one of his armory of weapons. He began battle with the lance used for unhorsing the enemy, while from his belt hung a two-handed sword at one side and an eighteen-inch dagger on the other. He also had available, either attached to his saddle or carried by his squire, a longer sword for thrusting like a lance, a battle-ax fitted with a spike behind the curved blade, and a club-headed mace with sharpened, ridged edges, a weapon favored by martial bishops and abbots on the theory that it did not come under the rule forbidding clerics 'to smite with the edge of the sword.'"

— A Distant Mirror, Barbara W. Tuchman

Like the medieval knight, gram-positive bacteria harbor an impressive array of offensive and defensive weapons. For protection, they utilize a thick and rigid cell wall. From behind this armor, they brandish an imposing number of toxins designed to subdue the host. These attributes make them formidable foes in their battles against the defenses of the human body.

After a period of relative calm, gram-positive bacteria have burst upon the scene in recent decades to once again garner notoriety as causes of serious and difficult-to-treat infections. Much of this is due to marked increases in antibiotic resistance among these bacteria, most notably methicillin resistance in *Staphylococcus aureus*, decreased susceptibility to penicillin in *S. pneumoniae*, and vancomycin resistance in the enterococci. In this section, we review some of the major gram-positive pathogens: staphylococci, pneumococci, other streptococci, enterococci, and *Listeria monocytogenes*. We focus on the appropriate antimicrobial treatment for infections caused by each of these organisms.

Excerpt(s) from *A Distant Mirror: The Calamitous 14th Century* by Barbara W. Tuchman, copyright © 1978 by Barbara W. Tuchman. Used by permission of Alfred A. Knopf, an imprint of the Knopf Doubleday Publishing Group, a division of Penguin Random House LLC. All rights reserved.

Staphylococci

Three species of staphylococci are of major medical importance: *S. aureus*, *Staphylococcus epidermidis*, and *Staphylococcus saprophyticus*. *S. aureus* is the "workaholic" of bacterial pathogens. Not only is this organism a frequent cause of human infections, but it also brings about a remarkable variety of disease manifestations, including bacteremia, endocarditis, skin and soft tissue infections, osteomyelitis, pneumonia, and toxic shock syndrome (Figure 10-1). It does so by producing a plethora of toxins that damage the host or manipulate its immune response. *S. aureus* is a gram-positive coccus that grows in grape-like clusters and often forms golden-colored colonies on agar plates (hence the name *aureus*, which means gold). *S. epidermidis* is the most important member of a larger group of bacteria referred to as *coagulase-negative staphylococci*. These bacteria are morphologically similar to *S. aureus* but are less virulent and less versatile. They are mainly associated with infections involving foreign objects, such as intravenous catheters, prosthetic heart valves, and prosthetic joints. *S. saprophyticus* is a member of the coagulase-negative staphylococci that causes community-acquired urinary tract infections.

A historical overview of the attempts to treat *S. aureus* infections is illustrative of the ability of bacteria to counter our best efforts at antimicrobial containment (Figure 10-2). In the 1940s and 1950s, infections caused by *S. aureus* were treated with **penicillin**, which was active against the thick cell wall of this bacterium. Resistance, however, soon developed in the form of bacteria producing β-lactamases that efficiently cleaved penicillin (step 1 in Figure 10-2). Now, relatively few strains remain susceptible to penicillin. Fortunately, antistaphylococcal penicillins, which are modified to resist

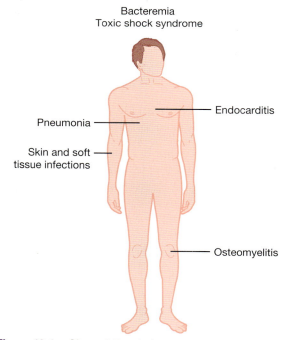

Figure 10-1. Sites of *Staphylococcus aureus* infections.

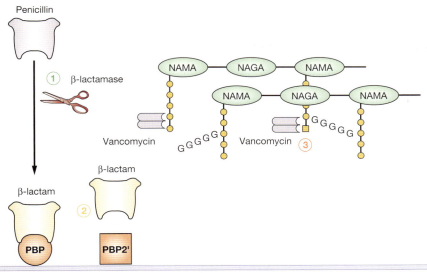

Figure 10-2. Mechanisms by which *Staphylococcus aureus* resists the action of antibiotics. (1) Although penicillin was initially effective against this bacterium, most strains now produce β-lactamases that cleave penicillin. For this reason, antistaphylococcal penicillins that are resistant to cleavage by staphylococcal β-lactamases were developed. (2) Methicillin-resistant *S. aureus* strains, however, produce an altered penicillin-binding protein (PBP) (referred to as PBP2′) that is not recognized by these compounds or other β-lactam agents. Vancomycin, a glycopeptide, overcomes this difficulty by binding to the terminal alanine-alanine group of the peptide side chain of peptidoglycan and thus inhibits peptidoglycan cross-linking without binding to PBPs. (3) Vancomycin-resistant strains of *S. aureus* are now being identified. Some of these strains have become resistant to vancomycin by altering the structure of the peptide side chain of newly formed peptidoglycan subunits so that they are not recognized by vancomycin. NAGA, *N*-acetylglucosamine; NAMA, *N*-acetylmuramic acid.

cleavage by staphylococcal β-lactamases, became available and were highly active against *S. aureus*. This group of agents includes **nafcillin, oxacillin**, and methicillin (the last of which is no longer available in the United States) (Table 10-1). Because of their narrow spectra and potency, these antibiotics remain the drugs of choice for many infections caused by *S. aureus*. In addition, cephalosporins resistant to cleavage by the staphylococcal β-lactamases were also developed. First- and fourth-generation cephalosporins (eg, **cefazolin, cefepime**) and some second-generation cephalosporins (eg, **cefuroxime**) are quite potent in this regard, whereas third-generation cephalosporins (eg, **ceftriaxone, cefotaxime**) are less potent. Later, the β-lactamase inhibitors clavulanate, sulbactam, and tazobactam, which inactivate the staphylococcal β-lactamases, were developed. Thus, β-lactam/β-lactamase inhibitor combinations, such as **ampicillin-sulbactam** and **piperacillin-tazobactam**, may be used to treat infections caused by *S. aureus*. Likewise, some carbapenems (**imipenem, meropenem**) are not hydrolyzed by these β-lactamases and are also useful in the treatment of infections caused by this bacterium.

The ever-resourceful *S. aureus* again countered, however, by altering one of its penicillin-binding proteins (PBPs) (step 2 in Figure 10-2). The variant PBP is called

Table 10-1. Antimicrobial Agents for Treatment of Infections Caused by *Staphylococcus aureus*

Antibiotic Class	Antibiotic
Antistaphylococcal penicillins	Nafcillin, oxacillin
First-generation cephalosporins	Cefazolin
Second-generation cephalosporins	Cefuroxime
Third-generation cephalosporins	Ceftriaxone, cefotaxime
Fourth-generation cephalosporins	Cefepime
β-Lactam/β-lactamase inhibitor combinations	Ampicillin-sulbactam, piperacillin-tazobactam
Carbapenems	Imipenem, meropenem
Also sometimes active	
Clindamycin	
Sulfa drugs	Trimethoprim-sulfamethoxazole
Quinolones	Ciprofloxacin, levofloxacin, moxifloxacin
Tetracyclines	Minocycline, doxycycline
Macrolides	Azithromycin
Rifamycins	Rifampin
Aminoglycosides	Gentamicin (synergistic doses)
If methicillin-resistant *Staphylococcus aureus*	
Glycopeptides	Vancomycin, dalbavancin, oritavancin, telavancin
Oxazolidinones	Linezolid, tedizolid
Quinolones	Delafloxacin
Daptomycin	
Tetracyclines	Omadacycline
Fifth-generation cephalosporins	Ceftaroline

PBP2′, and it does not bind any of the β-lactam compounds. Thus, PBP2′-producing strains of *S. aureus*, referred to as methicillin-resistant *S. aureus* (MRSA) for historical reasons, are actually resistant to all penicillins (including all antistaphylococcal penicillins), cephalosporins, and carbapenems. These strains are a serious and common problem in most intensive care units and are now a frequent cause of community-acquired infections. They are usually treated with vancomycin or **daptomycin**. Unfortunately, vancomycin-resistant *S. aureus* (VRSA) strains have recently been reported. Some of these strains have acquired the ability to alter the part of peptidoglycan normally bound by **vancomycin**, thus preventing this antibiotic from exerting its effect (step 3 in Figure 10-2). Other antibiotics that may be considered for specific types of MRSA infections include the oxazolidinones, **ceftaroline**, and some relatively new antibiotics, such as the long-acting glycopeptides, **delafloxacin**, and omadacycline. Thus,

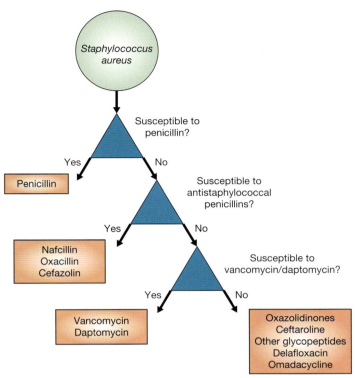

Figure 10-3. Simplified flowchart for deciding upon antibiotics for *Staphylococcus aureus* infections.

successful treatment of *S. aureus* infections requires close attention to antibiotic susceptibility results (Figure 10-3).

PEARL

Traditionally, MRSA strains were isolated from hospitalized patients or individuals exposed to health care systems. This has changed, however, and infections caused by MRSA strains are now commonly acquired in the community. One study noted that 12% of community-acquired *S. aureus* infections were caused by MRSA strains, and in some regions, this percentage is dramatically higher.

From Naimi TS, LeDell KH, Como-Sabetti K, et al. Comparison of community- and health care-associated methicillin-resistant Staphylococcus aureus infection. *JAMA.* 2003;290:2976-2984.
National Nosocomial Infections Surveillance System. National Nosocomial Infections Surveillance (NNIS) System Report, data summary from January 1992 through June 2004, issued October 2004. *Am J Infect Control.* 2004;32:470-485.

Other antibiotics, such as **clindamycin**, the older quinolones (**ciprofloxacin, levofloxacin, moxifloxacin**), **trimethoprim-sulfamethoxazole**, the older tetracyclines (**minocycline, doxycycline**), and the macrolides (**azithromycin**), are sometimes active against *S. aureus*, but in general, these agents should only be used if susceptibilities are known or the use of first-line agents is not possible (Table 10-1). **Rifampin** or synergistic doses of **gentamicin** are sometimes used along with β-lactams or **vancomycin** in the treatment of endocarditis or osteomyelitis caused by *S. aureus*. Rifampin is thought to facilitate clearance of this bacterium from the surface of prosthetic devices, such as artificial heart valves and joints.

S. epidermidis infections are treated similarly to *S. aureus* infections. Nearly all strains are resistant to penicillin, and many are resistant to the antistaphylococcal penicillins. Thus, **vancomycin** is often used to treat these infections.

QUESTIONS

1. Two antistaphylococcal penicillins used for intravenous therapy are _____ and _____.
2. *S. aureus* strains resistant to antistaphylococcal penicillins are called _____.
3. In addition to being resistant to methicillin, MRSA strains are also resistant to all other _____.
4. MRSA strains are usually susceptible to _____.

ANSWERS

1. oxacillin, nafcillin
2. MRSA
3. β-lactams
4. vancomycin

ADDITIONAL READINGS

Cong Y, Yang S, Rao X. Vancomycin resistant *Staphylococcus aureus* infections: a review of case updating and clinical features. *J Advanc Res*. 2020;21:169-176.

David MZ, Daum RS. Community-associated methicillin-resistant *Staphylococcus aureus*: epidemiology and clinical consequences of an emerging epidemic. *Clin Microbiol Rev*. 2010;23:616-687.

Liu C, Bayer A, Cosgrove SE, et al. Clinical practice guidelines by the Infectious Disease Society of America for the treatment of methicillin-resistant *Staphylococcus aureus* infections in adults and children: executive summary. *Clin Infect Dis*. 2011;52:285-292.

Tong SY, Davis JS, Eichenberger E, et al. *Staphylococcus aureus* infections: epidemiology, pathophysiology, clinical manifestations, and management. *Clin Microbiol Rev*. 2015;28:603-661.

Pneumococci

Pneumococci are frequent causes of community-acquired pneumonia, otitis media, sinusitis, and meningitis (Figure 10-4). These bacteria, which are formally designated *S. pneumoniae*, do not act covertly. Rather than avoid detection and cause disease by subversion, pneumococci boldly and forcefully attack the human body and cause significant amounts of tissue damage. As a result, pneumococcal infections are associated with extensive inflammatory responses that contribute to host tissue injury.

For many years, the treatment of infections caused by *S. pneumoniae* was straightforward: **Penicillin** or **ampicillin** was given. Physicians now recall those days with nostalgia because the choice of therapy has become somewhat more complex. An increasing percentage of pneumococcal strains produces PBPs that are poorly recognized by the natural penicillins and aminopenicillins, resulting in relative resistance. Approximately 4% of *S. pneumoniae* isolates in the United States now have intermediate or high levels of resistance to these agents. In many cases, however, this relative resistance can be overcome by giving higher doses of penicillin or ampicillin, which leads to higher drug concentrations and, as a result, sufficient binding to PBPs to cause bacterial killing.

This situation becomes more complicated when one appreciates that many β-lactams, such as the penicillins, achieve approximately 100-fold higher concentrations in plasma and the lungs than they do in cerebrospinal fluid. Thus, a "penicillin-resistant" strain of *S. pneumoniae* may be killed by the high penicillin concentrations present in the lung but persist in the relatively low concentrations found in the cerebrospinal fluid.

Over the same period, resistance to cephalosporins traditionally used to treat pneumococcal infections has increased as well. These cephalosporins include **cefuroxime**,

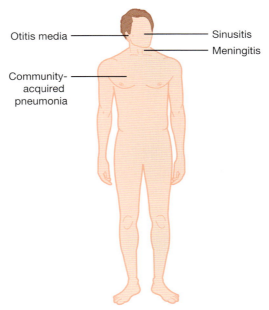

Figure 10-4. Sites of *Streptococcus pneumoniae* infections.

Table 10-2 Agents for Treatment of Infections Caused by *Streptococcus pneumoniae*

Antibiotic Class	Antibiotic
Natural penicillins	Penicillin G
Aminopenicillins	Ampicillin
Also sometimes active	
Clindamycin	
Sulfa drugs	Trimethoprim-sulfamethoxazole
Macrolides	Azithromycin
Tetracyclines	Doxycycline
If penicillin-resistant	
Second-generation cephalosporin	Cefuroxime
Third-generation cephalosporin	Ceftriaxone
Fourth-generation cephalosporin	Cefepime
Fifth-generation cephalosporin	Ceftaroline
Quinolones	Moxifloxacin, levofloxacin, gemifloxacin
Glycopeptide	Vancomycin
Alternatives	
Oxazolidinones	Linezolid, tedizolid
Carbapenems	Imipenem, meropenem

ceftriaxone, and **cefepime**. Like penicillin, cephalosporins achieve much higher concentrations in plasma and pulmonary tissues than within the central nervous system. Thus, similar arguments apply to both cephalosporin and penicillin resistance.

So, how is one to treat these infections? In general, the following guidelines apply in the treatment of *S. pneumoniae* infections with penicillin (Table 10-2). Pneumonia, otitis media, sinusitis, and bacteremia caused by all but the most resistant strains of *S. pneumoniae* should be treated with high doses of **penicillin** or **ampicillin**. These agents, however, should not be used to treat meningitis caused by strains that have even an intermediate level of resistance. Likewise, third-generation cephalosporins such as **ceftriaxone** can be used to treat most kinds of pneumococcal infections regardless of their sensitivities with the exception of meningitis caused by highly resistant strains. For these infections, **vancomycin** is recommended.

The difficulties in treating infections caused by penicillin-resistant pneumococci are compounded by the fact that these bacteria are also frequently resistant to several other antibiotics. Acquired genetic material that encodes for penicillin resistance also often carries genes that result in loss of susceptibility to many other antibiotics commonly used for pneumococcal infections. These include macrolide-like agents (**azithromycin**), tetracyclines (**doxycycline**), **clindamycin**, and sulfa drugs (**trimethoprim-sulfamethoxazole**). For infections caused by highly resistant strains, several options are available (Table 10-2). Certain quinolones (**moxifloxacin, gemifloxacin,** and **levofloxacin,** but not ciprofloxacin) and fifth-generation cephalosporins (**ceftaroline**) remain active against penicillin-resistant pneumococci, as does **vancomycin**. Less frequently used alternatives include oxazolidinones (**linezolid, tedizolid**) or carbapenems (**imipenem, meropenem**).

QUESTIONS

5. Prior to the emergence of resistant strains, *S. pneumoniae* infections were routinely treated with _____ or _____.
6. Currently, many pneumococcal strains are resistant to penicillins because they produce _____ that are poorly recognized by these agents.
7. Antibiotics commonly used to treat highly penicillin-resistant *S. pneumoniae* strains include _____, _____, and _____.
8. Penicillin-resistant strains of *S. pneumoniae* are often also resistant to other antibiotics used to treat infections caused by this bacterium, including _____, _____, _____, and _____.

ANSWERS

5. penicillin, ampicillin
6. PBPs
7. quinolones, ceftaroline, vancomycin
8. clindamycin, macrolides, tetracyclines, trimethoprim-sulfamethoxazole

ADDITIONAL READINGS

Feldman C, Anderson R. Recent advances in our understanding of *Streptococcus pneumoniae* infection. *F1000 Prime Rep*. 2014;6:82. doi:10.12703/P6-82

Garau J. Treatment of drug-resistant pneumococcal pneumonia. *Lancet Infect Dis*. 2002;2:404-415.

Musher DM, Bartlett JG, Doern GV. A fresh look at the definition of susceptibility of *Streptococcus pneumoniae* to beta-lactam antibiotics. *Arch Intern Med*. 2001;161:2538-2544.

Other Streptococci

S. pneumoniae is only one of many medically important streptococcal species. Bacteria classified as *Streptococcus pyogenes* (also called group A streptococci) are a frequent cause of pharyngitis ("strep throat"), skin and soft tissue infections, and streptococcal toxic shock syndrome (Figure 10-5). *Streptococcus agalactiae* strains (also called group B streptococci) colonize the female genital tract and cause sepsis and meningitis in neonates and infants less than 3 months of age. Viridans group streptococci, a large heterogeneous group of streptococci defined by their hemolysis pattern when grown on blood agar, colonize the human gastrointestinal and urogenital tracts and are the etiologic agents of several severe infections, including infective endocarditis and abscesses.

Traditional treatment of infections caused by these streptococci has consisted of the natural penicillins or aminopenicillins, and many of these bacteria remain susceptible to these agents (Table 10-3). Infections caused by *S. pyogenes* are routinely treated with **penicillin** or **ampicillin**. Alternatives include a first-generation cephalosporin (eg, **cefazolin**) or a macrolide (eg, **azithromycin**), although macrolide resistance is becoming more common. In severe invasive group A streptococcal infections, such as necrotizing fasciitis, **clindamycin** is added to a regimen of high-dose penicillin. Theoretically, clindamycin, which inhibits protein translation, blocks the production of some of the streptococcal toxins that contribute to the pathogenesis of these diseases. Intravenous immune globulin (IVIG) is also frequently given in these situations because it may contain antibodies that bind and neutralize these toxins. *S. agalactiae* is

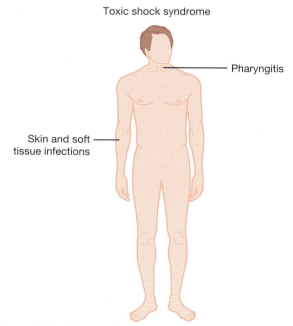

Figure 10-5. Sites of *Streptococcus pyogenes* infections.

Table 10-3 Antimicrobial Agents for Treatment of Infections Caused by Streptococcal Species Other Than *Streptococcus pneumoniae*

Antibiotic Class	Antibiotic
Natural penicillins	Penicillin G
Aminopenicillins	Ampicillin
Aminoglycosides are sometimes added for synergy	Gentamicin
Clindamycin is added for severe invasive *Streptococcus pyogenes* infections	
Alternatives	
First-generation cephalosporin	Cefazolin
Macrolide	Azithromycin
If penicillin resistant	
Glycopeptide	Vancomycin
Second-generation cephalosporin	Cefuroxime
Third-generation cephalosporin	Ceftriaxone

uniformly sensitive to **penicillin** and **ampicillin**. Synergistic doses of an aminoglycoside such as **gentamicin** are often initially added to regimens for serious infections. Although **penicillin** is still the agent of choice for infections caused by viridans group streptococci, resistance to this agent is increasingly common. As with *S. pneumoniae*, resistance is due to altered PBPs. Glycopeptides or cephalosporins (eg, **ceftriaxone**) are used to treat these resistant strains. An aminoglycoside (eg, **gentamicin**) is sometimes added to these agents for synergism.

QUESTIONS

9. Unlike *S. pneumoniae*, *S. pyogenes* continues to be nearly universally susceptible to _____.
10. In the treatment of serious invasive group A streptococcal infections, _____ should be used in conjunction with penicillin.
11. Viridans group streptococci differ from group A and group B streptococci in that they are more frequently resistant to _____.
12. In the treatment of infections caused by *S. agalactiae* and viridans group streptococci, _____ are sometimes used with penicillins because of synergy between these agents.

ANSWERS

9. penicillin
10. clindamycin
11. penicillin
12. aminoglycosides

ADDITIONAL READINGS

Carapetis JR, Jacoby P, Carville K, et al. Effectiveness of clindamycin and intravenous immunoglobulin, and risk of disease in contacts, in invasive group A streptococcal infections. *Clin Infect Dis*. 2014;59:358-365.

Doern GV, Ferraro MJ, Brueggemann AB, et al. Emergence of high rates of antimicrobial resistance among viridans group streptococci in the United States. *Antimicrob Agents Chemother*. 1996;40:891-894.

Parks T, Barrett L, Jones N. Invasive streptococcal disease: a review for clinicians. *Br Med Bull*. 2015;115:77-89.

Richter SS, Heilmann KP, Beekmann SE, et al. Macrolide-resistant *Streptococcus pyogenes* in the United States, 2002–2003. *Clin Infect Dis*. 2005;41:599-608.

Enterococci

Enterococci can be viewed as fickle residents of the human gastrointestinal tract. Normally, they innocuously inhabit this environmental niche, growing and multiplying in the nutritionally rich intestinal contents but causing no problems for their host. If, however, an individual becomes compromised in some way, these traitorous bacteria may turn against their host and cause serious infections. Compromise may take many forms, including the placement of a vascular or urinary catheter, abdominal surgery, or organ transplantation. Enterococcal disease manifests itself as urinary tract infections, bacteremia, endocarditis, wound infections, or intra-abdominal infections (Figure 10-6). The enterococcal species most commonly encountered in human disease are *Enterococcus faecalis* and *Enterococcus faecium*.

A truly remarkable aspect of the enterococci is their resistance to many antibiotics (Figure 10-7). These bacteria are intrinsically resistant to cephalosporins due to the production of altered PBPs. They have the ability to utilize folic acid derivatives from the environment, making them resistant to trimethoprim-sulfamethoxazole. Even penicillins and vancomycin, which are bactericidal against most susceptible bacteria, are only bacteriostatic against enterococci.

PEARL

All enterococci are not created equal. *E. faecium* tends to be much more resistant to antibiotics than *E. faecalis*. For example, in one study, 52% of *E. faecium* strains were resistant to vancomycin and 83% to ampicillin, whereas only 2% of *E. faecalis* strains were resistant to these agents.

From Huycke MM, Sahm DF, Gilmore MS. Multiple-drug resistant enterococci: the nature of the problem and an agenda for the future. *Emerg Infect Dis*. 1998;4:239-249.

The first-line antibiotics used for the treatment of enterococcal infections are the penicillins, in particular **penicillin G**, **ampicillin**, and **piperacillin** (Table 10-4). Note that cephalosporins are not active against enterococci. The carbapenems **imipenem** and **meropenem** are sometimes active. Unfortunately, enterococci are increasingly resistant to all these antibiotics, often because of the production of altered PBPs that do not bind β-lactams. In such strains, **vancomycin** is used in place of β-lactam antibiotics. Resistance to vancomycin, however, has also become common. Vancomycin-resistant enterococci (VRE) produce peptidoglycan containing an altered peptide side chain. The terminal portion of the peptide side chain is changed from D-alanine-D-alanine to D-alanyl-D-lactate. Whereas D-alanine-D-alanine is bound and sequestered by vancomycin, D-alanyl-D-lactate is not and thus renders the bacterium resistant to this antibiotic. Unless penicillin susceptible, VRE must be treated with **oxazolidinones**, **daptomycin**, or one of the newer tetracyclines.

The interaction between enterococci and aminoglycosides is complex. Enterococci do not normally take up aminoglycosides very well, resulting in universal

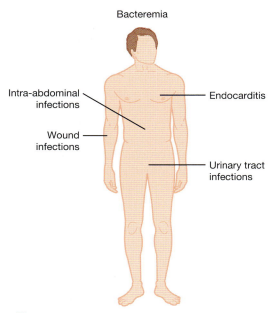

Figure 10-6. Sites of enterococcal infections.

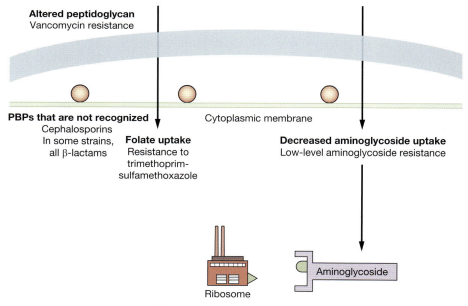

Figure 10-7. Mechanisms by which enterococci resist the actions of antibiotics. In some strains, altered peptidoglycan prevents binding by vancomycin. Enterococcal penicillin-binding proteins (PBPs) are not recognized by cephalosporins, and in some strains are not bound by any β-lactam agents. Enterococci do not need to synthesize folate because they assimilate this factor from the host, resulting in resistance to trimethoprim-sulfamethoxazole. Decreased uptake of aminoglycosides causes low-level resistance, whereas aminoglycoside modification and ribosome mutation result in high-level resistance.

Table 10-4. Antimicrobial Agents for Treatment of Infections Caused by Enterococci

Antibiotic Class	Antibiotic
Natural penicillins	Penicillin G
Aminopenicillins	Ampicillin
Extended-spectrum penicillins	Piperacillin
Also sometimes active	
Carbapenems	Imipenem, meropenem
For serious infections, add an aminoglycoside for synergy or use double β-lactam regimen.	Ampicillin plus gentamicin Ampicillin plus ceftriaxone
If penicillin resistant	
Glycopeptide	Vancomycin
If also vancomycin resistant	
Oxazolidinones	Linezolid, tedizolid
Tetracycline	Tigecycline
Also sometimes active	
Daptomycin	

"low-level" resistance to these agents and rendering them ineffective when used alone against these bacteria. However, aminoglycosides do penetrate these bacteria when used in conjunction with an appropriate antibiotic capable of disrupting the cell wall (eg, penicillin or vancomycin) and thus have synergistic activity against enterococci. This synergism converts the activity of penicillins and vancomycin from bacteriostatic to bactericidal. The significance of this change is that many experts prefer bactericidal activity for serious enterococcal infections, such as endocarditis. Unfortunately, several factors limit the usefulness of the synergistic activity of the aminoglycosides. All *E. faecium* strains contain a chromosomally encoded acetyltransferase that modifies tobramycin and prevents it from having even a synergistic effect. Thus, only **gentamicin** is usually recommended for use against enterococci. In addition, increasing rates of "high-level" resistance to aminoglycosides among enterococci are now being observed. This occurs when enterococci acquire genetic material that encodes for the production of aminoglycoside-modifying enzymes that abrogate even synergistic activity. Mutations may also occur that result in modification of the aminoglycoside binding site of the enterococcal ribosome, preventing aminoglycoside binding. In either case, synergistic activity is abolished. Finally, long-term administration of aminoglycosides, which is required for the treatment of some enterococcal infections such as endocarditis, is associated with a high incidence of toxicities. For these reasons, alternative antibiotic regimens, such as **ampicillin** plus **ceftriaxone**, are increasingly being used to treat these infections.

Pearl

Cephalosporins fail to bind the primary PBPs critical for the multiplication of enterococci and are, therefore, ineffective as monotherapy for these bacteria. The usefulness of ceftriaxone, a cephalosporin, in treating enterococcal infections is, therefore, somewhat surprising. The explanation is that secondary PBPs partially substitute for ampicillin-inactivated primary PBPs, causing ampicillin to be bacteriostatic rather than bactericidal when used as monotherapy. Ceftriaxone, however, inactivates these secondary PBPs. When ampicillin and ceftriaxone are used together, both primary and secondary PBPs are inactivated, which results in bactericidal activity.

_{Used with permission of American Society for Microbiology, from Mainardi JL, Gutmann L, Acar JF, et al. Synergistic effect of amoxicillin and cefotaxime against Enterococcus faecalis. Antimicrob Agents Chemother. 1995;39:1984-1987; permission conveyed through Copyright Clearance Center, Inc.}

Questions

13. The first-line antibiotics for enterococcal infections include the following β-lactams: _____, _____, and _____.
14. Penicillin-resistant enterococci are often treated with _____.
15. When used alone, cell wall–active agents such as β-lactams and vancomycin are only _____ for enterococci. To achieve _____ activity, gentamicin must be added.
16. The following antibiotics are used to treat penicillin-resistant VRE: _____, _____, and the newer _____.

Answers

13. penicillin G, ampicillin, piperacillin
14. vancomycin
15. bacteriostatic, bactericidal
16. oxazolidinones, daptomycin, tetracyclines

ADDITIONAL READINGS

Fernández-Hidalgo N, Almirante B, Gavaldà J, et al. Ampicillin plus ceftriaxone is as effective as ampicillin plus gentamicin for treating *Enterococcus faecalis* infective endocarditis. *Clin Infect Dis.* 2013;56:1261-1268.

Gold HS. Vancomycin-resistant enterococci: mechanisms and clinical observations. *Clin Infect Dis.* 2001;33:210-219.

Kohinke RM, Pakyz AL. Treatment of vancomycin-resistant enterococci: focus on daptomycin. *Curr Infect Dis Rep.* 2017;19(10):33. doi:10.1007/s11908-017-0589-2

Landman D, Quale JM. Management of infections due to resistant enterococci: a review of therapeutic options. *J Antimicrob Chemother.* 1997;40:161-170.

Listeria monocytogenes

L. monocytogenes is a gram-positive bacillus that is widespread in nature. It is commonly found in soil and the fecal flora of many animals. Ingestion of a large inoculum of these bacteria can lead to gastroenteritis in otherwise healthy people, whereas the very young, the old, and the immunocompromised may develop bacteremia that leads to meningitis (Figure 10-8). Pregnant women are also prone to systemic infections, which may cause fetal demise.

Ampicillin is the antibiotic of choice for infections caused by *L. monocytogenes* (Table 10-5). At first glance, this appears counterintuitive because *L. monocytogenes* is considered an intracellular pathogen, and ampicillin penetrates poorly into cells. The likely explanation for this paradox is that although *L. monocytogenes* invades and survives within the cytoplasm of many cell types, it is largely extracellular in the meninges

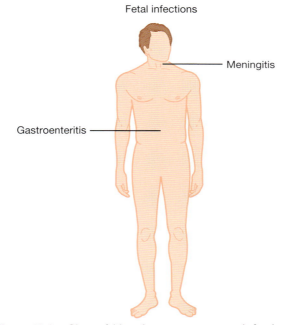

Figure 10-8. Sites of *Listeria monocytogenes* infections.

Table 10-5	Antimicrobial Agents for Treatment of Infections Caused by *Listeria monocytogenes*
Ampicillin plus gentamicin	
If penicillin allergic	
Trimethoprim-sulfamethoxazole	

and cerebral spinal fluid. Ampicillin alone is only bacteriostatic against *L. monocytogenes*. The addition of **gentamicin** results in synergistic bactericidal activity, so this antibiotic is usually used in conjunction with ampicillin. Gentamicin penetrates poorly into cerebrospinal fluid, but the small amounts that do accumulate in this compartment are apparently sufficient to cause synergistic killing. *L. monocytogenes* is intrinsically resistant to some commonly used antibiotics. For example, *L. monocytogenes* is not susceptible to cephalosporins because its PBPs are not bound by these agents. Because cephalosporins are frequently used alone as empiric therapy for meningitis, one must remember to add ampicillin to the treatment regimens of patients at risk for *L. monocytogenes* infections. Even vancomycin, which is active against most gram-positive bacteria, may not effectively treat individuals with *L. monocytogenes* meningitis. Patients who cannot tolerate ampicillin should be treated with **trimethoprim-sulfamethoxazole**.

QUESTIONS

17. _____ is active against *L. monocytogenes*, but _____ is usually given with it to achieve synergistic bacterial killing.
18. *L. monocytogenes* is resistant to _____, which are frequently used to empirically treat bacterial meningitis.
19. In patients who cannot tolerate penicillins because of allergy, _____ is used to treat infections caused by *L. monocytogenes*.

ANSWERS

17. Ampicillin, gentamicin
18. cephalosporins
19. trimethoprim-sulfamethoxazole

ADDITIONAL READINGS

Charlier C, Perrodeau E, Leclercq A, et al. Clinical features and prognostic factors of listeriosis: the MONALISA national prospective cohort study. *Lancet Infect Dis*. 2017;17:510-519.

Dryden MS, Jones NF, Phillips I. Vancomycin therapy failure in *Listeria monocytogenes* peritonitis in a patient on continuous ambulatory peritoneal dialysis. *J Infect Dis*. 1991;164:1239.

Hof H, Nichterlein T, Kretschmar M. Management of listeriosis. *Clin Microbiol Rev*. 1997;10:345-357.

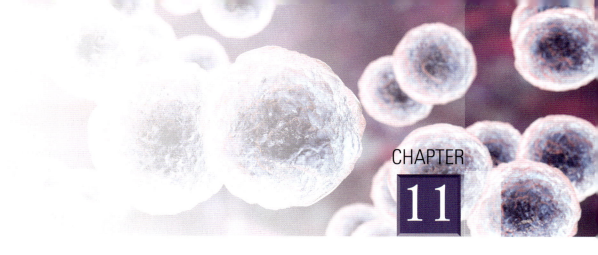

CHAPTER 11

Gram-Negative Bacteria

"Mail left the wearer vulnerable to crushing blows, and could be pierced by arrows or crossbow bolts.... Mail was supplemented by pieces of plate armour from the thirteenth century.... By the fifteenth century it is clear that the fully articulated suit of plate-armour had emerged, the wearer's pride in it such that the cloth coverings of earlier periods were abandoned and the armour worn 'white', polished and shining."
— **Armies and Warfare in the Middle Ages: The English Experience, Michael Prestwich**

Gram-negative bacteria are characterized by a cell envelope structure that supplements the cross-linked mail-like peptidoglycan cell wall with an additional layer of protection. Just as medieval knights had their mail covered with plate armor, gram-negative bacteria surround the peptidoglycan cell wall with a lipopolysaccharide (LPS)-rich outer membrane. The outer membrane forms a dense barrier that restricts penetration of many antibiotics into the periplasmic space and cytosol of the bacterium. Thus, to be effective against gram-negative bacteria, antibiotics must penetrate one additional layer of protection.

Gram-negative bacteria are among the most common causes of infections in humans. This group includes Enterobacterales (formerly called the Enterobacteriaceae), a large family of bacteria responsible for many gastrointestinal, urinary, and opportunistic infections. Another frequent cause of hospital-acquired infections is the pseudomonad *Pseudomonas aeruginosa*, which is noteworthy for its resistance to many different classes of antibiotics. *Neisseria* spp., the curved gram-negative bacilli *Helicobacter pylori* and *Campylobacter jejuni*, and the respiratory bacteria *Haemophilus influenzae* and *Bordetella pertussis* are also problematic human pathogens. In this section, we discuss the treatment of each of these organisms.

Enterobacterales

The Enterobacterales is a large order of gram-negative bacilli, most of which inhabit the human gastrointestinal tract. For this reason, they are often referred to as "enteric" gram-negative rods. Many members of this group are part of the normal flora of humans and only cause disease in the context of a compromised host. As such, they are "opportunistic" pathogens. Other members of the Enterobacterales, however, are strict pathogens, and isolation of these bacteria from a stool culture usually indicates a causal role in disease. Some species of bacteria fall into both groups. For example, although most *Escherichia coli* bacteria live harmlessly in the colon, some strains have acquired exogenous genetic material that allows them to cause urinary tract infections or diarrhea even in normal hosts.

ESCHERICHIA COLI, KLEBSIELLA SPP., AND PROTEUS SPP.

E. coli, *Klebsiella* spp., and *Proteus* spp. are versatile pathogens that commonly cause community-acquired infections in healthy individuals and also frequently lead to hospital-acquired infections. Bacteria from all three genera cause community-acquired urinary tract infections, with *E. coli* being the most frequent etiology of this disease (Figure 11-1). In the normal host, certain strains of *E. coli* are capable of causing gastroenteritis, including traveler's diarrhea and diarrhea associated with hemolytic uremic syndrome. In neonates, it is the leading cause of meningitis. All three genera of pathogens are frequent causes of hospital-acquired infections such as urinary tract

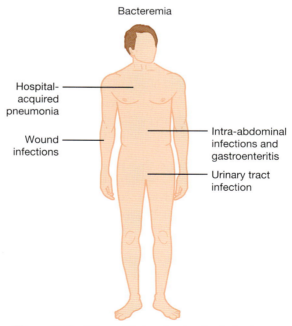

Figure 11-1. Sites of Enterobacterales infections.

infections in patients with urinary catheters, hospital-acquired pneumonia, bacteremia, wound infections, and intra-abdominal infections.

One cannot understand the treatment of infections caused by the Enterobacterales without understanding β-lactamases. For example, some community-acquired *E. coli* and *Proteus* strains remain susceptible to aminopenicillins, such as **ampicillin** (Table 11-1). However, many strains now harbor plasmids encoding the TEM-1 β-lactamase (see "Pearl" box), which allows them to resist killing by ampicillin, but not by first-generation cephalosporins, such as **cefazolin**. In contrast, all strains of *Klebsiella* express a chromosomally encoded β-lactamase that confers resistance to ampicillin. Most community-acquired infections caused by *E. coli*, *Proteus* spp., and *Klebsiella* spp. can be treated with quinolones (**ciprofloxacin, levofloxacin, moxifloxacin**), **trimethoprim-sulfamethoxazole**, or, sometimes, first-generation cephalosporins (**cefazolin**). One notable exception is *Proteus vulgaris*, which produces a chromosomally encoded β-lactamase that confers resistance to aminopenicillins and the first-generation cephalosporins. Third-generation cephalosporins, such as **ceftriaxone**, are frequently used to treat severe pyelonephritis caused by these bacteria. **Aztreonam** may also be used.

Hospital-acquired infections are much more difficult to treat because the strains of *E. coli*, *Klebsiella* spp., and *Proteus* spp. that cause them are frequently multidrug resistant. Potentially useful agents include third- and fourth-generation cephalosporins (eg, **ceftriaxone, cefepime**); cephalosporin plus β-lactamase inhibitors (eg, **ceftazidime-avibactam**); extended-spectrum penicillins plus β-lactamase inhibitors (**piperacillin-tazobactam**); carbapenems (eg, **imipenem, meropenem, ertapenem**); and carbapenems plus β-lactamase inhibitors (**imipenem-relebactam, meropenem-vaborbactam**), but treatment must be individualized and based on the susceptibilities of each isolate (Table 11-1). *E. coli*, *Klebsiella* spp., and *Proteus* spp. are often susceptible to aminoglycosides, such as **gentamicin, tobramycin, amikacin**, and **plazomicin**. However, these agents are usually not used as monotherapy but in conjunction with another agent in life-threatening infections such as sepsis.

Especially powerful β-lactamases, called extended-spectrum β-lactamases (ESBLs) and *Klebsiella pneumoniae* carbapenemases (KPCs), are of particular concern in *Klebsiella* strains and some isolates of *E. coli*. Strains that express these β-lactamases are resistant to most antibiotics (see "Pearl" box). Successful treatment of these strains requires careful attention to the results of susceptibility testing (Figure 11-2).

ENTEROBACTER, SERRATIA, CITROBACTER, PROVIDENCIA, AND MORGANELLA SPP.

Most of these bacteria are capable of colonizing the human gastrointestinal tract without causing disease but can cause pneumonia, urinary tract infections, intra-abdominal infections, wound infections, and bacteremia in compromised or hospitalized patients (see Figure 11-1).

Each of these bacterial species contains an inducible chromosomally encoded AmpC-type β-lactamase that confers resistance to penicillin, ampicillin/amoxicillin, and first-generation cephalosporins (see "Pearl" box). To further complicate matters, mutant strains that constitutively express high levels of this enzyme may be selected during therapy with some β-lactam antibiotics. These mutants are resistant to all β-lactams, except the carbapenems (**imipenem, meropenem, ertapenem**) and some

Table 11-1 Antimicrobial Agents for Treatment of Infections Caused by the Enterobacterales	
Antibiotic Class	**Antibiotic**
***Escherichia coli, Klebsiella* spp., *Proteus* spp.**	
Aminopenicillins (except *Klebsiella* spp. and *Proteus vulgaris*)	Ampicillin
First-generation cephalosporins (except for *P. vulgaris*)	Cefazolin
Sulfa drugs	Trimethoprim-sulfamethoxazole
Quinolones	Ciprofloxacin, levofloxacin, moxifloxacin
If resistant to the above antibiotics	
Third- and fourth-generation cephalosporins	Cefotaxime, ceftriaxone, cefepime
Cephalosporin plus β-lactamase inhibitor	Ceftazidime-avibactam
Monobactam	Aztreonam
Extended-spectrum penicillins plus β-lactamase inhibitor	Piperacillin-tazobactam
Carbapenems (with or without β-lactamase inhibitors)	Imipenem, meropenem, ertapenem Imipenem plus relebactam, meropenem plus vaborbactam
Add an aminoglycoside in serious infections	Gentamicin, tobramycin, amikacin, plazomicin
***Enterobacter, Serratia, Citrobacter, Providencia, Morganella* spp.**	
Carbapenems (with or without β-lactamase inhibitors)	Imipenem, meropenem, ertapenem Imipenem plus relebactam, meropenem plus vaborbactam
Sulfa drugs	Trimethoprim-sulfamethoxazole
Quinolones	Ciprofloxacin, levofloxacin, moxifloxacin
Fourth-generation cephalosporins	Cefepime
Add an aminoglycoside in serious infections	Gentamicin, tobramycin, amikacin, plazomicin
***Salmonella enterica, Shigella* spp.**	
Quinolones	Ciprofloxacin, levofloxacin
Third-generation cephalosporins	Cefotaxime, ceftriaxone, cefixime
Macrolides	Azithromycin
Sulfa drugs	Trimethoprim-sulfamethoxazole
Yersinia enterocolitica	
Aminoglycosides	Gentamicin
Tetracyclines	Doxycycline
Quinolones	Ciprofloxacin
Sulfa drugs	Trimethoprim-sulfamethoxazole

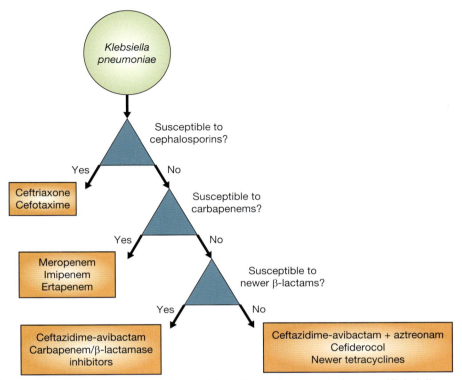

Figure 11-2. Antibiotics commonly considered in the treatment of severe *Klebsiella pneumoniae* infections.

β-lactam/β-lactamase inhibitor combinations such as **ceftazidime-avibactam**. Some experts feel that **cefepime** also has activity against these strains. A consequence of such selection is that a strain that initially appears susceptible to certain β-lactam antibiotics may become resistant during the course of therapy, resulting in treatment failure. Although many gram-negative bacteria encode AmpC β-lactamases, this phenomenon of selection of constitutively expressing mutants is particularly problematic in *Enterobacter*, *Citrobacter*, and *Klebsiella aerogenes* infections when treated with third-generation cephalosporins.

Pearl

Enterobacterales are particularly adept at producing β-lactamases to defend themselves against β-lactam antibiotics. Thus, a discussion of appropriate therapy for the Enterobacterales necessitates a basic understanding of the types of β-lactamases they produce and the β-lactams they degrade. Four such β-lactamases are TEM-1, AmpC, the ESBLs, and KPCs.

TEM-1: This β-lactamase is plasmid encoded and constitutively expressed. It confers resistance to ampicillin and amoxicillin.

AmpC: This β-lactamase is usually chromosomally encoded and inducible. When induced, AmpC β-lactamase confers resistance to penicillin, ampicillin/amoxicillin, and first-generation cephalosporins. Mutant strains that constitutively express large amounts of this enzyme are resistant to all β-lactam antibiotics except carbapenems and some β-lactam/β-lactamase inhibitor combinations such as ceftazidime-avibactam (and perhaps cefepime).

ESBL: β-Lactamases of this group are usually plasmid encoded and constitutively expressed. They are especially problematic because strains that produce them may appear susceptible to third-generation cephalosporins but are in fact resistant. These β-lactamases degrade all β-lactams except carbapenems and some β-lactam/β-lactamase inhibitor combinations. In addition, because the plasmids that carry *ESBL* genes also commonly encode resistance determinants for many other antibiotics, ESBL strains are often resistant to many non–β-lactam antibiotics as well.

KPC: KPCs are a relatively new class of β-lactamases that are increasingly being found in *K. pneumoniae* isolates. These β-lactamases degrade all β-lactams, including carbapenems. The genes encoding KPCs are carried on plasmids that also encode resistance to other antibiotics, making treatment exceedingly difficult. Aminoglycosides, some β-lactam/β-lactamase inhibitor combinations (eg, ceftazidime-avibactam), and the newer tetracyclines have been used with some success. The concern is that plasmids encoding KPCs will quickly disseminate to other genera of bacteria; examples of such spread have already been observed.

From Hirsch EB, Tam VH. Detection and treatment options for Klebsiella pneumoniae carbapenemases (KPCs): an emerging cause of multidrug-resistant infection. *J Antimicrob Chemother.* 2010;65:1119-1125.
From Jacoby GA, Munoz-Price LS. The new beta-lactamases. *N Engl J Med.* 2005;352:380-391.
From Lukac PJ, Bonomo RA, Logan LK. Extended-spectrum β-lactamase-producing Enterobacteriaceae in children: old foe, emerging threat. *Clin Infect Dis.* 2015;60:1389-1397.
From Pitout JDD, Laupland KB. Extended-spectrum beta-lactamase-producing Enterobacteriaceae: an emerging public-health concern. *Lancet Infect Dis.* 2008;8:159-166.

Strains of *Enterobacter*, *Serratia*, *Citrobacter*, *Providencia*, and *Morganella* spp. frequently harbor plasmids that confer resistance to other antibiotics as well, and treatment must be tailored to the susceptibilities of each individual strain. Quinolones (**ciprofloxacin, levofloxacin, moxifloxacin**) and **trimethoprim-sulfamethoxazole** may be effective. As with *E. coli*, *Klebsiella* spp., and *Proteus* spp., aminoglycosides (**gentamicin, tobramycin, amikacin, plazomicin**) are used in conjunction with another agent in life-threatening infections, such as sepsis.

SALMONELLA ENTERICA, SHIGELLA SPP., AND YERSINIA ENTEROCOLITICA

Most of the disease burden due to *Salmonella enterica*, *Shigella* spp., and *Yersinia enterocolitica* consists of gastroenteritis in otherwise healthy individuals (see Figure 11-1). In addition, some pathovars of *S. enterica* cause typhoid fever, a serious infection characterized by prolonged bacteremia.

Acute infectious diarrhea caused by *S. enterica* and *Y. enterocolitica* in the immunocompetent host usually does not require antibiotic therapy. Such therapy is recommended, however, if the infection has spread beyond the intestinal tract, if it is severe, or if the patient is immunocompromised. When antibiotics are indicated, *Salmonella* and *Shigella* infections should be treated with quinolones (eg, **ciprofloxacin,** levofloxacin), third-generation cephalosporins (eg, **ceftriaxone, cefixime**), or **azithromycin**. Some strains remain susceptible to **trimethoprim-sulfamethoxazole**. *Y. enterocolitica* is usually susceptible to aminoglycosides (**gentamicin**), tetracyclines (**doxycycline**), quinolones (**ciprofloxacin**), and **trimethoprim-sulfamethoxazole**.

QUESTIONS

1. Members of the Enterobacterales cause both _____- and _____-acquired infections.
2. Hospital-acquired infections caused by *E. coli* are often highly _____ to antibiotics.
3. ESBLs are most often produced by _____ or _____.
4. ESBLs confer resistance to all β-lactamases, except _____ and sometimes _____.
5. When produced in large amounts, AmpC β-lactamases are capable of degrading all β-lactams, except _____ (and perhaps cefepime).
6. In serious infections such as sepsis, an _____ is sometimes used in conjunction with a standard antibiotic to treat bacteria belonging to the Enterobacterales order.
7. Strains of *S. enterica* and *Shigella* spp. cause _____. These infections are treated with _____, _____, or _____.

ANSWERS

1. community, hospital
2. resistant
3. *E. coli, Klebsiella* spp.
4. carbapenems, β-lactam/β-lactamase inhibitor combinations
5. carbapenems
6. aminoglycoside
7. gastroenteritis, quinolones, third-generation cephalosporins, azithromycin

ADDITIONAL READINGS

Bajaj P, Singh NS, Virdi JS. *Escherichia coli* β-lactamases: what really matters. *Front Microbiol*. 2016;7:417. doi:10.3389/fmicb.2016.00417

Bush K. The ABCD's of β-lactamase nomenclature. *J Infect Chemother*. 2013;19:549-559.

Karami-Zarandi M, Rahdar HA, Esmaeili H, et al. *Klebsiella pneumoniae*: an update on antibiotic resistance mechanisms. *Future Microbiol*. 2023;18:65-81.

O'Hara CM, Brenner FW, Miller JM. Classification, identification, and clinical significance of *Proteus, Providencia*, and *Morganella*. *Clin Microbiol Rev*. 2000;13:534-546.

Podschun R, Ullmann U. *Klebsiella* spp. as nosocomial pathogens: epidemiology, taxonomy, typing methods, and pathogenicity factors. *Clin Microbiol Rev*. 1998;11:589-603.

Tamma PD, Aitken SL, Bonomo RA, et al. Infectious Diseases Society of America guidance on the treatment of AmpC β-lactamase–producing Enterobacterales, carbapenem-resistant *Acinetobacter baumannii*, and *Stenotrophomonas maltophilia* infections. *Clin Infect Dis*. 2022;74:2089-2114.

Pseudomonas aeruginosa

The genus *Pseudomonas* contains many species of gram-negative bacilli found in the environment, some of which occasionally cause serious infections in compromised individuals. By far, the most medically important of these opportunistic pathogens is *P. aeruginosa*. This bacterium is a frequent cause of hospital-acquired infections, especially pneumonia, urinary tract infections, and wound infections (Figure 11-3). In addition, the airways of many individuals with cystic fibrosis are chronically infected with *P. aeruginosa* by the time they are adults.

Treatment of *P. aeruginosa* infections is complicated by the array of resistance mechanisms that it harbors (Figure 11-4). This bacterium has a relatively impermeable outer membrane containing highly selective porins, produces multiple efflux pumps, and has a chromosome containing an inducible β-lactamase. For these reasons, aminopenicillins, macrolides, and most cephalosporins are ineffective against this bacterium. Nonetheless, several treatment options are available (Table 11-2). The extended-spectrum penicillin **piperacillin** does penetrate the outer membrane porins but at a relatively low rate. Therefore, this agent must be given in high doses to cause killing. Some members of the third-generation cephalosporins (eg, **ceftazidime**), fourth-generation cephalosporins (eg, **cefepime**), cephalosporin plus β-lactamase inhibitors (eg, **ceftolozane-tazobactam, ceftazidime-avibactam**), monobactams (**aztreonam**), carbapenems (eg, **imipenem, meropenem**), quinolones (eg, **ciprofloxacin, levofloxacin**), and aminoglycosides (eg, **tobramycin**) are active against *P. aeruginosa*. However, not all drugs within a class are equivalent regarding their antipseudomonal activity. For example, ciprofloxacin is more active than the other quinolones. Among the carbapenems, ertapenem should not be used to treat *P. aeruginosa* infections.

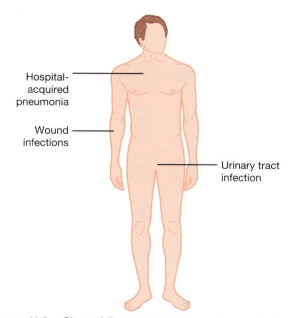

Figure 11-3. Sites of *Pseudomonas aeruginosa* infections.

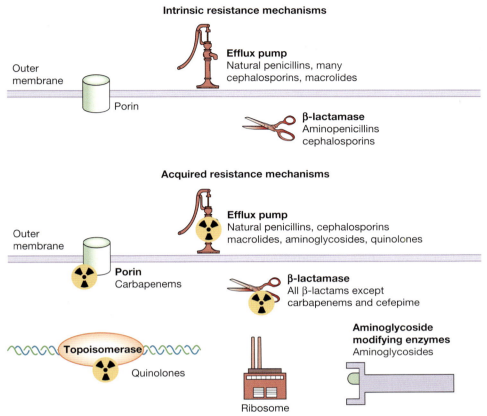

Figure 11-4. Intrinsic and acquired resistance mechanisms of *Pseudomonas aeruginosa*. Intrinsic resistance mechanisms are present in all strains of *P. aeruginosa*. Mutations and the acquisition of exogenous genetic material allow certain strains to acquire resistance to additional antibiotics through enhancement of intrinsic resistance mechanisms and production of new resistance determinants. The radioactivity symbol represents the acquisition of mutations that alter the production or characteristics of the indicated protein(s).

Unfortunately, *P. aeruginosa* is also especially adept at acquiring resistance to most antibiotics, so it is not reliably susceptible to any of these agents. Acquired resistance occurs by various mechanisms (see Figure 11-4). Mutations resulting in hyperproduction of the chromosomal β-lactamase result in resistance to all β-lactams except the carbapenems and cefepime. Likewise, mutations can cause the overproduction of efflux pumps, which may result in resistance to penicillins, cephalosporins, aminoglycosides, and quinolones. Mutations in the gene encoding one of the outer membrane porins may prevent penetration of the carbapenems, and the production of altered topoisomerases may result in loss of sensitivity to quinolones. Aminoglycoside resistance may also occur following the acquisition of genes that encode for the production of factors that acetylate or adenylate the aminoglycoside itself, preventing it from binding the ribosome.

As a result of intrinsic and acquired resistance, *P. aeruginosa* strains are frequently resistant to one or more antibiotics. For example, recent surveys indicate that 15% to

Table 11-2 Antimicrobial Agents for Treatment of Infections Caused by *Pseudomonas aeruginosa*

Antibiotic Class	Antibiotic
Extended-spectrum penicillins	Piperacillin
Third-generation cephalosporins	Ceftazidime
Fourth-generation cephalosporins	Cefepime
Cephalosporin plus β-lactamase inhibitor	Ceftolozane-tazobactam, ceftazidime-avibactam
Carbapenems	Imipenem, meropenem
Monobactams	Aztreonam
Quinolones	Ciprofloxacin, levofloxacin
Aminoglycosides	Tobramycin

25% of strains are resistant to piperacillin, 20% to 30% to ceftazidime, and 40% to 45% to aztreonam. Thus, no antibiotic regimen is uniformly effective against *P. aeruginosa*, and therapy must be guided by the susceptibility profiles of individual strains.

Even more disconcerting is the emergence of resistance *during* appropriate treatment of *P. aeruginosa* infections, which obviously leads to treatment failure. For these reasons, the treatment of serious *P. aeruginosa* infections can be challenging.

Pearl

Tazobactam does not have activity against common β-lactamases of *P. aeruginosa*. As a result, strains of *P. aeruginosa* that are resistant to piperacillin or ceftolozane are usually also resistant to piperacillin-tazobactam or ceftolozane-tazobactam, respectively.

From Acar JF, Goldstein FW, Kitzis MD. Susceptibility survey of piperacillin alone and in the presence of tazobactam. *J Antimicrob Chemother.* 1993;31(suppl A):23-28 by permission of Oxford University Press.

Questions

8. The following commonly used third- and fourth-generation cephalosporins have antipseudomonal activity: _____ and _____.
9. _____ is more active than the other quinolones against *P. aeruginosa*.
10. Because *P. aeruginosa* has a relatively high incidence of resistance, _____ antibiotic regimen is predictably effective against all *P. aeruginosa* strains.
11. Of the carbapenems, _____ does not have antipseudomonal activity.

ANSWERS

8. ceftazidime, cefepime
9. Ciprofloxacin
10. no
11. ertapenem

ADDITIONAL READINGS

Cunha BA. *Pseudomonas aeruginosa*: resistance and therapy. *Semin Respir Infect*. 2002;17:231-239.

El Zowalaty ME, Al Thani AA, Webster TJ, et al. *Pseudomonas aeruginosa:* arsenal of resistance mechanisms, decades of changing resistance profiles, and future antimicrobial therapies. *Future Microbiol*. 2015;10:1683-1706.

Hauser AR, Sriram P. Severe *Pseudomonas aeruginosa* infections. Tackling the conundrum of drug resistance. *Postgrad Med*. 2005;117:41-48.

Moore LS, Cunningham J, Donaldson H. A clinical approach to managing *Pseudomonas aeruginosa* infections. *Br J Hosp Med (Lond)*. 2016;77:C50-C54.

Neisseria spp.

The genus *Neisseria* includes two commonly encountered and medically important species: *Neisseria meningitidis* and *Neisseria gonorrhoeae*. *N. meningitidis* is a much-feared cause of meningitis and sepsis (Figure 11-5). Infections can progress at a remarkably rapid rate and lead to death of young, healthy individuals. *N. gonorrhoeae* causes the sexually transmitted illness gonorrhea. Infection with this bacterium usually leads to localized disease manifestations, such as cervicitis, urethritis, and pelvic inflammatory disease. The organism, however, may spread via the bloodstream to joints and the skin, resulting in disseminated gonococcal disease.

Strains of *N. meningitidis* are usually sensitive to **penicillin**, although resistance is becoming more common (Table 11-3). For this reason, third-generation cephalosporins, such as **ceftriaxone**, are the agents of choice prior to the availability of susceptibilities. Because meningitis and sepsis caused by this bacterium may be rapidly fatal,

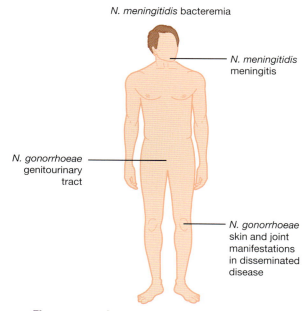

Figure 11-5. Sites of *Neisseria* spp. infections.

Table 11-3	Antimicrobial Agents for Treatment of Infections Caused by *Neisseria meningitidis*
Antibiotic Class	**Antibiotic**
Natural penicillins	Penicillin G
Third-generation cephalosporins	Ceftriaxone, cefotaxime
Postexposure prophylaxis	
Quinolone	Ciprofloxacin
Rifamycin	Rifampin

Table 11-4	Antimicrobial Agents for Treatment of Infections Caused by *Neisseria gonorrhoeae*
Antibiotic Class	**Antibiotic**
Third-generation cephalosporins	Ceftriaxone
Given in conjunction with doxycycline to empirically cover coinfection with *Chlamydia trachomatis*	

prophylaxis is given to close contacts of cases to prevent the acquisition of disease. **Ciprofloxacin** or **rifampin** is used for this purpose.

In the past, *N. gonorrhoeae* infections were also routinely treated with penicillin. However, the gradual emergence of strains harboring resistance-conferring traits has resulted in the ineffectiveness of penicillin for most cases of gonorrhea. These traits include plasmids that encode β-lactamases, mutations that result in increased efflux and decreased penetration through porins, and modification of penicillin-binding proteins (PBPs). *N. gonorrhoeae* has also acquired resistance to other antibiotics such as quinolones and tetracyclines. As a result, third-generation cephalosporins (eg, ceftriaxone) remain the only commonly used agent effective against this bacterium. Unfortunately, *N. gonorrhoeae* isolates are slowly becoming more resistant to this agent. Thus, current recommendations for the treatment of uncomplicated gonorrhea in adults call for the use of an increased dose of **ceftriaxone** (500 mg intramuscularly) (Table 11-4). Note that gonorrhea is frequently complicated by coinfection with *Chlamydia trachomatis*, so doxycycline should also be given as empiric treatment for *Chlamydia*.

QUESTIONS

12. The treatment of choice for *N. meningitidis* infections is _____ or _____.

13. The treatment of choice for uncomplicated *N. gonorrhoeae* infections in adults is _____.

14. Because of the frequency of coinfection, doxycycline for _____ should also be given to anyone being treated for gonorrhea.

ANSWERS

12. ceftriaxone, cefotaxime
13. ceftriaxone
14. *C. trachomatis*

ADDITIONAL READINGS

Lyss SB, Kamb ML, Peterman TA, et al. *Chlamydia trachomatis* among patients infected with and treated for *Neisseria gonorrhoeae* in sexually transmitted disease clinics in the United States. *Ann Intern Med.* 2003;139:178-185.

Tunkel AR, Hartman BJ, Kaplan SL, et al. Practice guidelines for the management of bacterial meningitis. *Clin Infect Dis.* 2004;39:1267-1284.

Workowski KA, Bachmann LH, Chan PA, et al. Sexually transmitted infections treatment guidelines, 2021. *MMWR Recomm Rep.* 2021;70:1-187.

Workowski KA, Berman SM, Douglas JM Jr. Emerging antimicrobial resistance in *Neisseria gonorrhoeae*: urgent need to strengthen prevention strategies. *Ann Intern Med.* 2008;148:606-613.

Curved Gram-Negative Bacteria

C. jejuni, *H. pylori*, and *Vibrio cholerae* all share a similar morphology: a curved gram-negative rod. In addition, these bacteria all infect the human gastrointestinal tract. However, they each differ in their disease manifestations and the antimicrobial regimens used to treat them.

CAMPYLOBACTER JEJUNI

C. jejuni is one of the most common causes of acute bacterial gastroenteritis in the world. This organism colonizes many types of wild and domesticated animals; humans become infected following ingestion of contaminated food or water. Clinical manifestations include diarrhea, fever, and abdominal pain (Figure 11-6).

Antibiotic treatment is indicated for only a subset of patients infected with *C. jejuni*. These include individuals with high fevers, bloody or profuse diarrhea, prolonged symptoms, or a compromised immune system. Preferred treatments are macrolides (**azithromycin**, **clarithromycin**) or quinolones (**ciprofloxacin**, **levofloxacin**), although resistance rates to quinolones are increasing. Alternatives include tetracyclines (**tetracycline**, **doxycycline**) or aminoglycosides (**gentamicin**, **tobramycin**, **amikacin**) (Table 11-5).

HELICOBACTER PYLORI

The discovery of the role of *H. pylori* in peptic ulcer disease is one of the great paradigm shifts in medicine in which an infectious etiology was identified for a disease formerly

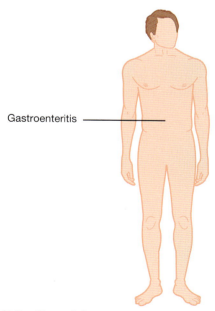

Figure 11-6. Sites of *Campylobacter jejuni* infections.

Table 11-5	Antimicrobial Agents for Treatment of Infections Caused by *Campylobacter jejuni*
Antibiotic Class	**Antibiotic**
Treatment of choice	
Macrolides	Azithromycin, clarithromycin
Quinolones	Ciprofloxacin, levofloxacin
Alternatives	
Tetracyclines	Tetracycline, doxycycline
Aminoglycosides	Gentamicin, tobramycin, amikacin

thought to be idiopathic in origin. *H. pylori* inhabits the human stomach, where it is associated with inflammation that predisposes to peptic ulcer disease (Figure 11-7). In the absence of antimicrobial therapy, infections tend to last for years, often for the lifetime of the individual.

H. pylori is susceptible to several antibiotics in vitro. These include **amoxicillin**, **clarithromycin**, **metronidazole**, **levofloxacin**, and **tetracycline** (Table 11-6). In addition, **bismuth subsalicylate**, more commonly known in the United States as Pepto-Bismol, is active against this bacterium. The bismuth component of this preparation disrupts the integrity of the *H. pylori* cell wall. Despite these in vitro susceptibilities, *H. pylori* is relatively difficult to eradicate with antibiotic therapy. Several factors may contribute to its recalcitrance. It is prone to develop resistance to antimicrobial agents, an especially problematic trait given that this organism causes chronic infections. A strain of *H. pylori* chronically inhabiting the stomach experiences the same cumulative

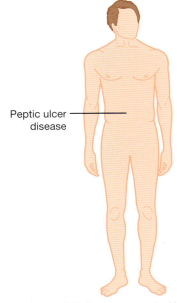

Figure 11-7. Sites of *Helicobacter pylori* infections.

Table 11-6	Antimicrobial Agents for Treatment of Infections Caused by *Helicobacter pylori*
Antibiotic Class	**Antibiotic**
Aminopenicillins	Amoxicillin
Macrolides	Clarithromycin
Metronidazole	
Tetracyclines	Tetracycline
Quinolones	Levofloxacin
Bismuth subsalicylate	
Recommended regimens	
Amoxicillin plus clarithromycin plus proton pump inhibitor	
Metronidazole plus clarithromycin plus proton pump inhibitor	
Bismuth subsalicylate plus metronidazole plus tetracycline plus proton pump inhibitor	

antibiotic exposure as its host, and each exposure increases the risk of resistance. In addition, the acidic environment of the stomach limits the efficacy of certain antibiotics, allowing *H. pylori* bacteria to survive for longer periods during therapy and further predisposing to antimicrobial resistance. Therefore, it is not surprising that 20% to 40% of isolates are resistant to metronidazole, and 10% are resistant to clarithromycin. Resistance to metronidazole results from mutations in the nitroreductase gene, which encodes a protein that reduces metronidazole to its active form. Mutations in one of the genes encoding a component of the 50S ribosomal subunit prevent binding of clarithromycin to the ribosome. For these reasons, eradication rates in infected individuals treated with a single antibiotic are quite low.

To counteract *H. pylori*'s predilection to develop resistance, combination regimens are used to treat this bacterium (see Table 11-6). These regimens each consist of at least two antimicrobial agents in conjunction with an antisecretory agent that blocks acid production. The antisecretory component of the regimen increases gastric pH, which allows for optimal activity of some antimicrobial agents and may also limit ongoing tissue damage due to acid exposure.

Pearl

In addition to peptic ulcer disease, *H. pylori* infection has been associated with a form of gastric malignancy called mucosa-associated lymphoid tissue (MALT) lymphoma. Interestingly, eradication of *H. pylori* has been associated with long-term remission of these cancers. This represents an example of the successful use of antibiotics to treat cancer.

Stolte M, Bayerdörffer E, Morgner A, et al. *Helicobacter* and gastric MALT lymphoma. *Gut.* 2002;50(suppl 3):III19-III24.

VIBRIO CHOLERAE

V. cholerae continues to be of global significance and causes pandemics of the diarrheal illness cholera. Patients with cholera often have profuse watery diarrhea that may lead to dehydration and death in a matter of hours (Figure 11-8). Antibiotics play an important role in decreasing the volume of stool and the duration of diarrhea in these patients. In the past, **tetracycline** and **doxycycline** were the agents of choice for cholera, but resistance is becoming increasingly common and occurs when strains acquire a plasmid that coexpresses resistance determinants to multiple antibiotics. Other active agents include a quinolone (**ciprofloxacin**) or a macrolide (**erythromycin**, **azithromycin**) (Table 11-7).

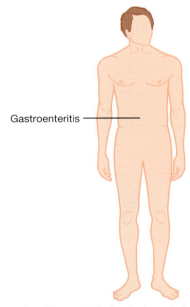

Figure 11-8. Sites of *Vibrio cholerae* infections.

Table 11-7 Antimicrobial Agents for Treatment of Infections Caused by *Vibrio cholerae*

Antibiotic Class	Antibiotic
Active agents	
Tetracyclines	Tetracycline, doxycycline
Quinolones	Ciprofloxacin
Macrolides	Erythromycin, azithromycin

QUESTIONS

15. Antimicrobial therapy for *C. jejuni* infections should _____ be given for uncomplicated diarrhea in a normal host.
16. First-line agents for the treatment of *C. jejuni* infections include _____ and _____.
17. *H. pylori* is prone to developing resistance to antibiotics, so treatment regimens consisting of _____ agents are recommended.
18. Treatment of *H. pylori* infections consists of two parts: an _____ component and an _____ component.
19. Traditionally, _____ and _____ were the antibiotics of choice for cholera, but resistance is now becoming increasingly common.
20. Other antibiotics used to treat cholera include _____, _____, and _____.

ANSWERS

15. not
16. macrolides, quinolones
17. multiple
18. antibiotic, acid-blocking
19. tetracycline, doxycycline
20. ciprofloxacin, erythromycin, azithromycin

ADDITIONAL READINGS

Bhattacharya SK. An evaluation of current cholera treatment. *Expert Opin Pharmacother*. 2003;4:141-146.

Chey WD, Leontiadis GI, Howden CW, et al. ACG clinical guideline: treatment of *Helicobacter pylori* infection. *Am J Gastroenterol*. 2017;112:212-239.

Lariviere LA, Gaudreau CL, Turgeon FF. Susceptibility of clinical isolates of *Campylobacter jejuni* to twenty-five antimicrobial agents. *J Antimicrob Chemother*. 1986;18:681-685.

Shane AL, Mody RK, Crump JA, et al. 2017 Infectious Diseases Society of America clinical practice guidelines for the diagnosis and management of infectious diarrhea. *Clin Infect Dis*. 2017;65:e45-e80.

Shiota S, Reddy R, Alsarraj A, et al. Antibiotic resistance of *Helicobacter pylori* among male United States veterans. *Clin Gastroenterol Hepatol*. 2015;13:1616-1624.

Yamamoto T, Nair GB, Albert MJ, et al. Survey of in vitro susceptibilities of *Vibrio cholerae* O1 and O139 to antimicrobial agents. *Antimicrob Agents Chemother*. 1995;39:241-244.

Other Gram-Negative Bacteria

Many other gram-negative bacterial species are also common causes of infections in humans. Here, we discuss four of them: *H. influenzae*, *B. pertussis*, *Moraxella catarrhalis*, and *Acinetobacter* spp.

HAEMOPHILUS INFLUENZAE

H. influenzae is a small pleomorphic (of variable morphology) gram-negative bacterium that is associated with mild as well as life-threatening infections. This organism causes otitis media, sinusitis, community-acquired pneumonia, conjunctivitis, meningitis, epiglottitis, and septic arthritis (Figure 11-9). *H. influenzae* strains with type B capsules are especially virulent and historically were a major cause of invasive infections, such as meningitis. However, they have become less common with the widespread use of the conjugate vaccine composed in part of type B capsular antigen.

For years, ampicillin or amoxicillin was routinely used to treat infections caused by *H. influenzae*. However, approximately 30% of strains now produce a β-lactamase that degrades these agents. Fortunately, this β-lactamase is inhibited by clavulanate and sulbactam, so aminopenicillin/β-lactamase inhibitor combinations (**amoxicillin plus clavulanate**, **ampicillin plus sulbactam**) remain effective (Table 11-8). Likewise, second- and third-generation cephalosporins (**cefuroxime**, **ceftriaxone**, **cefotaxime**) are stable in the presence of this β-lactamase. Other useful antibiotics include quinolones (**ciprofloxacin**, **levofloxacin**, **moxifloxacin**), macrolides (**azithromycin**), tetracyclines (**tetracycline**, **doxycycline**), and carbapenems (**imipenem**, **meropenem**, **ertapenem**). **Trimethoprim-sulfamethoxazole** is also active, although resistance is

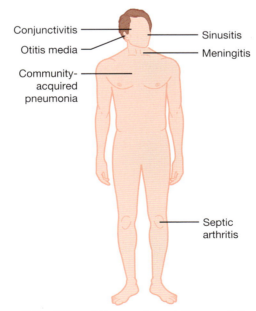

Figure 11-9. Sites of *Haemophilus influenzae* infections.

Table 11-8	Antimicrobial Agents for Treatment of Infections Caused by *Haemophilus influenzae*
Antibiotic Class	**Antibiotic**
Treatment of choice	
Aminopenicillins plus β-lactamase inhibitor	Amoxicillin/clavulanate, ampicillin/sulbactam
Second-generation cephalosporins	Cefuroxime
Third-generation cephalosporins	Ceftriaxone, cefotaxime
Also active	
Tetracyclines	Tetracycline, doxycycline
Macrolides	Azithromycin
Quinolones	Ciprofloxacin, levofloxacin, moxifloxacin
Carbapenems	Imipenem, meropenem, ertapenem
Sometimes active	
Sulfa drugs	Trimethoprim-sulfamethoxazole
Prophylaxis for serotype B	
Rifamycins	Rifampin

increasing. Close contacts of patients infected with serotype B *H. influenzae* should receive prophylaxis with **rifampin**.

BORDETELLA PERTUSSIS

B. pertussis is a small coccobacillary bacterium that causes pertussis, or whooping cough (Figure 11-10). In children, this disease is characterized by a series of short, rapid coughs followed by a gasp for air, causing a "whoop." Although traditionally viewed as a disease of children, whooping cough is increasingly being recognized as a frequent cause of cough lasting several weeks or longer in adults.

Antimicrobial treatment of pertussis is controversial but is usually recommended early in disease because it may shorten the course of the illness and limit transmission. Macrolides (**azithromycin, clarithromycin, erythromycin**) are the drugs of choice for both children and adults based on their in vitro activity and the results of clinical trials (Table 11-9). Other active agents include quinolones (**ciprofloxacin, levofloxacin, moxifloxacin**), **trimethoprim-sulfamethoxazole**, and tetracyclines (**tetracycline, doxycycline**). Postexposure prophylaxis with a macrolide should be considered in close contacts of contagious individuals with pertussis.

MORAXELLA CATARRHALIS

M. catarrhalis is a gram-negative diplococcus that commonly causes otitis media, pneumonia, and sinusitis (Figure 11-11). Nearly all strains produce a β-lactamase that confers resistance to amoxicillin and ampicillin. Antibiotics with some efficacy against this

CHAPTER 11 — Gram-Negative Bacteria

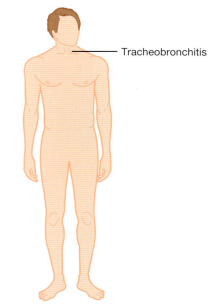

Figure 11-10. Sites of *Bordetella pertussis* infections.

Table 11-9	Antimicrobial Agents for Treatment of Infections Caused by *Bordetella pertussis*
Antibiotic Class	**Antibiotic**
Treatment of choice	
Macrolides	Azithromycin, clarithromycin, erythromycin
Other active agents	
Sulfa drugs	Trimethoprim-sulfamethoxazole
Quinolone[a]	Ciprofloxacin, levofloxacin, moxifloxacin
Tetracyclines[a]	Tetracycline, doxycycline
Postexposure prophylaxis	
Macrolides	Azithromycin, clarithromycin, erythromycin

[a]Quinolones and tetracyclines are contraindicated in children and pregnant women.

bacterium include extended-spectrum penicillins (**piperacillin**), β-lactam/β-lactamase inhibitor combinations (**amoxicillin plus clavulanate, ampicillin plus sulbactam**), second- and third-generation cephalosporins (**cefuroxime, ceftriaxone, cefotaxime**), aminoglycosides (**gentamicin, tobramycin, amikacin**), **trimethoprim-sulfamethoxazole**, tetracyclines (**tetracycline, doxycycline**), macrolides (**azithromycin, clarithromycin**), and quinolones (**ciprofloxacin, levofloxacin, moxifloxacin**) (Table 11-10).

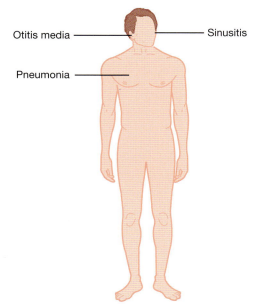

Figure 11-11. Sites of *Moraxella catarrhalis* infections.

Table 11-10	Antimicrobial Agents for Treatment of Infections Caused by *Moraxella catarrhalis*
Antibiotic Class	**Antibiotic**
Extended-spectrum penicillins	Piperacillin
Aminopenicillins plus β-lactamase inhibitor	Amoxicillin/clavulanate, ampicillin/sulbactam
Second-generation cephalosporins	Cefuroxime
Third-generation cephalosporins	Ceftriaxone, cefotaxime
Macrolides	Azithromycin, clarithromycin
Aminoglycosides	Gentamicin, tobramycin, amikacin
Sulfa drugs	Trimethoprim-sulfamethoxazole
Quinolones	Ciprofloxacin, levofloxacin, moxifloxacin
Tetracyclines	Tetracycline, doxycycline

ACINETOBACTER SPP.

Acinetobacter spp. are gram-negative rod-shaped and coccobacillary bacteria that cause several hospital- and community-acquired infections. These include pneumonia, bacteremia, and wound infections (Figure 11-12). Treatment can be problematic because many strains are highly antibiotic resistant. Interestingly, the β-lactamase inhibitor **sulbactam** has intrinsic bactericidal activity against this bacterium, and as expected, **ampicillin-sulbactam** has proven effective in treating infections caused by some of

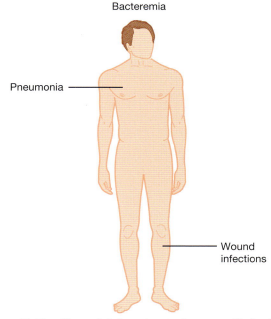

Figure 11-12. Sites of *Acinetobacter baumannii* infections.

Table 11-11	Antimicrobial Agents for Treatment of Infections Caused by *Acinetobacter* spp.
Antibiotic Class	**Antibiotic**
Aminopenicillins plus β-lactamase inhibitor	Ampicillin/sulbactam
Carbapenems	Imipenem, meropenem
Rifamycins	Rifampin
Aminoglycosides	Amikacin
Polymyxins	Polymyxin B, colistin
Tetracyclines	Tigecycline

these organisms (Table 11-11). Likewise, carbapenems (**imipenem**, **meropenem**, but not ertapenem), **rifampin**, and **amikacin** may be active. The latter two agents are usually used in combination with other antibiotics. However, resistance to each of these agents is increasing. **Polymyxins** and **tigecycline** are sometimes used for strains resistant to other antibiotics.

Questions

21. The use of ampicillin and amoxicillin for the treatment of *H. influenzae* infections is now limited by the production of a _____ by many strains.
22. The agents of choice for *H. influenzae* infections are _____, _____, _____, or _____.

23. The agents of choice for *B. pertussis* infections are _____, _____, and _____.
24. Other antibiotics active against *B. pertussis* include _____, _____, and _____.
25. Nearly all strains of *M. catarrhalis* produce a _____ that confers resistance to amoxicillin and ampicillin.
26. The β-lactamase inhibitor _____ has activity against some strains of *Acinetobacter baumannii*.

Answers

21. β-lactamase
22. aminopenicillin plus β-lactamase inhibitor combinations, second-generation cephalosporins, third-generation cephalosporins, tetracyclines
23. azithromycin, clarithromycin, erythromycin
24. trimethoprim-sulfamethoxazole, quinolones, tetracyclines
25. β-lactamase
26. sulbactam

ADDITIONAL READINGS

Doern GV, Brueggemann AB, Pierce G, et al. Antibiotic resistance among clinical isolates of *Haemophilus influenzae* in the United States in 1994 and 1995 and detection of beta-lactamase-positive strains resistant to amoxicillin-clavulanate: results of a national multicenter surveillance study. *Antimicrob Agents Chemother*. 1997;41:292-297.

Gordon KA, Fusco J, Biedenbach DJ, et al. Antimicrobial susceptibility testing of clinical isolates of *Bordetella pertussis* from Northern California: report from the SENTRY antimicrobial surveillance program. *Antimicrob Agents Chemother*. 2001;45:3599-3600.

Hewlett EL, Edwards KM. Clinical practice. Pertussis—not just for kids. *N Engl J Med*. 2005;352:1215-1222.

Ladhani S, Slack MP, Heath PT, et al. Invasive *Haemophilus influenzae* disease, Europe, 1996-2006. *Emerg Infect Dis*. 2010;16:455-463.

Munoz-Price LS, Weinstein RA. *Acinetobacter* infection. *N Engl J Med*. 2008;358:1271-1281.

Murphy TF, Parameswaran GI. *Moraxella* catarrhalis, a human respiratory tract pathogen. *Clin Infect Dis*. 2009;49:124-131.

Tamma PD, Aitken SL, Bonomo RA, et al. Infectious Diseases Society of America guidance on the treatment of AmpC β-lactamase–producing Enterobacterales, carbapenem-resistant *Acinetobacter baumannii*, and *Stenotrophomonas maltophilia* infections. *Clin Infect Dis*. 2022;74:2089-2114.

von König CH. Use of antibiotics in the prevention and treatment of pertussis. *Pediatr Infect Dis J*. 2005;24:S66-S68.

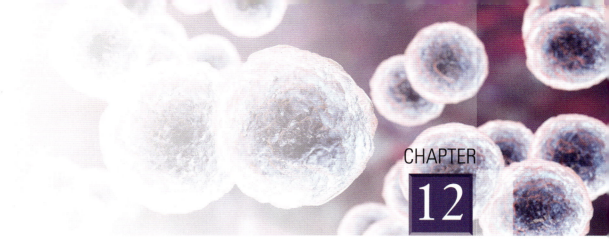

CHAPTER 12

Anaerobic Bacteria

"The trebuchet was a lever on a fulcrum, and proved very effective... Heavy weights were suspended from the forward end and these, when the rear portion was released, swung it into the air with its missile.... In 1345 a captured messenger was launched back into Auberoche."

—**Sieges of the Middle Ages, Philip Warner**

Just as medieval attackers shattered the defensive walls of castles using trebuchets and other assault weapons, many anaerobes injure the human body by elaborating powerful toxins. Some of these toxins, such as those made by several clostridial species, are among the most potent bacterial toxins known.

Anaerobes are bacteria unable to grow in physiologic concentrations of oxygen. Many of these organisms are normal inhabitants of the human oral cavity, gastrointestinal tract, and female genital tract. Infections often occur following disruption of mucosal surfaces in regions where large numbers of anaerobic bacteria reside. *Bacteroides*, *Porphyromonas*, and *Prevotella* spp. are anaerobic gram-negative bacteria that are frequently encountered in such scenarios. Other anaerobic bacteria are found in the environment and cause infections following inadvertent inoculation into the human body. *Clostridium* spp. that cause tetanus, botulism, and gas gangrene are examples of such anaerobic bacteria. In this section, we discuss these organisms, with particular emphasis on effective antimicrobial therapies used to treat the infections they cause.

Clostridium spp.

Clostridium spp. are gram-positive spore-forming anaerobic bacilli. They cause several well-known and feared diseases in humans, such as tetanus, botulism, and gas gangrene. In addition, a bacterium closely related to this group, *Clostridioides difficile*, is an important cause of iatrogenic gastrointestinal infections. Although these diseases are quite distinct, they have in common that each is mediated by a potent toxin or toxins.

Clostridium tetani is the etiologic agent of tetanus (Figure 12-1). This disease is characterized by persistent tonic spasm usually involving the masseter muscles ("lockjaw") and the musculature of the trunk. Symptoms follow inoculation of *C. tetani* spores into a deep wound. The devitalized tissue creates an anaerobic environment that allows germination of the spores and subsequent release of tetanus toxin. This toxin is transported to the brain and spinal cord through nerve axons and causes generalized muscle spasms and autonomic dysfunction. Treatment of tetanus consists of intensive supportive care, with a focus on the respiratory and neuromuscular systems. Antitoxin is given to neutralize circulating tetanus toxin. **Metronidazole** and **penicillin** are the antimicrobial agents of choice, with some data indicating that metronidazole is associated with better outcomes (Table 12-1).

Classically, botulism is acquired by ingestion of food contaminated with *Clostridium botulinum* spores, although it can also follow contamination of wounds (Figure 12-1). *C. botulinum*, like *C. tetani*, produces a neurotoxin that causes systemic effects. Botulinum toxin, however, leads to cranial neuropathies, weakness, and flaccidity rather than muscular spasm. Thus, the signs and symptoms of botulism differ significantly from those of tetanus. Patients with botulism also require intensive supportive care and the administration of antitoxin. **Penicillin** is the therapy of choice, and **metronidazole** is a useful alternative (Table 12-1).

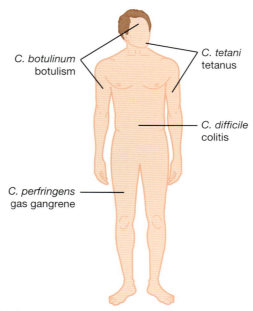

Figure 12-1. Sites of infections caused by *Clostridium* and *Clostridioides* spp.

Table 12-1. Antimicrobial Agents for Treatment of Infections Caused by *Clostridium* spp.

Antibiotic Class	Antibiotic
Treatment of choice	
Natural penicillins	Penicillin G[a]
Metronidazole	

[a] Exception: *Clostridioides difficile* infections should not be treated with penicillin. Oral vancomycin or fidaxomicin should be used. For infections caused by *Clostridium perfringens*, clindamycin should be used with penicillin.

Clostridium perfringens is the cause of gas gangrene, a life-threatening and rapidly progressive infection of the soft tissues, muscles, and deeper structures of the body (see Figure 12-1). Therapy consists of surgical debridement in conjunction with antimicrobial therapy. **Penicillin** plus **clindamycin** is recommended (Table 12-1).

Unlike the other members of this group of bacteria, *C. difficile* causes disease that is not associated with trauma or ingestion but rather with antibiotic use. The normal flora of the human colon appears to be sufficient to prevent high levels of colonization by *C. difficile*. Following administration of antibiotics, however, many components of the normal flora are suppressed, allowing overgrowth by *C. difficile*. Infection by this bacterium is associated with a wide spectrum of disease, from minimal diarrhea to fulminant and life-threatening pseudomembranous colitis (Figure 12-1). First-line treatment includes stopping the causative antibiotic if possible and administering an anticlostridial antibiotic. These agents include oral vancomycin or oral fidaxomicin. Oral **vancomycin** is not appreciably absorbed and achieves high levels in the gastrointestinal tract (Table 12-1). **Fidaxomicin** is a niche macrocyclic antibiotic approved for the treatment of *C. difficile* infections that may be associated with lower rates of recurrence. This agent inhibits transcription by RNA polymerase.

PEARL

Historically, the antibiotics most often associated with the development of *C. difficile* disease were thought to be clindamycin, ampicillin, and cephalosporins. A more recent analysis, however, found that second- and third-generation cephalosporins and carbapenems were associated with the greatest risk of developing *C. difficile* disease.

From Hensgens MPM, Goorhuis A, Dekkers OM, et al. Time interval of increased risk for Clostridium difficile infection after exposure to antibiotics. *J Antimicrob Chemother.* 2012;67:742-748 by permission of Oxford University Press.

PEARL

Fidaxomicin, like rifamycins, inhibits bacterial RNA synthesis. Its usefulness in the treatment of *C. difficile* infections is the consequence of two factors: (1) It has potent activity against *C. difficile* and (2) it has a narrow spectrum of activity, leaving much of the gastrointestinal microbiome undisturbed. This microbiome acts to prevent the reemergence of *C. difficile* following treatment of an initial infection.

From Johnson AP, Wilcox MH. Fidaxomicin: a new option for the treatment of Clostridium difficile infection. *J Antimicrob Chemother*. 2012;67:2788-2792 by permission of Oxford University Press.

QUESTIONS

1. *Clostridium* spp. are _____, _____-forming, gram-_____ bacilli.
2. For most clostridial infections, _____ and _____ are the agents of choice.
3. *C. difficile* colitis is treated with oral _____ or oral _____.

ANSWERS

1. anaerobic, spore, positive
2. penicillin, metronidazole
3. vancomycin, fidaxomicin

ADDITIONAL READINGS

Ahmadsyah I, Salim A. Treatment of tetanus: an open study to compare the efficacy of procaine penicillin and metronidazole. *Br Med J (Clin Res Ed)*. 1985;291:648-650.

Alexander CJ, Citron DM, Brazier JS, et al. Identification and antimicrobial resistance patterns of clinical isolates of *Clostridium clostridioforme*, *Clostridium innocuum*, and *Clostridium ramosum* compared with those of clinical isolates of *Clostridium perfringens*. *J Clin Microbiol*. 1995;33:3209-3215.

Bagdasarian N, Rao K, Malani PN. Diagnosis and treatment of *Clostridium difficile* in adults: a systematic review. *JAMA*. 2015;313:398-408.

Cohen SH, Gerding DN, Johnson S, et al. Clinical practice guidelines for *Clostridium difficile* infection in adults: 2010 update by the Society for Healthcare Epidemiology of America (SHEA) and the Infectious Diseases Society of America (IDSA). *Infect Control Hosp Epidemiol*. 2010;31:431-455.

Darke SG, King AM, Slack WK. Gas gangrene and related infection: classification, clinical features and aetiology, management and mortality. A report of 88 cases. *Br J Surg*. 1977;64:104-112.

Sobel J. Botulism. *Clin Infect Dis*. 2005;41:1167-1173.

Stevens DL, Bisno AL, Chambers HF, et al. Practice guidelines for the diagnosis and management of skin and soft tissue infections: 2014 update by the Infectious Diseases Society of America. *Clin Infect Dis*. 2014;59:e10-e52.

Anaerobic Gram-Negative Bacilli

The oral cavity, gastrointestinal tract, and vagina of humans are colonized with high numbers by several anaerobic gram-negative bacilli, including *Bacteroides* (most importantly, the *Bacteroides fragilis* group), *Prevotella*, and *Porphyromonas* spp. Under appropriate circumstances, these bacteria can contribute to periodontal disease, pleuropulmonary infections, pelvic inflammatory disease, and intra-abdominal abscesses (Figure 12-2). It has been postulated that their virulence is enhanced by other bacterial species, and thus these organisms are usually associated with polymicrobial infections.

Anaerobic gram-negative bacilli, particularly the *B. fragilis* group of bacteria, frequently produce β-lactamases that destroy many penicillins and cephalosporins. Carbapenems and some cephalosporins (the cephamycins cefotetan and cefoxitin), however, are usually not substrates for these β-lactamases. Likewise, these enzymes are inactivated by β-lactamase inhibitors.

Treatment of anaerobic infections is often empirical and based on the observation that anaerobic gram-negative bacilli are susceptible to several β-lactam/β-lactamase inhibitor combinations (eg, **ampicillin-sulbactam**, **piperacillin-tazobactam**), carbapenems (**imipenem**, **meropenem**, **ertapenem**), and **metronidazole** (Table 12-2). Other agents with relatively good activity against anaerobic gram-negative bacilli are **clindamycin**, **piperacillin**, **tigecycline**, and certain members of the cephalosporin (**cefotetan**, **cefoxitin**) and quinolone (**moxifloxacin**) classes.

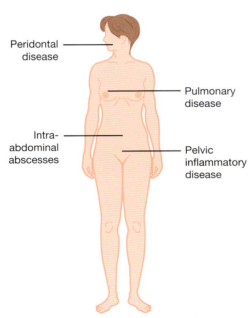

Figure 12-2. Sites of infections caused by anaerobic gram-negative bacilli.

Table 12-2 Antimicrobial Agents for Treatment of Infections Caused by *Bacteroides*, *Prevotella*, and *Porphyromonas* spp.

Antibiotic Class	Antibiotic
First-line agents	
β-Lactam/β-lactamase inhibitor combinations	Ampicillin-sulbactam, piperacillin-tazobactam
Carbapenems	Imipenem, meropenem, ertapenem
Metronidazole	
Second-line agents	
Clindamycin	
Second-generation cephalosporins	Cefotetan, cefoxitin
Extended-spectrum penicillins	Piperacillin
Quinolones	Moxifloxacin
Tetracycline-like agents	Tigecycline

QUESTIONS

4. _____, _____, and _____ spp. are clinically important anaerobic gram-negative bacilli.

5. The three types of antibiotics that have excellent activity against anaerobic gram-negative bacilli are _____, _____, and _____.

6. Other antibiotics that have good activity against anaerobic gram-negative bacilli include _____, _____, _____, _____, and certain members of the _____.

ANSWERS

4. *Bacteroides*, *Prevotella*, *Porphyromonas*
5. β-lactam/β-lactamase inhibitor combinations, carbapenems, metronidazole
6. clindamycin, piperacillin, moxifloxacin, tigecycline, cephalosporins

ADDITIONAL READINGS

Boyanova L, Kolarov R, Mitov I. Recent evolution of antibiotic resistance in the anaerobes as compared to previous decades. *Anaerobe*. 2015;31:4-10.

Brook I, Wexler HM, Goldstein EJ. Antianaerobic antimicrobials: spectrum and susceptibility testing. *Clin Microbiol Rev*. 2013;26:526-546.

Snydman DR, Jacobus NV, McDermott LA, et al. National survey on the susceptibility of *Bacteroides fragilis* group: report and analysis of trends for 1997–2000. *Clin Infect Dis*. 2002;35(suppl 1):S126-S134.

Vedantam G, Hecht DW. Antibiotics and anaerobes of gut origin. *Curr Opin Microbiol*. 2003;6:457-461.

CHAPTER 13

Atypical Bacteria

"On the next day Cestius, at the head of a large force of picked men and all the archers, began to assault the Temple from the north. The Jews resisted from the roof of the colonnade, and repeatedly drove back those who approached the wall, but at length they were overwhelmed by the hail of missiles and withdrew. The front rank of the Romans then rested their shields against the wall, and on these the second row rested theirs and so on, till they formed a protective covering known to them as a 'tortoise.' When the missiles fell on this they glanced off harmlessly, so that the soldiers received no hurt as they undermined the wall...."

—**The Jewish War, Josephus**

As mentioned previously, several bacteria do not conveniently fall into the categories of gram-positive bacteria, gram-negative bacteria, anaerobic bacteria, spirochete, or mycobacteria. These organisms are discussed here and referred to as "atypical bacteria" because many of them are hard to visualize by routine methods such as Gram staining or are difficult to grow on laboratory media. Although this classification is not perfect, it does allow for a way of thinking about this diverse group of bacteria regarding antimicrobial therapy. The following bacteria are discussed in this group: *Chlamydia* spp., *Mycoplasma* spp., *Legionella pneumophila*, *Brucella* spp., *Francisella tularensis*, and *Rickettsia* spp.

Many of the bacteria in this group kill or damage human cells by actually living and multiplying within them. In this way, they are similar to the medieval miners who tunneled under formidable defensive walls to allow an assault on the castle from within. A practical implication of this intracellular lifestyle is that the antibiotics used to treat infections caused by these bacteria usually must penetrate well into host cells.

Excerpt from *The Jewish War* by Josephus published by Penguin Classics. Copyright © 1986. Reprinted by permission of Penguin Books Limited.

Chlamydia

Bacteria of the genus *Chlamydia* are obligate intracellular organisms that have an interesting biphasic life cycle. These bacteria exist as either an inert but transmissible extracellular form called an elementary body (EB) or a metabolically active and multiplicative intracellular form called a reticulate body (RB). The *Chlamydia* genus consists of three clinically important species: *Chlamydia trachomatis*, *Chlamydia pneumoniae*, and *Chlamydia psittaci*. *C. trachomatis* is the cause of one of the most common sexually transmitted illnesses and also a leading cause of blindness in some parts of the world. *C. pneumoniae* is a common etiology of community-acquired pneumonia, and *C. psittaci* causes psittacosis, a rare type of pneumonia that is acquired from exotic birds (Figure 13-1).

Because *Chlamydia* spp. are metabolically active only within host cells, antibiotics that penetrate to high levels within cells are required to treat infections caused by these bacteria. Agents of choice include some macrolides (**azithromycin**), tetracyclines (**doxycycline**), and some quinolones (Table 13-1). Doxycycline is the treatment of choice for *C. trachomatis* infections, and azithromycin is an alternative. β-Lactams are in general ineffective against *Chlamydia* spp., but for unclear reasons, **amoxicillin** retains some activity. Because of its long history of safe use during pregnancy, it is used in this situation for *C. trachomatis* infections. Note that **clindamycin** has some activity against *C. trachomatis* and is used in some antibiotic regimens for the treatment of pelvic inflammatory disease.

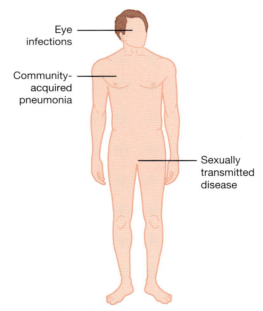

Figure 13-1. Sites of infections caused by *Chlamydia* spp.

Table 13-1	Antimicrobial Agents for Treatment of Infections Caused by *Chlamydia* spp.
Antibiotic Class	**Antibiotic**
Tetracyclines	Doxycycline
Macrolides	Azithromycin
Quinolones	Levofloxacin (*Chlamydia trachomatis*), moxifloxacin (*Chlamydia pneumoniae*)
During pregnancy	
Macrolides	Azithromycin
Aminopenicillins	Amoxicillin

QUESTIONS

1. The three classes of antibiotics with the best activity against *Chlamydia* spp. are _____, _____, and _____.
2. *Chlamydia* spp. are in general resistant to most _____, although for unclear reasons _____ has some activity against *C. trachomatis*.

ANSWERS

1. macrolides, tetracyclines, quinolones
2. β-lactams, amoxicillin

ADDITIONAL READINGS

Adimora AA. Treatment of uncomplicated genital *Chlamydia trachomatis* infections in adults. *Clin Infect Dis*. 2002;35(suppl 2):S183-S186.

Hammerschlag MR. Pneumonia due to *Chlamydia pneumoniae* in children: epidemiology, diagnosis, and treatment. *Pediatr Pulmonol*. 2003;36:384-390.

Stewardson AJ, Grayson ML. Psittacosis. *Infect Dis Clin North Am*. 2010;24:7-25.

Workowski KA, Bachmann LH, Chan PA, et al. Sexually transmitted infections treatment guidelines, 2021. *MMWR Recomm Rep*. 2021;70:1-187.

Mycoplasma

Members of the *Mycoplasma* genus share the property of being among the smallest known free-living organisms. Although several species are capable of causing disease in humans, *Mycoplasma pneumoniae* is the most commonly encountered. These bacteria, which can only grow when intimately associated with host cells or on highly supplemented laboratory media, are a frequent cause of community-acquired pneumonia (Figure 13-2). Effective treatments include a macrolide (**azithromycin**) or a tetracycline (**doxycycline**) (Table 13-2). Other active agents include quinolones (**levofloxacin, moxifloxacin**). Mycoplasmas lack cell walls, so β-lactams have no activity against them.

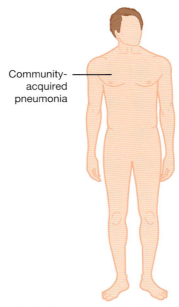

Figure 13-2. Sites of infections caused by *Mycoplasma pneumoniae*.

Table 13-2	Antimicrobial Agents for Treatment of Infections Caused by *Mycoplasma pneumoniae*
Antibiotic Class	**Antibiotic**
Macrolides	Azithromycin
Tetracyclines	Doxycycline
Quinolones	Levofloxacin, moxifloxacin

QUESTIONS

3. The three classes of antibiotics with the best activity against *M. pneumoniae* are _____, _____, and _____.
4. *M. pneumoniae* bacteria lack a cell wall, so _____ are not active against them.

ANSWERS

3. macrolides, tetracyclines, quinolones
4. β-lactams

ADDITIONAL READINGS

Metlay JP, Waterer GW, Long AC, et al. Diagnosis and treatment of adults with community-acquired pneumonia: an official clinical practice guideline of the American Thoracic Society and Infectious Diseases Society of America. *Am J Respir Crit Care Med*. 2019;200:e45-e67.

Taylor-Robinson D, Bébéar C. Antibiotic susceptibilities of mycoplasmas and treatment of mycoplasmal infections. *J Antimicrob Chemother*. 1997;40:622-630.

Legionella

Legionella spp. are environmental bacteria that inhabit natural and man-made water systems. Several species of *Legionella* are capable of causing disease in humans, but *L. pneumophila* is the most common. These bacteria cause Legionnaires disease, a severe form of pneumonia following inhalation or aspiration of this environmental organism, as well as Pontiac fever, which is a milder form of the disease that lacks respiratory features (Figure 13-3). *Legionella* may cause either community- or hospital-acquired pneumonia. Once in the lung, *Legionella* organisms are taken up by macrophages and multiply within them. The net result of this process is the development of pneumonia that is frequently severe and often accompanied by systemic signs and symptoms, including high fever, chills, nausea, vomiting, diarrhea, and confusion. Laboratory studies may show evidence of hepatic or renal dysfunction and hyponatremia.

Because *Legionella* resides within macrophages during infection, treatment consists of antibiotics that penetrate into and are active within these phagocytes. Such antibiotics include macrolides, tetracyclines, and quinolones. Agents of choice are **azithromycin** and **levofloxacin** (Table 13-3). Other active agents include **ciprofloxacin**, **moxifloxacin**, and **clarithromycin**.

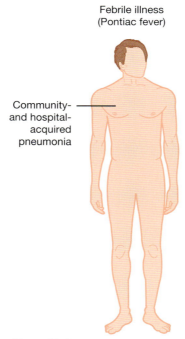

Figure 13-3. Sites of infections caused by *Legionella* spp.

Table 13-3	Antimicrobial Agents for Treatment of Infections Caused by *Legionella* spp.
Antibiotic Class	**Antibiotic**
First-line agents	
Macrolides	Azithromycin
Quinolones	Levofloxacin
Second-line agents	
Macrolides	Clarithromycin
Quinolones	Ciprofloxacin, moxifloxacin

QUESTIONS

5. The agents of choice for *Legionella* infections are _____ and _____.

6. During infection, *Legionella* bacteria reside primarily within _____, so antibiotics must penetrate into these cells to kill these bacteria.

ANSWERS

5. azithromycin, levofloxacin
6. macrophages

ADDITIONAL READINGS

Blázquez Garrido RM, Espinosa Parra FJ, Alemany Francés L, et al. Antimicrobial chemotherapy for Legionnaires disease: levofloxacin versus macrolides. *Clin Infect Dis*. 2005;40:800-806.

Phin N, Parry-Ford F, Harrison T, et al. Epidemiology and clinical management of Legionnaires' disease. *Lancet Infect Dis*. 2014;14:1011-1021.

Roig J, Rello J. Legionnaires' disease: a rational approach to therapy. *J Antimicrob Chemother*. 2003;51:1119-1129.

Yu VL, Greenberg RN, Zadeikis N, et al. Levofloxacin efficacy in the treatment of community-acquired legionellosis. *Chest*. 2004;125:2135-2139.

Brucella

Brucella spp. are small gram-negative coccobacilli and cause brucellosis, a disease of animals that is occasionally transmitted to humans. Species most commonly associated with human disease include *Brucella melitensis*, *Brucella abortus*, *Brucella suis*, and *Brucella canis*. Close contact with animals and ingestion of unpasteurized milk or cheese are risk factors for acquisition. Symptoms include fever, sweats, malaise, anorexia, and fatigue (Figure 13-4). Brucellosis is difficult to diagnose and, if untreated, may last for weeks or months. Prolonged infections tend to cause localized manifestations, such as osteoarthritis, sacroiliitis, or epididymo-orchitis.

During infection, *Brucella* bacteria survive and multiply within phagocytic cells. Therefore, the antibiotic regimens for brucellosis contain doxycycline, an agent that penetrates well into cells. The preferred regimens are **doxycycline** plus **rifampin** or **doxycycline** plus either **gentamicin** or **streptomycin** (Table 13-4). (The latter agent is a rarely used aminoglycoside.) Quinolones (**ciprofloxacin**, **levofloxacin**, **moxifloxacin**) are also effective when used in conjunction with other agents such as **rifampin**, but experience is more limited. **Trimethoprim-sulfamethoxazole** plus **rifampin** is recommended for small children and **trimethoprim-sulfamethoxazole** plus **rifampin** or **rifampin** alone for pregnant women, in whom doxycycline and quinolones are contraindicated. Infections must be treated for extended periods (eg, 6 weeks), and relapses may occur.

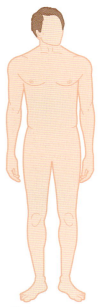

Figure 13-4. Sites of infections caused by *Brucella* spp.

Table 13-4	Antimicrobial Agents for Treatment of Infections Caused by *Brucella* spp.
Antibiotic Class	**Antibiotic**
First-line regimens	
Tetracyclines plus rifamycins	Doxycycline plus rifampin
Tetracyclines plus aminoglycosides	Doxycycline plus gentamicin, doxycycline plus streptomycin
Alternative agents	
Sulfa drugs	Trimethoprim-sulfamethoxazole
Quinolones	Ciprofloxacin, levofloxacin, moxifloxacin

Questions

7. The four antibiotics most commonly used in treatment regimens for brucellosis are _____, _____, _____, and _____.
8. Combination therapy is usually used to treat brucellosis. Three common regimens are doxycycline plus _____, doxycycline plus _____, and doxycycline plus _____.
9. Because doxycycline and quinolones are not recommended for pregnant women, _____ with or without _____ is used for these individuals when they acquire brucellosis.

Answers

7. doxycycline, gentamicin, streptomycin, rifampin
8. rifampin, gentamicin, streptomycin
9. rifampin, trimethoprim-sulfamethoxazole

Additional Readings

Ariza J, Gudiol F, Pallares R, et al. Treatment of human brucellosis with doxycycline plus rifampin or doxycycline plus streptomycin. A randomized, double-blind study. *Ann Intern Med*. 1992;117:25-30.

Franco MP, Mulder M, Gilman RH, et al. Human brucellosis. *Lancet Infect Dis*. 2007;7:775-786.

Pappas G, Akritidis N, Bosilkovski M, et al. Brucellosis. *N Engl J Med*. 2005;352:2325-2336.

Solís García del Pozo J, Solera J. Systematic review and meta-analysis of randomized clinical trials in the treatment of human brucellosis. *PLoS ONE*. 2012;7(2):e32090. doi:10.1371/journal.pone.0032090

HISTORY

Brucellosis has been blamed for one of the worst peacetime naval disasters, the collision between the HMS Victoria and the HMS Camperdown in 1893 off the coast of Syria. This collision resulted in the sinking of the Victoria, the flagship of the British Mediterranean Fleet, and the death of 358 of her crew. Some authorities believe that the commanders of these ships were suffering from brucellosis, which was endemic in parts of the Mediterranean region at that time. This may have led to impairment of their judgment and performance, leading to the collision.

From Vassallo DJ. The centenary of the sinking of the Mediterranean Fleet flagship, HMS Victoria. What was the role of Malta fever? *J R Nav Med Serv.* 1993;79:91-99.

Francisella tularensis

F. tularensis, a gram-negative coccobacillus that primarily infects animals, causes tularemia. Humans acquire the infection from animals either directly through contact with contaminated animals or animal products or indirectly through the bite of an insect, exposure to contaminated water or mud, or inhalation of aerosolized organisms.

Tularemia presents as one of several syndromes: ulceroglandular, glandular, typhoidal, pneumonic, oropharyngeal, and oculoglandular disease (Figure 13-5). In ulceroglandular disease, patients typically have a skin lesion at the site of inoculation and

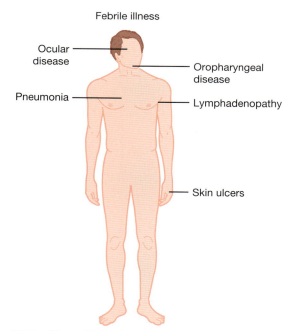

Figure 13-5. Sites of infections caused by *Francisella tularensis*.

Table 13-5 — Antimicrobial Agents for Treatment of Infections Caused by *Francisella tularensis*

Antibiotic Class	Antibiotic
Aminoglycosides	Streptomycin, gentamicin
Quinolones	Ciprofloxacin
Tetracyclines	Doxycycline

tender regional lymphadenopathy involving one or more draining lymph nodes. Glandular tularemia is similar, except that there is no apparent portal of entry. Patients with typhoidal tularemia present with a febrile illness and sepsis. Those with pneumonic disease have the signs and symptoms of pneumonia. In oropharyngeal tularemia, individuals have an ulcerative pharyngitis with enlarged cervical lymph nodes. Finally, oculoglandular disease is characterized by conjunctival erythema following inoculation of the organism into the eye.

Although *F. tularensis* is a facultative intracellular bacterium, the use of the aminoglycoside **streptomycin** has yielded the best results in the treatment of tularemia (Table 13-5). The reasons for this are unclear but may indicate that antimicrobial killing of the extracellular phase of infection is sufficient for cure. **Gentamicin** is frequently used in place of streptomycin because it is more readily available, although outcomes may not be quite as good. Quinolones (**ciprofloxacin**) and tetracyclines (**doxycycline**) are also used.

QUESTIONS

10. *F. tularensis* is usually acquired through direct or indirect exposure to _____.

11. Aminoglycoside antibiotics used to treat tularemia include _____ and _____.

12. Other antibiotics useful in the treatment of tularemia include _____ and _____.

ANSWERS

10. animals
11. streptomycin, gentamicin
12. ciprofloxacin, doxycycline

ADDITIONAL READINGS

Ellis J, Oyston PC, Green M, et al. Tularemia. *Clin Microbiol Rev*. 2002;15:631-646.
Enderlin G, Morales L, Jacobs RF, et al. Streptomycin and alternative agents for the treatment of tularemia: review of the literature. *Clin Infect Dis*. 1994;19:42-47.
Harik NS. Tularemia: epidemiology, diagnosis, and treatment. *Pediatr Ann*. 2013;42:288-292.

Rickettsia

A large number of *Rickettsia* spp. are capable of causing disease in humans. These bacteria are small, have a gram-negative–like cell envelope structure, and are obligate intracellular pathogens. Although the particular features of the rickettsial diseases differ somewhat, most consist of fever, headache, and rash, and most are acquired from arthropod vectors (Figure 13-6). Many of these diseases will also have characteristic black eschars at the site where the organism was inoculated by the vector. Examples of rickettsial diseases include Rocky Mountain spotted fever (*Rickettsia rickettsii*), Mediterranean spotted fever (*Rickettsia conorii*), rickettsialpox (*Rickettsia akari*), epidemic typhus (*Rickettsia prowazekii*), murine typhus (*Rickettsia typhi*), and scrub typhus (caused by the closely related bacterium *Orientia tsutsugamushi*).

Most rickettsial diseases are treated with **doxycycline**, which penetrates well into cells where the obligate intracellular *Rickettsia* bacteria reside (Table 13-6). This

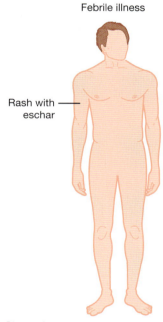

Figure 13-6. Sites of infections caused by *Rickettsia* spp.

Table 13-6. Antimicrobial Agents for Treatment of Infections Caused by *Rickettsia*

Antibiotic Class	Antibiotic
First-line agent	
Tetracyclines	Doxycycline, tetracycline
Alternatives	
Quinolones	Ciprofloxacin

antibiotic is even recommended for children with some rickettsial diseases because the short course required for treatment is unlikely to harm bone or teeth. **Tetracycline** may also be used. Some experts feel that **ciprofloxacin** may also be used to treat Rocky Mountain spotted fever, Mediterranean spotted fever, and rickettsialpox.

QUESTIONS

13. The treatment of choice for rickettsial infections is _____.
14. Other agents with activity against *Rickettsia* spp. are _____ and _____.

ANSWERS

13. doxycycline
14. tetracycline, ciprofloxacin

ADDITIONAL READINGS

Biggs HM, Behravesh CB, Bradley KK, et al. Diagnosis and management of tickborne rickettsial diseases: Rocky Mountain spotted fever and other spotted fever group rickettsioses, ehrlichioses, and anaplasmosis—United States. *MMWR Recomm Rep.* 2016;65:1-44.

Parola P, Paddock CD, Raoult D. Tick-borne rickettsioses around the world: emerging diseases challenging old concepts. *Clin Microbiol Rev.* 2005;18:719-756.

Walker DH. Rickettsiae and rickettsial infections: the current state of knowledge. *Clin Infect Dis.* 2007;45(suppl 1):S39-S44.

HISTORY

It has been speculated that louse-borne rickettsial diseases greatly weakened Napoleon's army during its retreat from Russia. Recently, investigators have verified this by detecting the DNA of *R. prowazekii* in dental pulp from the remains of soldiers buried in Lithuania.

From Raoult D, Dutour O, Houhamdi L, et al. Evidence for louse-transmitted diseases in soldiers of Napoleon's grand army in Vilnius. *J Infect Dis.* 2006;193:112-120 by permission of Oxford University Press.

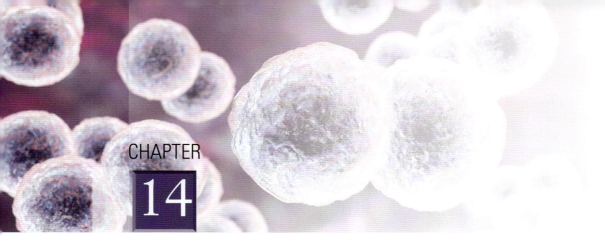

CHAPTER 14

Spirochetes

"So they sent Robert Fitz Hildebrand, a man of low birth indeed but also of tried military qualities, and, what disgraces and sullies the prime and the fame of soldiers, he was likewise a lustful man, drunken and unchaste. On arriving with a fine body of knights he obtained a most cordial reception, became extremely intimate with William, and could go in and out of his castle as he liked. Then, stung by desire, he seduced his wife, and afterwards, when a vile and abominable plan had been formed by agreement between him and the wife, he fettered William very tightly and imprisoned him in a dungeon, and enjoying his castle, wealth, and wife he likewise abandoned and rejected the countess, who had proudly sent him there, and made a pact with the king and the bishop. Nor did that reckless seducer escape punishment, as I have already said, for daring to devise such a villainous and treacherous plot, since, God most justly avenging his injustice, a worm was born at the time when the traitorous corrupter lay in the unchaste bosom of the adulteress and crept through his vitals, and slowly eating away his entrails it gradually consumed the scoundrel, and at length, in affliction of many complaints and the torment of many dreadful sufferings, it brought him to his end by a punishment he richly deserved."

—**Gesta Stephani, edited and translated by K. R. Potter**

Spirochetes are spiral- or corkscrew-shaped bacteria. Several types of bacteria within this group are medically important, but two in particular are commonly encountered by clinicians. These are *Treponema pallidum*, the cause of the sexually transmitted disease syphilis, and *Borrelia burgdorferi*, the etiologic agent of Lyme disease. *Leptospira interrogans* causes a less common but potentially serious disease called leptospirosis. In this section, these bacteria and the antimicrobial treatment of the infections they cause are discussed.

Treponema pallidum

Syphilis is a sexually transmitted disease that is caused by the spirochete *T. pallidum*. Acute infection, known as primary syphilis, is usually manifested by the presence of a chancre at the site of inoculation (Figure 14-1). The chancre spontaneously heals, but several weeks later, the signs and symptoms of secondary syphilis may develop. These include skin rashes, mucous patches, fever, malaise, and lymphadenopathy. The manifestations of secondary syphilis usually resolve but are prone to recur. At some point, individuals enter a disease phase known as *latent syphilis*, during which there is no overt evidence of infection. Latent syphilis is divided into two parts: *early latent syphilis*, which is defined by the initial infection having occurred within the previous year, and *late latent syphilis*, which is defined by the initial infection having occurred greater than 1 year earlier. This distinction is important because antibiotic treatment regimens differ for these two phases of illness. Long after the initial infection, some individuals will develop tertiary syphilis, a clinical illness that presents as chronically progressive disease. Tertiary syphilis usually manifests as cardiovascular abnormalities or gumma formation in the skin or internal organs. To further complicate matters, invasion of the central nervous system by *T. pallidum* may occur during any stage of syphilis. This results in neurosyphilis, which may take the form of meningeal or meningovascular disease, ocular involvement, general paresis, tabes dorsalis, or gummatous central nervous system disease.

Because *T. pallidum* cannot be grown in vitro, most of what is known about its susceptibility to antibiotics is based on human trials. These trials indicate that **penicillin** is quite effective against this organism (Table 14-1). The route of administration and

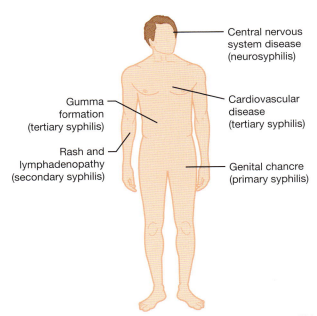

Figure 14-1. Sites of infections caused by *Treponema pallidum*.

Table 14-1	Antimicrobial Agents for Treatment of Infections Caused by *Treponema pallidum*
Antibiotic Class	**Antibiotic**
Agent of choice	
Natural penicillins	Penicillin G (including benzathine penicillin)
Alternatives	
Tetracyclines	Tetracycline, doxycycline
Third-generation cephalosporins	Ceftriaxone

the duration of treatment vary with the stage and type of syphilis as well as host factors. For example, primary, secondary, and early latent syphilis are treated with a single intramuscular injection of benzathine penicillin (see "Pearl" box). In contrast, late latent and tertiary syphilis are treated with three injections of benzathine penicillin given at 1-week intervals. Neurosyphilis is treated with 10 to 14 days of intravenous penicillin G. Alternatives for patients with allergies to penicillin include **tetracycline, doxycycline**, or **ceftriaxone**. Supportive data for the use of these alternative agents are lacking for certain clinical situations; as a result, desensitization and subsequent treatment with penicillin is considered optimal therapy in some penicillin-allergic patients, such as pregnant women.

QUESTIONS

1. The antibiotic of choice for syphilis is _____.
2. The route of administration and the duration of treatment for syphilis depend on the _____ of disease.
3. Intramuscular _____ _____ allows for slow release of penicillin into the circulation over several days.

ANSWERS

1. penicillin
2. stage
3. benzathine penicillin

ADDITIONAL READINGS

Golden MR, Marra CM, Holmes KK. Update on syphilis: resurgence of an old problem. *JAMA*. 2003;290:1510-1514.

Workowski KA, Bachmann LH, Chan PA, et al. Sexually transmitted infections treatment guidelines, 2021. *MMWR Recomm Rep*. 2021;70:1-187.

Pearl

Benzathine penicillin is a repository form of penicillin consisting of the benzathine tetrahydrate salt of penicillin G. In vivo, the compound is hydrolyzed to slowly release penicillin G. Thus, low but long-lasting levels of penicillin can be achieved following a single intramuscular dose. Depending on the dose, levels can be detected from 1 to 4 weeks following injection. Thus, this form of penicillin is useful in treating bacteria that are exquisitely sensitive to penicillin (ie, have low minimal inhibitory concentrations) but require prolonged exposure. *T. pallidum* is one example of such an organism.

From Kaplan EL, Berrios X, Speth J, et al. Pharmacokinetics of benzathine penicillin G: serum levels during the 28 days after intramuscular injection of 1,200,000 units. *J Pediatr.* 1989;115:146-150.

Borrelia burgdorferi

B. burgdorferi causes Lyme disease, the most common vector-borne illness in the United States and Europe. Similar to syphilis, Lyme disease progresses in stages. Stage 1 disease occurs shortly after inoculation of the bacterium into the host via a tick bite. This results in a characteristic annular skin rash known as erythema migrans, which appears at the site of the tick bite (Figure 14-2). Stage 2 disease occurs days to weeks later, when the organism has disseminated. Patients may have secondary skin rashes, lymphadenopathy, meningitis and neurologic findings, or evidence of cardiac involvement. Months to years later, patients may develop stage 3 disease, which is characterized by arthritis or chronic neurologic abnormalities such as cognitive impairment.

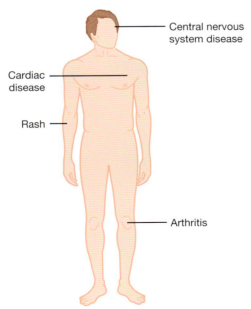

Figure 14-2. Sites of infections caused by *Borrelia burgdorferi*.

Table 14-2. Antimicrobial Agents for Treatment of Infections Caused by *Borrelia burgdorferi*

Antibiotic Class	Antibiotic
First-line agent	
Tetracyclines	Doxycycline
Second-line agent	
Aminopenicillins	Amoxicillin
Alternatives	
Second-generation cephalosporins	Cefuroxime
Serious neurologic and cardiac involvement	
Third-generation cephalosporins	Ceftriaxone

The treatment of choice for most manifestations of Lyme disease in people aged 8 years or above and in nonpregnant women is oral **doxycycline** (Table 14-2). The best studied alternative agents are oral **amoxicillin** and oral **cefuroxime**. Individuals with severe neurologic or cardiac involvement or with arthritis who fails to respond to oral agents should be treated with intravenous **ceftriaxone**. In vitro and in vivo observations indicate that rifampin, quinolones, aminoglycosides, and first-generation cephalosporins are ineffective against this organism.

QUESTIONS

4. The antibiotic of choice for Lyme disease is _____.
5. Other antibiotics used for the treatment of stage 1 Lyme disease include _____ and _____.
6. Lyme disease with serious neurologic or cardiac involvement should be treated with intravenous antibiotics such as _____.

ANSWERS

4. doxycycline
5. amoxicillin, cefuroxime
6. ceftriaxone

ADDITIONAL READINGS

Steere AC. Lyme disease. *N Engl J Med*. 2001;345:115-125.

Wormser GP, Dattwyler RJ, Shapiro ED, et al. The clinical assessment, treatment, and prevention of Lyme disease, human granulocytic anaplasmosis, and babesiosis: clinical practice guidelines by the Infectious Diseases Society of America. *Clin Infect Dis*. 2006;43:1089-1134.

Leptospira interrogans

L. interrogans is a thin spirochete that causes the zoonotic infection leptospirosis. This bacterium is shed in the urine of many types of domestic and wild animals; acquisition by humans occurs following direct or indirect exposure to contaminated water, mud, or animal tissues. Individuals with leptospirosis may present with disease severity ranging from subclinical illness to multiorgan failure leading to death. Those with severe disease often have a biphasic illness consisting of initial fever, headaches, conjunctival suffusion, and myalgias, followed by defervescence and subsequent recrudescence with liver, renal, or meningeal involvement (Figure 14-3).

Mild leptospirosis is usually treated with oral antibiotics, such as **doxycycline** or **amoxicillin**. Moderate or severe disease is treated with intravenous agents, such as **penicillin G**, **ceftriaxone**, or **ampicillin** (Table 14-3).

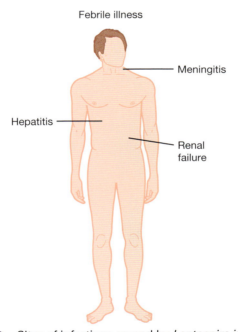

Figure 14-3. Sites of infections caused by *Leptospira interrogans*.

Table 14-3	Antimicrobial Agents for Treatment of Infections Caused by *Leptospira interrogans*
Antibiotic Class	**Antibiotic**
Mild disease	
Tetracyclines	Doxycycline
Aminopenicillins	Amoxicillin
Moderate and severe disease	
Natural penicillins	Penicillin G
Aminopenicillins	Ampicillin
Third-generation cephalosporins	Ceftriaxone

Questions

7. Like the other spirochetes, *L. interrogans* is susceptible to penicillin/amoxicillin and _____.

8. _____ and _____ are the agents of choice for mild leptospirosis.

9. For severe leptospirosis, intravenous _____, _____, or _____ is recommended.

Answers

7. doxycycline
8. Doxycycline, amoxicillin
9. penicillin, ampicillin, ceftriaxone

Additional Readings

Bharti AR, Nally JE, Ricaldi JN, et al;. Leptospirosis: a zoonotic disease of global importance. *Lancet Infect Dis.* 2003;3:757-771.

Haake DA, Levett PN. Leptospirosis in humans. *Curr Top Microbiol Immunol.* 2015;387:65-97.

CHAPTER 15

Mycobacteria

"My dear lords, you are very gallant knights with much experience of war, and you know that the King of France whom we serve sent us to this place (Calais) to hold the town and castle for as long as our honour and his interests might require it. We have done everything in our power, but now our help has failed us and you are pressing us so hard that we have nothing left to eat. We must all die or go mad with hunger if the noble king whom you serve does not take pity on us. So I ask you, dear lords, to beg him humbly to have mercy on us and allow us to go away just as we are, taking for himself the town and citadel and all the things in them. He will find enough to satisfy him."

—Chronicles, Jean Froissart

The mycobacteria are, in general, slow-growing organisms that cause chronic diseases. Often, individuals afflicted with mycobacterial infections succumb after prolonged infections that slowly and progressively weaken the body and result in emaciation and debilitation. In this regard, mycobacterial disease is akin to a protracted siege on the body rather than an all-out assault that rapidly overruns its defenses.

The *Mycobacteria* are a group of organisms that produce cell envelopes rich in lipids and fatty acids. One fatty acid, mycolic acid, is particularly abundant and makes up 60% of the cell wall mass of these bacteria. Although mycobacteria have a gram-positive cell envelope structure, their high lipid content does not allow penetration of Gram stain, preventing visualization of these organisms by this technique. Rather, a method called "acid-fast" staining must be used to detect them.

Excerpt from *Chronicles* by Jean Froissart published by Penguin Classics. Copyright © Geoffrey Bereton, 1968, 1978. Reprinted by permission of Penguin Books Limited.

In this section, we discuss *Mycobacterium tuberculosis*, the cause of tuberculosis; *Mycobacterium avium* complex (MAC), a frequent cause of lung disease and lymphadenitis; and *Mycobacterium leprae*, the etiologic agent of leprosy. Although the unique lipid-rich cell envelopes of mycobacteria allow these pathogens to cause severe disease, they are also their Achilles heels in that certain antibiotics, such as isoniazid and pyrazinamide, target the production of these molecules. Thus, these agents tend to be quite specific for mycobacteria. Other agents used to treat mycobacteria, such as rifampin and streptomycin, have more general antimicrobial mechanisms and can also be used to treat other bacteria.

Mycobacterium tuberculosis

M. tuberculosis is the etiologic agent of tuberculosis, which, on a global level, is the leading cause of death by a single infectious agent. Inhalation of these bacteria may lead directly to overt disease or more commonly results in latent infection, in which the individual is asymptomatic but still harbors the mycobacteria. In latent infection, the bacteria may overcome the host's containment at a later time, resulting in reactivation disease. This most frequently occurs during the 2-year period following initial infection or at a later time when the host's immune system becomes weakened as a result of increasing age or other forms of immunosuppression. Reactivation disease predominantly affects the lungs, but virtually any organ may be involved (Figure 15-1). In pulmonary disease, the lung apices are classically affected, and the formation of cavitary lesions is common. Extrapulmonary disease may involve lymph nodes, the pleural space, bone, the genitourinary system, or the central nervous system. Disseminated disease, referred to as "miliary tuberculosis," also occurs. Regardless of the organ systems involved, disease tends to be chronic, debilitating, and associated with the formation of necrotizing granulomas.

M. tuberculosis is prone to develop resistance to antimicrobial agents. As a result, most drug regimens for active disease contain multiple agents. A typical initial regimen is **isoniazid**, **rifampin**, **pyrazinamide**, and **ethambutol** (Table 15-1). All four drugs are continued for 2 months, after which the regimen is usually narrowed to isoniazid plus rifampin if the infecting strain is susceptible to these agents. Isoniazid and rifampin are then continued for an additional 4 months to complete therapy. **Rifabutin** is

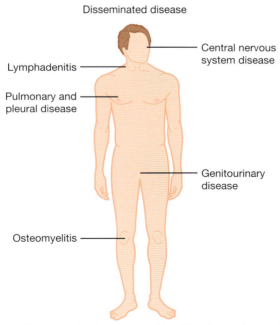

Figure 15-1. Sites of infections caused by *Mycobacterium tuberculosis*.

Table 15-1	Antimicrobial Agents for Treatment of Infections Caused by *Mycobacterium tuberculosis*
Active Disease	
(Isoniazid plus rifampin plus pyrazinamide plus ethambutol) × 2 mo, followed by (isoniazid plus rifampin) × 4 mo	
Latent Infection	
Rifapentine plus isoniazid × 3 mo (weekly dosing) or Rifampin plus isoniazid × 3 mo (daily dosing) or Rifampin × 4 mo (daily dosing)	

frequently substituted for rifampin in patients simultaneously being treated for human immunodeficiency virus (HIV) infection because it interferes less with the metabolism of antiretroviral agents.

If the infecting strain is resistant to isoniazid and rifampin, the patient is said to have multidrug-resistant (MDR) tuberculosis. Treatment of MDR tuberculosis is difficult and often requires the use of several second-line agents, such as bedaquiline, linezolid, levofloxacin, moxifloxacin, delamanid, or pretomanid. These agents tend to be less active than first-line agents, or their use is associated with an increased frequency of adverse effects. Current guidelines for the treatment of MDR tuberculosis recommend that at least five drugs to which the mycobacterial strain is susceptible in vitro be used for the first 5 to 7 months, followed by four drugs to complete a 15- to 21-month total treatment course.

Because individuals with latent infections (as opposed to active disease) have a much lower bacterial burden, the likelihood of spontaneous mutations that lead to antibiotic resistance is much lower. Thus, these individuals can be successfully treated with fewer agents, such as **rifampin** for 4 months, **isoniazid** plus **rifampin** for 3 months, or **isoniazid** plus **rifapentine** for 3 months. The latter regimen is given once per week, which facilitates directly observed therapy.

QUESTIONS

1. Because *M. tuberculosis* is prone to develop resistance to antimicrobial agents, most initial treatment regimens for active disease consist of _____ drugs.
2. The most commonly used treatment regimen for active tuberculosis consists of _____, _____, _____, and _____.
3. Treatment of drug-resistance tuberculosis differs from that of drug-susceptible tuberculosis in that _____ drugs are used for a _____ duration.
4. Agents used to treat latent tuberculosis include _____, _____, or _____.

Answers

1. four
2. isoniazid, rifampin, pyrazinamide, ethambutol
3. more, longer
4. rifampin, rifapentine, isoniazid

History

Tuberculosis is indeed a very old disease. Polymerase chain reaction amplification of samples from mummified remains has confirmed its presence in ancient Egypt and in the Americas before the arrival of Columbus.

From Mackowiak PA, Blos VT, Aguilar M, et al. On the origin of American tuberculosis. *Clin Infect Dis*. 2005;41:515-518.
From Zink AR, Sola C, Reischl U, et al. Characterization of Mycobacterium tuberculosis complex DNAs from Egyptian mummies by spoligotyping. *J Clin Microbiol*. 2003;41:359-367.

Additional Readings

Garcia-Prats AJ, Starke JR, Waning B, et al. New drugs and regimens for tuberculosis disease treatment in children and adolescents. *J Ped Infect Dis Soc*. 2022;11(suppl 3):S101-S109.

Nahid P, Dorman SE, Alipanah N, et al. Official American Thoracic Society/Centers for Disease Control and Prevention/Infectious Diseases Society of America clinical practice guidelines: treatment of drug-susceptible tuberculosis. *Clin Infect Dis*. 2016;63:e147-e195.

Seaworth BJ, Griffith DE. Therapy of multidrug-resistant and extensively drug-resistant tuberculosis. *Microbiol Spectr*. 2017;5(2). doi:10.1128/microbiolspec.TNMI7-0042-2017

Sterling TR, Njie G, Zenner D, et al. Guidelines for the treatment of latent tuberculosis infection: recommendations from the National Tuberculosis Controllers Association and CDC, 2020. *MMWR Recomm Rep*. 2020;69(1):1-11.

Mycobacterium avium Complex

MAC consists of two closely related mycobacterial species: *M. avium* and *Mycobacterium intracellulare*. These pathogens cause pulmonary disease in adults, especially in those with predisposing lung abnormalities (Figure 15-2). In contrast, cervical lymphadenitis caused by MAC most often occurs in children. Disseminated disease is almost exclusively seen in severely immunocompromised individuals, especially those with acquired immunodeficiency syndrome (AIDS). As with illnesses caused by other mycobacterial species, each of these diseases is chronic in nature and tends to have an insidious onset.

MAC disease, like tuberculosis, must be treated with multiple agents for prolonged periods to prevent the emergence of resistance and accomplish clinical cure. In addition, immunocompromised individuals must be placed on maintenance therapy for life or until immune reconstitution is achieved to prevent relapse. The recommended treatment regimen for MAC disease consists of **azithromycin** plus **rifampin** plus **ethambutol** (Table 15-2). **Amikacin** is sometimes added to this regimen in the presence of severe pulmonary disease or macrolide resistance. Alternative agents include **clarithromycin**, **rifabutin**, and **clofazimine**.

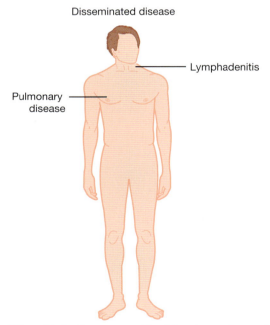

Figure 15-2. Sites of infections caused by *Mycobacterium avium* complex.

Table 15-2	Antimicrobial Agents for Treatment of Infections Caused by *Mycobacterium avium* Complex
Antibiotic Class	**Antibiotic**
Azithromycin plus rifampin plus ethambutol	
Alternative Agents	
Macrolides	Clarithromycin
Aminoglycosides	Amikacin
Clofazimine	

QUESTIONS

5. Infections caused by MAC are often initially treated with _____ antibiotics.
6. Most treatment regimens for MAC infections include _____, _____, and _____.
7. _____ is sometimes included in antibiotic regimens for the treatment of *M. avium* infections if infection is severe or macrolide resistance is present.

ANSWERS

5. three
6. azithromycin, rifampin, ethambutol
7. Amikacin

ADDITIONAL READINGS

Daley CL, Iaccarino JM, Lange C, et al. Treatment of nontuberculous mycobacterial pulmonary disease: an official ATS/ERS/ESCMID/IDSA clinical practice guideline. *Clin Infect Dis.* 2020;71:e1-e36.

Panel on Guidelines for the Prevention and Treatment of Opportunistic Infections in Adults and Adolescents with HIV. Guidelines for the prevention and treatment of opportunistic infections in adults and adolescents with HIV. National Institutes of Health, Centers for Disease Control and Prevention, HIV Medicine Association, and Infectious Diseases Society of America. Accessed November 20, 2023. https://clinicalinfo.hiv.gov/en/guidelines/adult-and-adolescent-opportunistic-infection

Mycobacterium leprae

M. leprae causes one of the oldest and most stigmatized human diseases: leprosy or Hansen disease. Recognition of leprosy dates back to biblical times, when afflicted individuals were shunned for fear of spreading the dreaded disease. This illness is chronic and is characterized by infiltrative skin lesions and progressive neuropathy that may lead to disfigurement (Figure 15-3). It is now clear that leprosy can have a spectrum of disease manifestations, from paucibacillary (tuberculoid) to multibacillary (lepromatous). In paucibacillary leprosy, examination of affected tissues shows evidence of a robust immune response but few bacteria. In multibacillary leprosy, bacteria are numerous and appear to elicit little or no immune response.

A three-antibiotic regimen is recommended for the treatment of leprosy: **dapsone**, **rifampin**, and **clofazimine** (Table 15-3). As is seen with other mycobacterial

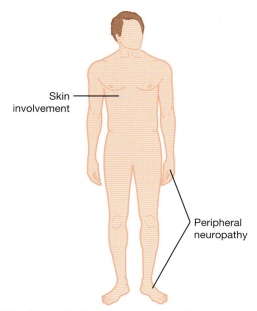

Figure 15-3. Sites of infections caused by *Mycobacterium leprae*.

Table 15-3. Antimicrobial Agents for Treatment of Infections Caused by *Mycobacterium leprae*

Antibiotic Class	Antibiotic
Dapsone plus rifampin plus clofazimine	
Alternative Agents	
Tetracyclines	Minocycline
Quinolones	Levofloxacin Moxifloxacin
Macrolides	Clarithromycin

infections, the emergence of resistance occurs when a single antibiotic is used, so combination therapy is recommended. The duration of therapy differs with the type of leprosy. Multibacillary leprosy is usually treated for 12-24 months, whereas paucibacillary leprosy is treated for 6-12 months. Alternative agents, for which there is less clinical experience, include **minocycline**, **clarithromycin**, and **quinolones**.

QUESTIONS

8. Leprosy can have a spectrum of disease manifestations, ranging from _____ leprosy to _____ leprosy.
9. Like other mycobacterial infections, leprosy requires treatment with _____ antibiotics for _____ periods.
10. The standard treatment regimen for leprosy is _____, _____, and _____.

ANSWERS

8. multibacillary, paucibacillary
9. multiple, prolonged
10. dapsone, rifampin, clofazimine

HISTORY

Beginning in 1866 and continuing for the next 103 years, people living in Hawaii and diagnosed with leprosy were exiled to arguably the most famous leprosy colony in the world: Molokai. It is estimated that more than 8,000 people were forcibly moved to this island in an attempt to limit the spread of leprosy among the people of Hawaii. In the early days of the colony, inhabitants were provided only minimal food and shelter and virtually no medical care. As a consequence, the mortality rate for individuals during their first 5 years at Molokai was nearly 50%.

From Tayman J. *The Colony. The Harrowing True Story of the Exiles of Molokai.* Scribner; 2006.

ADDITIONAL READINGS

Kar HK, Gupta R. Treatment of leprosy. *Clin Dermatol*. 2015;33:55-65.
Smith CS, Aerts A, Saunderson P, et al. Multidrug therapy for leprosy: a game changer on the path to elimination. *Lancet Infect Dis*. 2017;17(9):e293-e297. doi:10.1016/S1473-3099(17)30418-8
World Health Organization. *Guidelines for the diagnosis, treatment and prevention of leprosy.* 2018. https://apps.who.int/iris/bitstream/handle/10665/274127/9789290226383-eng.pdf?ua=1

PART 4

Empiric Therapy

"I must say that to die with one's sword still sheathed is most regrettable."
— The Book of Five Rings, Miyamoto Musashi

"All action in War, as we have already said, is directed on probable, not on certain, results. Whatever is wanting in certainty must always be left to fate, or chance, call it which you will. We may demand that what is so left should be as little as possible...."
— On War, Carl von Clausewitz

Choosing the correct antibiotic is relatively straightforward when the causative bacterium has been identified, but what does one do when the microbiologic etiology of an infection is unknown? In severely ill patients, antibiotics must be administered empirically, before culture results are available. That is, antibiotics are prescribed based on what is known about the usual bacterial causes of such infections and their anticipated susceptibilities.

In the preceding chapter, we discussed the major pathogenic bacteria and the infectious syndromes they cause. The antibiotics that are effective against each of these bacteria were then listed. In this section, we discuss the major infectious syndromes and the bacteria that commonly cause them. Based on this information and what was learned in the preceding section, the antimicrobial agents that adequately target the most likely etiologic bacteria for each disease are listed.

Rather than being arbitrary, recommended empiric antibiotic choices make sense when one understands the common bacterial causes of infectious syndromes and the antibiotics that are active against these bacteria. Thus, by the end of this section, you should be able to easily list the appropriate antibiotic regimens for the treatment of these common infectious diseases.

A word of caution: Although in this section we focus on choosing antibiotics with activity against the expected bacterial pathogens for each disease, in clinical practice, other factors enter into these decisions. Local patterns of antibiotic resistance must be taken into account, as should the history of infections and the agents used to treat them in each individual patient. Cost is an important factor in choosing antibiotics. A patient's allergic profile and comorbidities must also be considered. Finally, agents proven to be effective in clinical trials are given preference over agents that are indicated on theoretical grounds alone.

CHAPTER 16

Pneumonia

In the war between bacteria and the human body, the lungs are a common battlefield. Frequent bacterial incursions from the heavily colonized oropharynx and nasopharynx are facilitated by the relatively straight, short, and open conduits of the trachea and bronchi. Fortunately, many bacteria that successfully enter the lungs are quickly and imperceptibly eradicated. However, all too often, the protective mechanisms of the respiratory tract are overwhelmed, and the features of pneumonia become apparent. The patient develops fever, chills, rigors, cough, pleurisy, and, sometimes, dyspnea. On physical examination, tachycardia, tachypnea, and abnormalities on chest auscultation are noted. Laboratory abnormalities include an elevated peripheral blood leukocyte count, often with a left shift representing immature neutrophils being marginated into the blood. Chest radiographs show pulmonary infiltrates.

Pneumonia occurs in two major forms: community-acquired pneumonia (CAP) and hospital-acquired pneumonia (HAP). As suggested by their names, these entities are defined by where the infectious agent is acquired. Whereas CAP typically occurs in individuals residing in their homes, HAP afflicts those who are in a hospital. The importance of this distinction is that the circumstances under which the pneumonia was acquired dictate to a large extent the type of pathogens that may cause it and, therefore, the most appropriate empiric therapy.

COMMUNITY-ACQUIRED PNEUMONIA

Acute CAP has been divided into two categories: typical and atypical. Although these classifications are useful in understanding the etiology of pneumonia, significant overlap occurs between them, and the clinical presentations of typical and atypical pneumonia are not distinct enough to be useful in decisions about therapy.

Typical CAP usually presents with the sudden onset of fever, chills, pleuritic chest pain, and a productive cough. Afflicted individuals are usually older than 50 years of age. Radiographic examination shows a lobar or subsegmental infiltrate. The usual suspects in cases of typical CAP are *Streptococcus pneumoniae* and *Haemophilus influenzae* (Table 16-1). Other aerobic gram-negative bacteria and *Staphylococcus aureus* are less common.

Table 16-1. Bacterial Causes of Community-Acquired Pneumonia

Bacteria	Incidence (%)
Streptococcus pneumoniae	36-42
Haemophilus influenzae	9-40
Mycoplasma pneumoniae	2-19
Chlamydia pneumoniae	0-10
Legionella spp.	1-4
Other aerobic gram-negative bacteria	7-34

From Gadsby NJ, Russell CD, McHugh MP, et al. Comprehensive molecular testing for respiratory pathogens in community-acquired pneumonia. *Clin Infect Dis*. 2016;62:817-823; Jones RN. Microbial etiologies of hospital-acquired bacterial pneumonia and ventilator-associated bacterial pneumonia. *Clin Infect Dis*. 2010;51(suppl 1):581-587.

In contrast, atypical CAP is often preceded by a mild respiratory illness manifested by pharyngitis and rhinorrhea. The pneumonia is often, but not always, mild and is accompanied by a nonproductive cough. Patients may be younger than those with typical CAP, and chest radiographs may show interstitial infiltrates instead of lobar or subsegmental infiltrates. *Legionella* spp., *Mycoplasma pneumoniae*, and *Chlamydia pneumoniae* are frequent bacterial causes of atypical pneumonia (see Table 16-1). Viral infections such as influenza and COVID-19 also cause this type of pneumonia.

Optimal empiric therapy for CAP is controversial but in all cases is based on the most common etiologic bacteria, host predisposing factors, and the severity of illness (Figure 16-1 and Table 16-2).

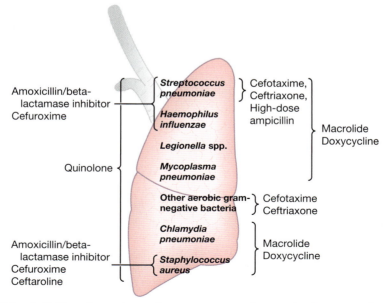

Figure 16-1. Activities of agents used to treat community-acquired pneumonia.

Table 16-2 Empiric Antimicrobial Therapy for Community-Acquired Pneumonia

Antibiotic Class	Antibiotic
Mild disease (outpatient therapy)	
Previously healthy (no comorbidities)	
Oral β-lactam given in high doses	Amoxicillin
or	
Oral tetracycline	Doxycycline
With comorbidities	
Oral quinolone	Moxifloxacin, levofloxacin
or	
Oral β-lactam given in high doses	Amoxicillin/clavulanate, cefuroxime
plus	
Oral macrolide	Azithromycin, clarithromycin
or	
Oral β-lactam given in high doses	Amoxicillin/clavulanate, cefuroxime
plus	
Oral tetracycline	Doxycycline
Moderately severe disease (patient admitted to the hospital)	
β-Lactam	Cefotaxime, ceftriaxone, ceftaroline, ampicillin/sulbactam
plus	
Macrolide	Azithromycin, clarithromycin
or	
Quinolone	Moxifloxacin, levofloxacin
Severe disease (patient admitted to an intensive care unit)	
β-Lactam	Cefotaxime, ceftriaxone, ceftaroline, ampicillin/sulbactam
plus either	
Macrolide	Azithromycin
or	
Antistreptococcal quinolone	Moxifloxacin, levofloxacin
If *Pseudomonas aeruginosa* is suspected, add	
Antipseudomonal agent	
If methicillin-resistant *Staphylococcus aureus* is suspected, add	
Glycopeptide	Vancomycin
or	
Oxazolidinone	Linezolid

For individuals with mild disease that can be treated in the outpatient setting, experts recommend high-dose **amoxicillin** or **doxycycline** unless the patient has comorbidities. If there are comorbidities, treatment should be with (1) an oral antistreptococcal quinolone (**moxifloxacin, levofloxacin**) or (2) an oral β-lactam agent (**amoxicillin/clavulanate, cefuroxime**) plus either a macrolide (**azithromycin, clarithromycin**) or **doxycycline**. Macrolides and doxycycline are effective against atypical pathogens, *H. influenzae*, and some strains of *S. pneumoniae*. In contrast, the strength of the β-lactams is their activity against *S. pneumoniae*. When given in high doses, β-lactam antibiotics achieve levels within the lung that are sufficient to kill all strains of *S. pneumoniae*, except those that are highly resistant to these agents. The β-lactams amoxicillin/clavulanate and cefuroxime also have excellent activity against *H. influenzae*. Given the complementary strengths of these agents, experts feel that they should be used together to treat CAP in patients with comorbidities that place them at higher risk for poor outcomes and for antibiotic-resistant pathogens. Oral antistreptococcal quinolones are highly effective against penicillin-resistant *S. pneumoniae*, *H. influenzae*, and atypical pathogens and are also efficacious for the treatment of CAP in the outpatient setting in the presence of comorbidities. Obviously, quinolones and doxycycline should be avoided in small children.

For patients with moderately severe CAP requiring admission to the hospital, intravenous therapy is usually given. It is recommended that these patients receive either (1) a combination of a macrolide (**azithromycin, clarithromycin**) and β-lactam (**cefotaxime, ceftriaxone, ceftaroline, ampicillin/sulbactam**) or (2) monotherapy with an antistreptococcal quinolone (**moxifloxacin, levofloxacin**). Either of these regimens is effective against *S. pneumoniae* (including most penicillin-resistant strains), *H. influenzae*, *Legionella* spp., and atypical pathogens. If risk factors for methicillin-resistant *S. aureus* or *Pseudomonas aeruginosa* infection are present (eg, prior isolation of these bacteria or recent hospitalization or antibiotic use), an appropriate antistaphylococcal agent (**vancomycin, linezolid**) or antipseudomonal agent (**piperacillin-tazobactam, cefepime, ceftazidime, aztreonam, meropenem, imipenem**) should be added.

Patients with severe CAP requiring admission to an intensive care unit should receive a combination of a β-lactam (**cefotaxime, ceftriaxone, ceftaroline, ampicillin/sulbactam**) plus either an **azithromycin** or an antistreptococcal quinolone (**moxifloxacin, levofloxacin**). If patients have risk factors for methicillin-resistant *S. aureus* or *P. aeruginosa*, antibiotics to cover these pathogens should be added.

HOSPITAL-ACQUIRED PNEUMONIA

The presence of the endotracheal tube compromises the innate defenses of the lung and facilitates infection in mechanically ventilated patients. It is, therefore, not surprising that 80% of HAP is "ventilator-associated pneumonia" (VAP), defined as pneumonia that develops after 48 hours of endotracheal intubation. The common causes of VAP are quite different than those of CAP and include *S. aureus*, *P. aeruginosa*, *Acinetobacter baumannii*, and members of the Enterobacterales (Table 16-3).

The choice of initial empiric therapy for VAP is particularly important because inappropriate treatment regimens (eg, antibiotics that are not effective against the causative bacteria) are associated with increased mortality, even when subsequently adjusted after culture and susceptibility data become available. Obviously, inappropriate antimicrobial therapy is more likely when infection is caused by a

Table 16-3	Bacterial Causes of Ventilator-Associated Pneumonia
Bacteria	Incidence (%)
Staphylococcus aureus	12-42
Pseudomonas aeruginosa	21-61
Acinetobacter spp.	5-37
Enterobacterales	5-19

From Guillamet CV, Kollef MH. Update on ventilator-associated pneumonia. *Curr Opin Crit Care*. 2015;21:430-438.

multidrug-resistant organism because these organisms are more likely to be resistant to empirically prescribed treatment regimens. Therefore, patients with risk factors for multidrug-resistant bacteria are treated with more potent empiric antibiotic regimens than those who lack these risk factors. These risk factors include prior intravenous antibiotic use within 90 days, septic shock, prior acute respiratory distress syndrome, 5 or more days of hospitalization prior to the onset of VAP, acute renal replacement therapy, and residence in an intensive care unit where multidrug-resistant VAP bacteria are frequently encountered. In patients without these risk factors, empiric antibiotic therapy consists of an antibiotic that is active against both methicillin-susceptible *S. aureus* and *P. aeruginosa* (eg, piperacillin-tazobactam or cefepime or imipenem). Treatment of VAP in patients with risk factors for multidrug-resistant organisms is more complex (Table 16-4 and Figure 16-2). Combination therapy using antibiotics

Table 16-4	Empiric Antimicrobial Therapy for Ventilator-Associated Pneumonia With Risk Factors for Multidrug Resistance
Antibiotic Class	Antibiotic
An agent with activity against methicillin-resistant *Staphylococcus aureus*	
Glycopeptide	Vancomycin
or	
Oxazolidinone	Linezolid
plus	
An antipseudomonal β-lactam	
Antipseudomonal penicillin/β-lactamase inhibitor	Piperacillin-tazobactam
or	
Antipseudomonal cephalosporin	Ceftazidime, cefepime
or	
Carbapenem	Imipenem, meropenem
or	
Monobactam	Aztreonam

(continued)

Table 16-4. Empiric Antimicrobial Therapy for Ventilator-Associated Pneumonia With Risk Factors for Multidrug Resistance (*Continued*)

Antibiotic Class	Antibiotic
plus	
A second antipseudomonal antibiotic	
Quinolone	Ciprofloxacin, levofloxacin
or	
Polymyxin	Colistin, polymyxin B

from at least three different classes is recommended to maximize the likelihood of giving at least one agent that is effective against these highly resistant bacteria. These regimens should include an agent with activity against MRSA such as a glycopeptide (**vancomycin**) or an oxazolidinone (**linezolid**). Two agents active against *P. aeruginosa* and other gram-negative bacteria are also recommended. The first gram-negative agent should be chosen from the following: an antipseudomonal penicillin (**piperacillin-tazobactam**), an antipseudomonal cephalosporin (**ceftazidime, cefepime**), a carbapenem (**imipenem, meropenem**) or a monobactam (**aztreonam**). The preferred second antipseudomonal agent is a fluoroquinolone (**ciprofloxacin, levofloxacin**), although a polymyxin (**colistin, polymyxin B**) may also be used (see Table 16-4 and Figure 16-2).

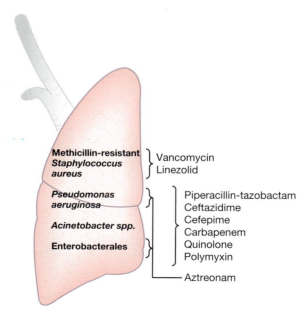

Figure 16-2. Activities of agents used to treat hospital-acquired pneumonia.

Two issues should be kept in mind when choosing antibiotics from this list for individual patients. First, it is best to use agents that the patient has not recently received because prior exposure to an antibiotic increases the risk of resistance. Second, local resistance patterns should be used to guide the choice of an agent. Finally, antibiotics should be chosen to minimize the chance of an allergic or adverse drug reaction.

QUESTIONS

1. Bacterial pathogens that cause atypical CAP include _____, _____, and _____.
2. The four drug classes most commonly used to treat CAP are the _____, _____, _____, and _____.
3. Empiric treatment for severe CAP is a _____ plus either a/an _____ or a _____.
4. The bacterial causes of VAP include _____, _____, _____, and the Enterobacterales.
5. An antibiotic with activity against methicillin-_____ *S. aureus* is not necessary in the empiric treatment of a patient with VAP and no risk factors for multidrug-resistant bacteria.
6. Treatment of VAP in a patient with risk factors for multidrug-resistant organisms includes one agent with activity against methicillin-resistant *S. aureus*, such as _____ or _____.

ANSWERS

1. *M. pneumoniae, C. pneumoniae, Legionella pneumophila*
2. macrolides, β-lactams, quinolones, tetracyclines
3. β-lactam, azithromycin, quinolone
4. *S. aureus, P. aeruginosa, A. baumannii*
5. resistant
6. vancomycin, linezolid

ADDITIONAL READINGS

File TM, Ramirez JA. Community-acquired pneumonia. *New Engl J Med.* 2023;389:632-641.

Kalil AC, Metersky ML, Klompas M, et al. Executive summary: management of adults with hospital-acquired and ventilator-associated pneumonia: 2016 clinical practice guidelines by the Infectious Diseases Society of America and the American Thoracic Society. *Clin Infect Dis.* 2016;63:575-582.

Metlay JP, Waterer GW, Long AC, et al. Diagnosis and treatment of adults with community-acquired pneumonia. An official clinical practice guideline of the American Thoracic Society and Infectious Diseases Society of America. *Am J Respir Crit Care Med.* 2019;200(7):e45-e67. doi:10.1164/rccm.201908-1581ST

Modi AR, Kovacs CS. Hospital-acquired and ventilator-associated pneumonia: diagnosis, management, and prevention. *Cleve Clin J Med.* 2020;87:633-639.

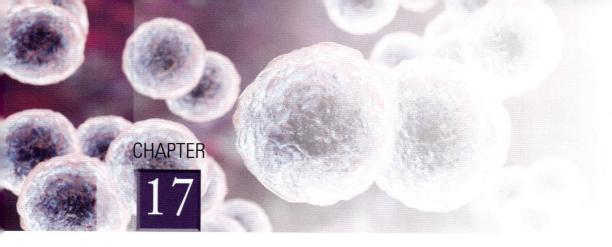

CHAPTER 17

Urinary Tract Infections

The urinary system is another portal between the outside environment and the interior of the human body, and it is frequently exploited by bacterial pathogens to cause infection. The vulnerability of this aspect of human anatomy is underscored by the incidence of urinary tract infections (UTIs); it is estimated that approximately 10% of women have a UTI each year. These infections may be relatively benign, involving only the urethra and the bladder, in which case they are referred to as *acute cystitis*. Alternatively, they may be more severe and involve the kidneys in the form of pyelonephritis. Individuals with acute bacterial cystitis often present with symptoms of dysuria, urinary frequency, and hematuria. The additional symptoms of fevers, chills, nausea, vomiting, and flank pain suggest pyelonephritis. Laboratory analysis shows pyuria, hematuria, and bacteriuria.

UTIs are classified as "uncomplicated" or "complicated." Uncomplicated UTIs are those that occur in young, healthy, nonpregnant women; complicated UTIs are all other UTIs. The typical complicated UTI would be an infection in a woman with diabetes or with a structural abnormality of her urinary system or who acquired her infection in the hospital. The differentiation between complicated and uncomplicated infections is important because it affects both the spectrum of bacteria involved and the duration of antibiotic treatment.

In uncomplicated acute cystitis and pyelonephritis, the causative bacteria are predictable. In most cases, *Escherichia coli* will be the etiologic organism (Table 17-1 and Figures 17-1 and 17-2). *Staphylococcus saprophyticus*, *Proteus mirabilis*, *Klebsiella* spp., and other Enterobacterales are also sometimes cultured. Unlike their hospital-acquired counterparts, these community-acquired bacteria are usually susceptible to many antibiotics. In complicated UTIs, bacteria that are more antibiotic resistant, such as *Pseudomonas aeruginosa*, *Enterobacter* spp., *Serratia* spp., *Citrobacter* spp., and *Staphylococcus aureus*, assume a more prominent role, as do enterococci (see Table 17-1; Figure 17-3).

Recommended empirical treatment of acute uncomplicated cystitis is a 5-day course of **nitrofurantoin** (Table 17-2). A 3-day course of oral **trimethoprim-sulfamethoxazole** was formerly the treatment of choice; but because of increasing resistance, it is now only recommended if local resistance rates of uropathogens do not exceed 20%, and this agent has not been used to treat a UTI in the preceding

Table 17-1. Bacterial Causes of Urinary Tract Infections

Bacteria	Incidence (%)
Uncomplicated	
Escherichia coli	53-79
Proteus mirabilis	4-5
Staphylococcus saprophyticus	3
Klebsiella spp.	2-3
Other Enterobacterales	3
Complicated	
E. coli	26-29
Enterococci	13-17
Pseudomonas aeruginosa	9-16
Klebsiella spp.	8-10
Other Enterobacterales	9-11

From Bronsema DA, Adams JR, Pallares R, et al. Secular trends in rates and etiology of nosocomial urinary tract infections at a university hospital. *J Urol*. 1993;150:414-416; Gaynes R, Edwards JR. Overview of nosocomial infections caused by gram-negative bacilli. *Clin Infect Dis*. 2005;41:848-854; Goldstein FW. Antibiotic susceptibility of bacterial strains isolated from patients with community-acquired urinary tract infections in France. Multicentre Study Group. *Eur J Clin Microbiol Infect Dis*. 2000;19:112-117; Kahlmeter G. An international survey of the antimicrobial susceptibility of pathogens from uncomplicated urinary tract infections: the ECO.SENS Project. *J Antimicrob Chemother*. 2003;51:69-76.

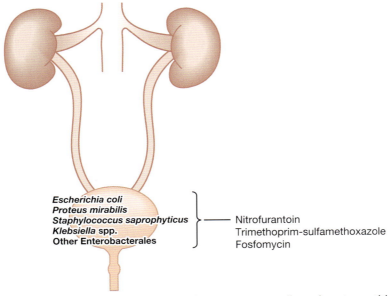

Figure 17-1. Activities of agents used to treat uncomplicated acute cystitis.

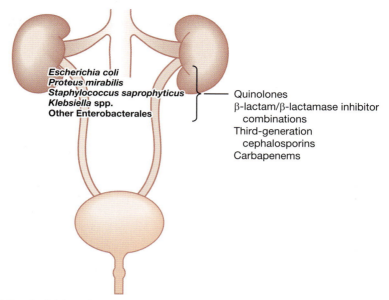

Figure 17-2. Activities of agents used to treat uncomplicated acute pyelonephritis.

3 months. Although somewhat less effective, a single dose of an older agent, fosfomycin, may also be used. These antibiotics are active against many of the *E. coli*, other Enterobacterales, and *S. saprophyticus* strains that cause these infections.

The same bacteria that cause uncomplicated cystitis also cause uncomplicated pyelonephritis (see Figure 17-2). The treatment recommendations, however, are different because nitrofurantoin does not achieve the high serum levels necessary to

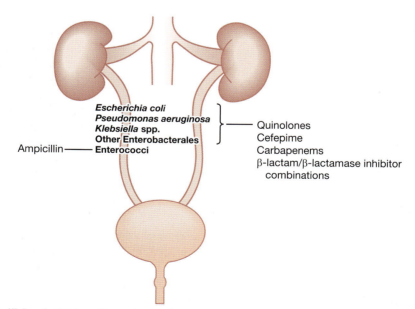

Figure 17-3. Activities of agents used to treat complicated urinary tract infections.

Table 17-2   Empiric Antimicrobial Therapy for Urinary Tract Infections

Antibiotic Class	Antibiotic
Uncomplicated acute cystitis	
Nitrofurantoin	
Oral trimethoprim-sulfamethoxazole	
Fosfomycin	
Uncomplicated acute pyelonephritis	
Quinolones	Ciprofloxacin, levofloxacin
β-lactam/β-lactamase inhibitor	Piperacillin-tazobactam
Third-generation cephalosporins	Ceftriaxone
Carbapenem	Meropenem, imipenem, ertapenem
Complicated urinary tract infections	
Quinolones	Ciprofloxacin, levofloxacin
Fourth-generation cephalosporins	Cefepime
Carbapenems	Imipenem, meropenem
β-lactam/β-lactamase inhibitor	Piperacillin/tazobactam
If gram-positive bacteria are seen in urine, add	
Aminopenicillin	Ampicillin, amoxicillin

treat pyelonephritis-associated bacteremia and because the consequences of inappropriate treatment of resistant organisms with trimethoprim-sulfamethoxazole are more severe with pyelonephritis. Recommended treatment regimens depend on the severity of the disease, with oral agents being used for mild disease and intravenous therapy for severe disease (see Table 17-2). For mild disease, oral quinolones (**ciprofloxacin**, **levofloxacin**) are often used empirically, although resistance and safety are now concerns. Therapy for severe disease is with a quinolone (**ciprofloxacin**, **levofloxacin**), a β-lactam/β-lactamase inhibitor combination (**piperacillin-tazobactam**), a third-generation cephalosporin (**ceftriaxone**), or a carbapenem (**imipenem, meropenem, ertapenem**). Antimicrobial treatment for acute pyelonephritis should be continued for 7 to 10 days. Note that moxifloxacin is not approved for use in the treatment of UTIs.

Antibiotic therapy for complicated UTIs must be effective against the more resistant organisms that sometimes cause these infections (see Figure 17-3 and Table 17-2). Typical regimens include a quinolone (**ciprofloxacin**, **levofloxacin**), **cefepime**, an antipseudomonal carbapenem (**imipenem, meropenem**), or β-lactam/β-lactamase inhibitor combination (**piperacillin/tazobactam**). If gram-positive bacteria are seen on Gram stain of the urine (suggesting the presence of enterococci), **ampicillin** or **amoxicillin** should be added. Treatment is usually continued for 7 to 10 days or longer.

QUESTIONS

1. The most common cause of uncomplicated acute cystitis is _____.
2. Recommended empiric antibiotic therapy for acute cystitis in a young healthy woman who is not pregnant is _____, _____, or _____.
3. If gram-positive bacteria are seen in the urine of a patient with a complicated UTI, one must be concerned about _____ as the etiologic organism.
4. Patients with diabetes, with structural abnormalities of their urinary systems, who acquired their infection in the hospital, or who have other conditions that predispose to infection by a broader range of bacteria, are said to have _____ UTIs.
5. Antibiotic treatment of complicated UTIs is with _____, _____, _____, or _____.

ANSWERS

1. E. coli
2. nitrofurantoin, trimethoprim-sulfamethoxazole, fosfomycin
3. enterococci
4. complicated
5. cefepime, quinolone, β-lactam/β-lactamase inhibitor combination, carbapenem

ADDITIONAL READINGS

Bagshaw SM, Laupland KB. Epidemiology of intensive care unit-acquired urinary tract infections. *Curr Opin Infect Dis.* 2006;19:67-71.

Barber AE, Norton JP, Spivak AM, et al. Urinary tract infections: current and emerging management strategies. *Clin Infect Dis.* 2013;57:719-724.

Gupta K, Hooton TM, Naber KG, et al. International clinical practice guidelines for the treatment of acute uncomplicated cystitis and pyelonephritis in women: a 2010 update by the Infectious Diseases Society of America and the European Society for Microbiology and Infectious Diseases. *Clin Infect Dis.* 2011;52:e103-e120.

Hooton TM. Clinical practice: uncomplicated urinary tract infection. *N Engl J Med.* 2012;366:1028-1037.

Rubenstein JN, Schaeffer AJ. Managing complicated urinary tract infections: the urologic view. *Infect Dis Clin North Am.* 2003;17:333-351.

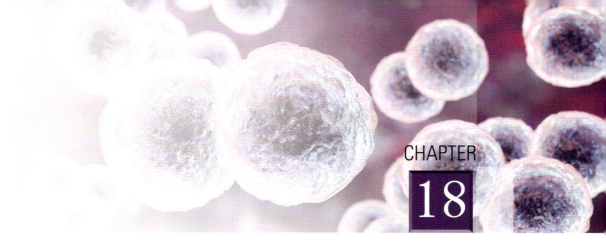

CHAPTER 18

Pelvic Inflammatory Disease

Pelvic inflammatory disease (PID) is the unfortunate consequence of the failure of successive barriers of the female reproductive system to check the invasion of sexually transmitted microbes. In PID, bacteria migrate from the cervix into the uterus and subsequently to the fallopian tubes, ovaries, and peritoneal cavity. Persistent inflammation may lead to abscess formation and scarring of these structures, which predisposes to infertility and ectopic pregnancy.

The patient with PID typically presents with abnormal bleeding, dyspareunia, vaginal discharge, lower abdominal pain, fever, and chills. Physical examination is often remarkable for fever, abnormal cervical or vaginal mucopurulent discharge, uterine or adnexal tenderness, and cervical motion tenderness. Laboratory examination may show an elevated peripheral white blood cell count, the presence of white blood cells in vaginal secretions, and elevated erythrocyte sedimentation rate and C-reactive protein measurements.

The pathogenesis of PID involves a complex interaction between sexually transmitted bacteria and normal flora, particularly anaerobes (Table 18-1 and Figure 18-1). As such, it is a polymicrobial infection. The sexually transmitted bacteria that are most often implicated are *Neisseria gonorrhoeae* and *Chlamydia trachomatis*. Components of the vaginal flora frequently isolated from PID lesions include the anaerobic *Bacteroides* and *Peptostreptococcus* spp. as well as facultative anaerobic bacteria such as *Escherichia coli*,

Table 18-1 Bacterial Causes of Pelvic Inflammatory Disease

Bacteria	Incidence (%)
Neisseria gonorrhoeae	27-56
Chlamydia trachomatis	22-31
Anaerobic and facultative anaerobic bacteria	20-78

From Jossens MO, Schachter J, Sweet RL. Risk factors associated with pelvic inflammatory disease of differing microbial etiologies. *Obstet Gynecol*. 1994;83:989-997; Sweet RL. Role of bacterial vaginosis in pelvic inflammatory disease. *Clin Infect Dis*. 1995;20(suppl 2):S271-S275.

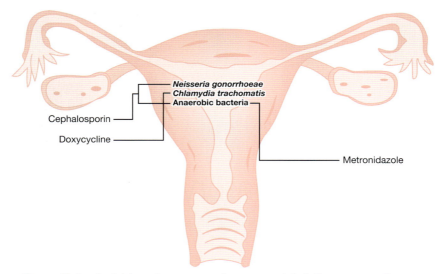

Figure 18-1. Activities of agents used to treat pelvic inflammatory disease.

Gardnerella vaginalis, *Haemophilus influenzae*, and group B streptococci. Currently, the extent to which each of these contributes to the progression of PID is unclear.

Empiric treatment of PID must take into account the spectrum of organisms that contribute to this infection as well as the severity of illness (Table 18-2 and Figure 18-1). All regimens should be effective against *N. gonorrhoeae* and *C. trachomatis*. Currently, the role of anaerobic bacteria in PID is controversial, but many experts

Table 18-2	Empiric Antimicrobial Therapy for Pelvic Inflammatory Disease
Mild-to-moderate disease	
Single IM dose of cephalosporin	Ceftriaxone, cefoxitin plus probenecid, cefotaxime
+ Oral doxycycline	
± Oral metronidazole	
Severe disease[a]	
Ceftriaxone	
+ Oral doxycycline	
+ Oral metronidazole	
or	
Cephalosporin	Cefotetan, cefoxitin
+ Oral doxycycline	

IM, intramuscular.
[a]Twenty-four to 48 hours after clinical improvement, intravenous antibiotics may be discontinued, and a total 14-day course of therapy completed with oral doxycycline combined with oral metronidazole.

feel that therapy should also be directed against these organisms. Individuals who have only mild-to-moderate disease should be treated as outpatients with oral antibiotics. Recommended regimens include a single intramuscular dose of a cephalosporin (eg, **ceftriaxone, cefoxitin** plus probenecid, **cefotaxime**) along with a 14-day course of oral doxycycline with or without **metronidazole**. (Concurrent administration of probenecid with cefoxitin delays excretion of this antibiotic, prolonging therapeutic serum levels.) Those who are severely ill should be admitted to the hospital and treated initially with intravenous agents. Common initial regimens include (1) **ceftriaxone** plus oral **doxycycline** plus oral **metronidazole** or (2) a cephalosporin with anaerobic activity (eg, **cefotetan, cefoxitin**) plus oral **doxycycline**. Intravenous antibiotics can be discontinued 24 to 48 hours after patients show clinical improvement and a total course of 14 days of therapy completed with oral doxycycline combined with oral metronidazole.

QUESTIONS

1. Antibiotic treatment of PID should include agents with activity against sexually transmitted bacteria such as _____ and _____ and perhaps also _____ bacteria.
2. The treatment regimen for mild PID is a single intramuscular dose of a _____ plus _____ with or without _____.
3. Two initial treatment regimens for severe PID are (1) _____ plus oral doxycycline plus oral metronidazole and (2) a _____ with anaerobic activity plus oral _____.
4. In the PID antibiotic regimen consisting of cefotetan plus doxycycline, cefotetan is effective against _____ as well as _____ bacteria, whereas doxycycline is effective against _____.

ANSWERS

1. *N. gonorrhoeae, C. trachomatis*, anaerobic
2. cephalosporin, doxycycline, metronidazole
3. ceftriaxone, cephalosporin, doxycycline
4. *N. gonorrhoeae*, anaerobic, *C. trachomatis*

ADDITIONAL READINGS

Brunham RC, Gottlieb SL, Paavonen J. Pelvic inflammatory disease. *N Engl J Med.* 2015;372: 2039-2048.
Bugg CW, Taira T. Pelvic inflammatory disease: diagnosis and treatment in the emergency department. *Emerg Med Pract.* 2016;18:1-24.
Ross JD. Pelvic inflammatory disease: how should it be managed? *Curr Opin Infect Dis.* 2003;16:37-41.
Workowski KA, Bachmann LH, Chan PA, et al. Sexually transmitted infections treatment guidelines, 2021. *MMWR Recomm Rep.* 2021;70:1-187.

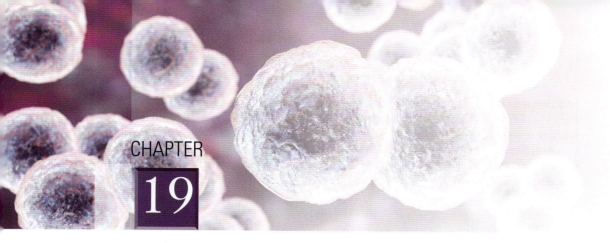

CHAPTER 19

Meningitis

The overwhelming pathogenic potential of bacteria is arguably most apparent in acute bacterial meningitis. This illness often evolves rapidly and is uniformly fatal in the absence of antimicrobial therapy. Even with modern medicine's sophisticated diagnostic techniques and array of highly potent antibiotics, approximately one in four adults with acute bacterial meningitis die. Obviously, there is little margin for error in choosing appropriate antibiotic therapy for this disease.

Individuals with acute bacterial meningitis present with headache, fever, neck stiffness, altered mental status, photophobia, nausea, vomiting, and seizures. Physical examination is often remarkable for nuchal rigidity and sometimes for neurologic deficits. Of critical diagnostic importance is examination of the cerebrospinal fluid (CSF). Patients with bacterial meningitis will have an elevated white blood cell count and protein concentration with a decreased glucose level in their CSF. In addition, bacteria are often visualized by Gram stain in a specimen of this fluid.

The typical bacterial causes of acute meningitis vary with the age of the patient (Table 19-1). In neonates, *Streptococcus agalactiae* and *Escherichia coli* predominate. Now that the *Haemophilus influenzae* type B vaccine is widely used, *Streptococcus pneumoniae*

Table 19-1	Bacterial Causes of Acute Bacterial Meningitis
Bacterium	Incidence (%)
Streptococcus pneumoniae	58-72
Streptococcus agalactiae	1-18
Neisseria meningitidis	11-14
Haemophilus influenzae	3-7
Listeria monocytogenes	3-5

From Thigpen MC, Whitney CG, Messonnier NE, et al. Bacterial meningitis in the United States, 1998–2007. *N Engl J Med.* 2011;364:2016-2025; From Bijlsma MW, Brouwer MC, Kasanmoentalib ES, et al. Community-acquired bacterial meningitis in adults in the Netherlands, 2006-14: a prospective cohort study. *Lancet Infect Dis.* 2016;16:339-347.

and *Neisseria meningitidis* have become the most common bacteria isolated from small children. *N. meningitidis* is the major cause of acute bacterial meningitis in older children and young adults, whereas *S. pneumoniae* is seen with the greatest frequency in older adults. In a minority of the very young, of older individuals, and of those who are immunocompromised, *Listeria monocytogenes* will be identified as the cause of acute bacterial meningitis. Aerobic gram-negative bacilli are also a concern in older individuals.

An understanding of the pathogenesis of acute bacterial meningitis aids one in choosing appropriate therapy. In this disease, bacteria multiply in the CSF, which often lacks antibodies and complement. Because of these deficiencies in the immune response, many experts feel that antibiotics that merely inhibit bacterial growth (ie, those that are bacteriostatic) are not optimal. Rather, antibiotics that actually kill the bacteria (ie, have bactericidal activity) provide the greatest chance of sterilizing the CSF. In addition, antibiotics must efficiently cross the blood-brain barrier to reach the CSF in concentrations sufficient for killing. As a result, many antibiotics are administered at higher doses to patients with meningitis relative to patients with other infections. Finally, a significant portion of the tissue damage associated with bacterial meningitis is thought to result from the inflammation provoked by the large numbers of bacteria in the CSF and meninges; this inflammatory response may be enhanced by the rapid lysis of these bacteria when they are initially exposed to bactericidal antibiotics. For this reason, some experts recommend the concomitant administration of corticosteroids with antimicrobial agents in specific situations.

In the absence of a diagnostic Gram stain of CSF, antimicrobial therapy for acute bacterial meningitis must be empiric (Table 19-2 and Figure 19-1). Third-generation cephalosporins (**ceftriaxone, cefotaxime**) are the backbone of most empiric antimicrobial regimens because they are bactericidal, penetrate relatively well into the CSF,

Table 19-2. Empiric Antimicrobial Therapy for Acute Bacterial Meningitis (Nondiagnostic or Delayed Gram Stain of Cerebrospinal Fluid)

Antibiotic Class	Antibiotic
Third-generation cephalosporin`	Ceftriaxone, cefotaxime
plus	
Glycopeptide	Vancomycin
If patient <3 mo or >50 y of age	
Add aminopenicillin	Ampicillin
If patient compromised	
Glycopeptide	Vancomycin
plus	
Cephalosporin	Cefepime
with or without	
Aminopenicillin	Ampicillin

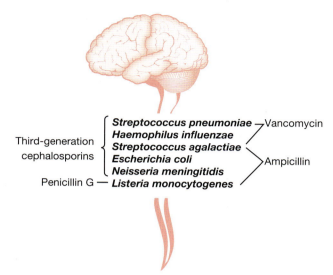

Figure 19-1. Activities of agents used to treat acute bacterial meningitis.

and are effective against most strains of *S. pneumoniae*, *N. meningitidis*, and *H. influenzae*. However, some *S. pneumoniae* strains are resistant to cephalosporins. Although cephalosporins achieve high levels in the lungs and are effective therapy for pneumonia caused by all but the most resistant strains, they fail to reach levels sufficient for killing of moderately resistant strains in the CSF. Thus, it is recommended that **vancomycin** be used in conjunction with a third-generation cephalosporin as empiric therapy for acute bacterial meningitis. **Ampicillin** is often added in infants younger than 3 months of age and in adults older than 50 years to provide coverage of *L. monocytogenes* and *S. agalactiae*. (Note that *L. monocytogenes* is one of the few gram-positive bacteria against which vancomycin is not effective—hence, the need for ampicillin.) In compromised patients, such as those who develop meningitis following neurosurgery, have CSF shunts, or recently received high doses of steroids, treatment should be broadened to cover staphylococci and antibiotic-resistant gram-negative bacilli.

In infants younger than 3 months of age, the Gram stain CSF findings are not often diagnostic, and these patients should all receive at least a third-generation cephalosporin plus vancomycin until culture results are available. Some experts suggest also giving ampicillin to empirically cover for *L. monocytogenes*. However, in adults, the results of a Gram stain specimen of CSF should guide the initial choice of antibiotics for acute bacterial meningitis. Because of the requirement for bactericidal activity and efficient penetration into the CSF, only a subset of potentially useful antibiotics is suitable for treating meningitis (Table 19-3). Gram-positive cocci in pairs in the CSF of an adult patient suggest *S. pneumoniae*, which should be treated with a third-generation cephalosporin (**ceftriaxone, cefotaxime**) plus **vancomycin** to ensure effective therapy against penicillin-resistant strains. In contrast, gram-positive cocci in a specimen from an infant younger than 3 months of age suggest *S. agalactiae*, for which **penicillin G** or **ampicillin** should be given. Some experts suggest also adding gentamicin. Gram-negative diplococci indicate *N. meningitidis*, which is usually treated with **ceftriaxone** or **cefotaxime**. Small pleomorphic gram-negative bacilli are consistent

Table 19-3	Specific Antimicrobial Therapy for Acute Bacterial Meningitis (Based on Gram Stain of Cerebrospinal Fluid)
Antibiotic Class	**Antibiotic**
Streptococcus pneumoniae	
Third-generation cephalosporin	Ceftriaxone, cefotaxime
plus	
Glycopeptide	Vancomycin
Neisseria meningitidis	
Third-generation cephalosporin	Ceftriaxone, cefotaxime
Haemophilus influenzae	
Third-generation cephalosporin	Ceftriaxone, cefotaxime
Listeria monocytogenes	
Natural penicillin	Penicillin G
or	
Aminopenicillin	Ampicillin
with or without	
Aminoglycoside	Gentamicin
Streptococcus agalactiae	
Aminopenicillin	Ampicillin
with or without	
Aminoglycoside	Gentamicin
Escherichia coli	
Third-generation cephalosporin	Ceftriaxone, cefotaxime

with *H. influenzae*, which is treated with a third-generation cephalosporin (**ceftriaxone**, **cefotaxime**). Larger gram-negative bacilli, especially in a neonate, suggest *E. coli*, which is treated with a third-generation cephalosporin (**ceftriaxone**, **cefotaxime**). Gram-positive bacilli suggest *L. monocytogenes* and require the use of **penicillin G** or **ampicillin**. Some experts would also add **gentamicin** for synergistic killing. In all cases, therapy should be adjusted accordingly once susceptibility results are available.

QUESTIONS

1. In adults, the most common bacterial causes of acute meningitis are _____, _____, and _____.
2. Appropriate empiric therapy for a 65-year-old patient with acute bacterial meningitis and a nondiagnostic Gram stain specimen of the CSF is a _____ plus _____ plus _____.
3. Appropriate therapy for a 19-year-old college student with acute meningitis and gram-negative diplococci in her CSF is a _____.

4. Appropriate therapy for a 2-month-old infant with acute meningitis and *S. agalactiae* growing from her CSF sample is _____. Some experts would also add _____.

ANSWERS

1. *S. pneumoniae, N. meningitidis, L. monocytogenes*
2. third-generation cephalosporin, vancomycin, ampicillin
3. third-generation cephalosporin
4. ampicillin, gentamicin

ADDITIONAL READINGS

Brouwer MC, McIntyre P, de Gans J, et al. Corticosteroids for acute bacterial meningitis. *Cochrane Database Syst Rev.* 2010;(9):CD004405.

Brouwer MC, Tunkel AR, van de Beek D. Epidemiology, diagnosis, and antimicrobial treatment of acute bacterial meningitis. *Clin Microbiol Rev.* 2010;23:467-492.

Tunkel AR, Hartman BJ, Kaplan SL, et al. Practice guidelines for the management of bacterial meningitis. *Clin Infect Dis.* 2004;39:1267-1284.

van de Beek D, Brouwer M, Hasbun R, et al. Community-acquired bacterial meningitis. *Nat Rev Dis Primer.* 2016;2:16074.

van Ettekoven CN, van de Beek D, Brouwer MC. Update on community-acquired bacterial meningitis: guidance and challenges. *Clin Microbiol Infect.* 2017;23:601-606.

CHAPTER 20

Cellulitis

Just as medieval castles had formidable walls designed to keep attackers out, our bodies are covered with a protective layer of skin that is deceptively effective in preventing bacteria from gaining access to the vulnerable deeper tissues. That our surrounding environment is filled with microorganisms held at bay by this barrier is evidenced by the high rates of infections associated with breaches in our skin, such as burn injuries or surgical wounds. One common type of infection that occurs when bacteria gain access to the dermis and subcutaneous tissues under the skin is cellulitis.

Individuals with cellulitis usually present with fever and local findings, such as a tender, warm, erythematous, swollen, and indurated area of skin, often surrounding the wound or abrasion that served as the portal of entry. In some cases, the disease may be severe, and signs of systemic toxicity including tachycardia and hypotension may be present.

The bacterial etiology of cellulitis depends on the location of the infection and any special exposures associated with its cause. For example, cellulitis following exposure to salt water suggests *Vibrio vulnificus* as an etiology. Cellulitis associated with foot ulcers in patients with diabetes is caused by a mixture of aerobic gram-positive, aerobic gram-negative, and anaerobic bacteria. However, most cellulitis cases in immunocompetent hosts result from inoculation of skin organisms through breaks or disruption in the epidermis. Thus, uncomplicated cellulitis in an immunocompetent patient without a history of unusual exposures is usually caused by *Staphylococcus aureus*, *Streptococcus pyogenes*, or other streptococci (Table 20-1). In cellulitis associated with pustules, abscesses, or purulent drainage, *S. aureus* is more likely.

Because it is difficult to determine the specific bacterial etiology of cellulitis in individual patients, treatment is usually empiric and consists of agents with potent activity against gram-positive bacteria (Table 20-2 and Figure 20-1). The increasing resistance of *S. aureus* and *S. pyogenes* to antibiotics, however, has complicated treatment choices. In general, severe infections should be treated in the hospital with intravenous antibiotics, whereas mild-to-moderate infections may be treated with oral antibiotics in the outpatient setting. If the likelihood of methicillin-resistant *S. aureus* (MRSA) is low, suitable choices for parenteral therapy include antistaphylococcal penicillins (**nafcillin**, **oxacillin**) and first-generation cephalosporins (**cefazolin**). Oral

Table 20-1	Bacterial Causes of Cellulitis
Bacterium	Incidence (%)
Staphylococcus aureus	13-37
Streptococcus pyogenes	4-17
Other streptococci	1-8

From Duvanel T, Auckenthaler R, Rohner P, et al. Quantitative cultures of biopsy specimens from cutaneous cellulitis. *Arch Intern Med*. 1989;149:293-296; Hook EW 3rd, Hooton TM, Hortoon CA, et al. Microbiologic evaluation of cutaneous cellulitis in adults. *Arch Intern Med*. 1986;146:295-297; Kielhofner MA, Brown B, Dall L. Influence of underlying disease process on the utility of cellulitis needle aspirates. *Arch Intern Med*. 1988;148:2451-2452; Sigurdsson AF, Gudmundsson S. The etiology of bacterial cellulitis as determined by fine-needle aspiration. *Scand J Infect Dis*. 1989;21:537-542.

agents include **dicloxacillin** and first-generation cephalosporins (**cephalexin**); **clindamycin**, **doxycycline**, and **trimethoprim-sulfamethoxazole** can also be used. When risk factors for MRSA are present (eg, previous MRSA infection, injection drug use), common parenteral options include **vancomycin** and **daptomycin**. Alternative agents include other glycopeptides (**telavancin, dalbavancin, oritavancin**), oxazolidinones

Table 20-2	Empiric Antimicrobial Therapy for Cellulitis
Antibiotic Class	Antibiotic
If methicillin-resistant *Staphylococcus aureus* is not suspected	
Antistaphylococcal penicillins	Dicloxacillin, nafcillin, oxacillin
First-generation cephalosporins	Cephalexin, cefazolin
Clindamycin	
Tetracyclines	Doxycycline
Sulfa drugs	Trimethoprim-sulfamethoxazole
If methicillin-resistant *S. aureus* is suspected	
Tetracyclines	Doxycycline, omadacycline
Clindamycin	
Sulfa drugs	Trimethoprim-sulfamethoxazole
Oxazolidinones	Linezolid, tedizolid
Glycopeptides	Vancomycin, telavancin, dalbavancin, oritavancin
Daptomycin	
Fifth-generation cephalosporins	Ceftaroline
Quinolones	Delafloxacin
If severely compromised	
Vancomycin plus cefepime	
Vancomycin plus either imipenem or meropenem	

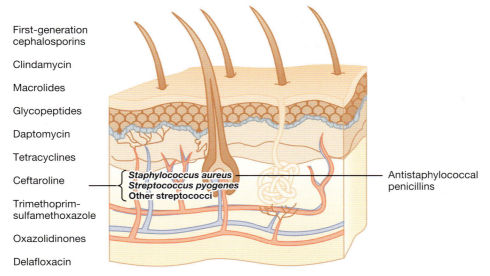

Figure 20-1. Activities of agents used to treat cellulitis.

(**linezolid**, **tedizolid**), **ceftaroline**, **delafloxacin**, and **omadacycline**. **Trimethoprim-sulfamethoxazole**, oxazolidinones (**linezolid**, **tedizolid**), and **clindamycin** are oral agents that can be considered. In severely compromised patients, gram-negative bacteria are also a concern, and broad empiric coverage is recommended (eg, **vancomycin** plus **cefepime** or **vancomycin** plus either **imipenem** or **meropenem**). In all situations, the actual choice should be guided by local resistance patterns.

QUESTIONS

1. In immunocompetent individuals without unusual exposures, the most common causes of cellulitis are _____, _____, and other _____.
2. Appropriate empiric oral therapy for an otherwise healthy 48-year-old roofer, who develops cellulitis on his arm at the site of an abrasion, who is not seriously ill, and who is at low risk for MRSA would be _____, _____, a _____-generation cephalosporin, _____, or _____.
3. In a patient at low risk for MRSA, appropriate parental therapy for cellulitis would be _____, _____, or _____.
4. Appropriate therapy for a 72-year-old woman known to be colonized with MRSA and who is now hypotensive and has cellulitis involving her left leg at the site where a saphenous vein had been harvested several years earlier would be _____ or _____.

ANSWERS

1. *S. aureus*, *S. pyogenes*, streptococci
2. dicloxacillin, clindamycin, first, doxycycline, trimethoprim-sulfamethoxazole

3. nafcillin, oxacillin, cefazolin
4. vancomycin, daptomycin

ADDITIONAL READINGS

Dryden MS. Complicated skin and soft tissue infection. *J Antimicrob Chemother.* 2010;65(suppl 3):iii35-iii44.

Stevens DL, Bisno AL, Chambers HF, et al. Practice guidelines for the diagnosis and management of skin and soft tissue infections: 2014 update by the Infectious Diseases Society of America. *Clin Infect Dis.* 2014;59:e10-e52.

Swartz MN. Clinical practice. Cellulitis. *N Engl J Med.* 2004;350:904-912.

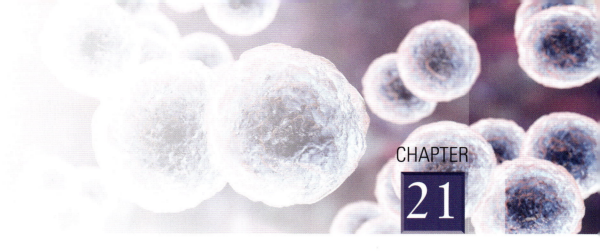

CHAPTER 21

Otitis Media

Among children in the United States, acute otitis media is the most common illness for which antibacterial agents are prescribed. The pathogenesis of this infection reflects the continuity of the middle ear with the upper respiratory tract via the eustachian tube. Typically, an antecedent event such as an upper respiratory infection or allergies causes congestion of the respiratory mucosa and blockage of the eustachian tube. As a result, fluid accumulates in the middle ear and subsequently becomes infected by organisms of the upper respiratory tract.

Children with acute otitis media may present with the rapid onset of otalgia (ear pain), hearing loss, irritability, anorexia, apathy, fever, swelling around the ear, and otorrhea (discharge from the affected ear). On otoscopic examination, findings include middle ear effusion and inflammatory changes.

Because the fluid of the middle ear is seeded by organisms of the upper respiratory tract, it is not surprising that the bacteria that commonly cause acute otitis media are *Streptococcus pneumoniae*, *Haemophilus influenzae*, and *Moraxella catarrhalis* (Table 21-1). Each of these bacteria has a mechanism by which it resists the action of penicillin. An increasing number of *S. pneumoniae* strains produce altered penicillin-binding proteins (PBPs) that do not bind penicillins. Approximately one-third to one-half of *H. influenzae* strains that cause acute otitis media produce β-lactamases, as do nearly all strains of *M. catarrhalis*. These mechanisms must be taken into account when treating acute otitis media.

Table 21-1	Bacterial Causes of Acute Otitis Media
Bacteria	**Incidence (%)**
Streptococcus pneumoniae	25-50
Haemophilus influenzae	15-32
Moraxella catarrhalis	3-63

From Klein JO. Otitis media. *Clin Infect Dis*. 1994;19:823-833; Pettigrew MM, Gent JF, Revai K, et al. Microbial interactions during upper respiratory tract infections. *Emerg Infect Dis*. 2008;14:1584-1591.

Table 21-2. Empiric Antimicrobial Therapy for Acute Otitis Media

Antibiotic Class	Antibiotic
First-line therapy	
Aminopenicillin	High-dose amoxicillin
If risk factors for amoxicillin resistance	
Penicillin/β-lactamase inhibitor	Amoxicillin/clavulanate
If mild allergy to penicillin	
Oral cephalosporin	Cefdinir, cefpodoxime, cefuroxime
IV or IM cephalosporin	Ceftriaxone
If type I hypersensitivity allergic reaction	
Macrolide	Azithromycin, clarithromycin
Clindamycin	

IM, intramuscular; IV, intravenous.

Currently, controversy exists regarding whether all children with acute otitis media should receive antimicrobial therapy. Some experts feel that children aged 2 years and above without severe symptoms at presentation may be treated symptomatically for 48 to 72 hours. If improvement occurs, these children may not require antibiotics. Other experts suggest that all children with acute otitis media should receive antibiotics. When treatment is indicated, it is empiric because cultures of middle ear fluid are infrequently obtained in uncomplicated acute otitis media.

High-dose **amoxicillin** is first-line therapy for acute otitis media (Table 21-2 and Figure 21-1). At first glance, this agent appears to be an odd choice for the treatment of an infection caused by bacteria that are often penicillin resistant. When given in high doses, however, amoxicillin achieves levels in the middle ear fluid that exceed the minimal inhibitory concentrations of all but the most highly penicillin-resistant *S. pneumoniae* strains. Although many strains of *H. influenzae* and *M. catarrhalis* produce β-lactamases that degrade amoxicillin, clinical studies have demonstrated resolution in many cases of amoxicillin-treated otitis media caused by these two pathogens.

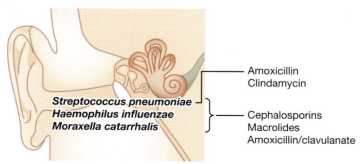

Figure 21-1. Activities of agents used to treat otitis media.

Some experts recommend that patients at risk for infection caused by amoxicillin-resistant bacteria (eg, children recently treated with β-lactam antibiotics; children with purulent conjunctivitis, which is usually caused by β-lactam–resistant *H. influenzae*) be treated with high-dose **amoxicillin/clavulanate**. In patients who have mild (non–type I hypersensitivity) allergic responses to amoxicillin, cephalosporins (oral **cefdinir**, **cefpodoxime**, **cefuroxime**, or intramuscular/intravenous **ceftriaxone**) may be used. In those with type I hypersensitivity reactions (urticaria or anaphylaxis) to penicillins, macrolides (**azithromycin**, **clarithromycin**) or **clindamycin** may be used.

History

Antibiotics such as amoxicillin are used so commonly today that we have grown accustomed to their healing power. In contrast, health care providers who witnessed the early injections of penicillin were astounded by what they saw. Charles Grossman's description of the first person in the United States to be treated with penicillin is such an example. The patient was a severely ill 33-year-old woman who was dying of β-hemolytic streptococcal bacteremia (most likely *Streptococcus pyogenes*) in 1941. She had fevers of 103 to 106°F for 4 weeks. Fortunately, her physician was also treating Dr John F. Fulton. Dr Fulton was a friend of Dr Howard Florey, who had pioneered the use of penicillin in Great Britain. In fact, Dr Florey's children were staying in the Fulton household to avoid the bombing of London. Dr Fulton and his associates were able to use their influence to obtain a small quantity of penicillin, and treatment of the patient was begun on a Saturday. Already by Monday, the patient was improving and "eating hearty meals." She recovered and lived to the age of 90 years.

From Grossman CM. The first use of penicillin in the United States. *Ann Intern Med*. 2008;149:135-136.

Questions

1. The most common bacterial causes of acute otitis media are _____, _____, and _____.
2. The antibiotic treatment of choice for acute otitis media is high-dose _____.
3. Amoxicillin is thought to be effective against penicillin-resistant _____ because at high doses, it achieves levels in the middle ear fluid that exceed the minimal inhibitory concentrations of all but the most highly penicillin-resistant strains.
4. You are asked to prescribe antibiotic therapy for a penicillin-allergic 5-year-old girl with acute otitis media who has failed to improve after 72 hours without antibiotics. Her mother states that the last time she received penicillin, she developed urticaria. Appropriate antibiotic therapies would be a _____ or _____.

Answers

1. *S. pneumoniae, H. influenzae, M. catarrhalis*
2. amoxicillin

3. *S. pneumoniae*

4. macrolide, clindamycin

ADDITIONAL READINGS

El Feghaly RE, Nedved A, Katz SE, et al. New insights into the treatment of acute otitis media. *Exp Rev Anti Infect Ther.* 2023;21:523-534.

Klein JO. Is acute otitis media a treatable disease? *N Engl J Med.* 2011;364:168-169.

Lieberthal AS, Carroll AE, Chonmaitree T, et al. The diagnosis and management of acute otitis media. *Pediatrics.* 2013;131:e964-e999.

Paradise JL. A 15-month-old child with recurrent otitis media. *JAMA.* 2002;288:2589-2598.

Venekamp RP, Damoiseaux RA, Schilder AG. Acute otitis media in children. *Am Fam Physician.* 2017;95:109-110.

Venekamp RP, Sanders SL, Glasziou PP, Rovers MM. Antibiotics for acute otitis media in children. *Cochrane Database Syst Rev.* 2023;11:CD000219. doi:10.1002/14651858.CD000219.pub5

CHAPTER 22

Infective Endocarditis

It has long been asserted that the heart is the most important organ in the human body. Our language is full of clichés that reflect this, for example, "get to the heart of the matter" and "heart-to-heart talk." If the heart falters for even a few minutes, life ceases. For this reason, a microbial attack on the heart has dire consequences. Such attacks may take the form of infective endocarditis, an infection of the endocardial surface of the heart, particularly the heart valves.

The etiology of infective endocarditis is straightforward. Typically, bacteria gain access to the bloodstream by various mechanisms, including inoculation during dental procedures, via a colonized intravenous catheter, or from injection of illicit drugs. The bacteria then attach to the surface of a heart valve, usually at a site of disrupted endothelium from anomalous blood flow patterns. Such patterns are often the consequence of valvular abnormalities caused by rheumatic fever or congenital defects. Vegetations—masses of fibrin, platelets, and bacteria attached to the endocardium—form at the site of infection and provide a protected haven for the multiplication and persistence of bacteria. The result of this process is the gradual destruction of the heart valve.

Although infective endocarditis has been recognized as a disease entity since the 1500s, its diagnosis remains difficult. Patients present with nonspecific complaints such as fatigue, malaise, weakness, weight loss, fever, chills, night sweats, and dyspnea on exertion. Physical examination findings may also be nonspecific and include fever and hematuria. Signs more suggestive of infective endocarditis include Osler nodes, Janeway lesions, Roth spots, and splinter hemorrhages, but these are less common. One clear clue to the presence of infective endocarditis is a new heart murmur, which should make the attentive clinician suspect the diagnosis. Laboratory evaluation may show an elevated erythrocyte sedimentation rate and C-reactive protein level, mild anemia, and an abnormal urinalysis with hematuria, pyuria, or proteinuria.

The most common etiologic agents of infective endocarditis vary somewhat with the population being studied; in general, though, viridans group streptococci, *Staphylococcus aureus*, and enterococci cause most cases of native valve endocarditis, whereas coagulase-negative staphylococci and *S. aureus* are the major pathogens cultured from patients with prosthetic valve endocarditis (Table 22-1). Among the viridans group

Table 22-1	Causes of Bacterial Endocarditis
Bacteria	Incidence (%)
Viridans group streptococci	18-48
Staphylococcus aureus	22-32
Enterococci	7-11
Coagulase-negative staphylococci	7-11
HACEK organisms	2-7

HACEK, *Haemophilus parainfluenzae*, *Aggregatibacter aphrophilus*, *Aggregatibacter actinomycetemcomitans*, *Cardiobacterium hominis*, *Eikenella corrodens*, and *Kingella kingae*.
Data from Fowler VG Jr, Miro JM, Hoen B, et al; for ICE Investigators. Staphylococcus aureus endocarditis: a consequence of medical progress. *JAMA*. 2005;293:3012-3021; Hoen E, Duval X. Clinical practice. Infective endocarditis. *N Engl J Med*. 2013;368:1425-1433; Tleyjeh IM, Steckelberg JM, Murad HS, et al. Temporal trends in infective endocarditis: a population-based study in Olmsted County, Minnesota. *JAMA*. 2005;293:3022-3028.

streptococci, *Streptococcus sanguinis*, *Streptococcus mutans*, and *Streptococcus mitis* are common. A small proportion of endocarditis cases are caused by a relatively obscure group of gram-negative bacilli referred to by the acronym HACEK: ***Haemophilus parainfluenzae***, ***Aggregatibacter aphrophilus***, ***Aggregatibacter actinomycetemcomitans***, ***Cardiobacterium hominis***, ***Eikenella corrodens***, and ***Kingella kingae***.

The protective environment provided by the vegetation makes bacterial endocarditis difficult to treat. Antibiotics must be given in high doses and for prolonged periods. Because the predominant causes of endocarditis are gram-positive bacteria, β-lactam agents are sometimes used with synergistic doses of gentamicin to enhance killing. Even intensive therapy, however, is not always sufficient, and surgical intervention is often required, so management of patients with endocarditis should include surgical consultation. Given the difficulty in treating these infections and the prolonged courses of antibiotics that are required, identifying the causative organism by obtaining multiple blood cultures is critical for defining optimal therapy.

Not infrequently, patients with bacterial endocarditis require antimicrobial therapy prior to the availability of blood culture results or with blood cultures that have been sterilized by prior use of antibiotics. In these situations, infectious disease consultation should be sought and therapy should be focused on the most likely causative organisms, including those for which the individual patient has epidemiologic risks. A typical antibiotic regimen for empiric treatment of native valve endocarditis is **vancomycin** plus **ceftriaxone** (Table 22-2 and Figure 22-1). Vancomycin is effective against *S. aureus* and viridans group streptococci and is active against most enterococcal strains. Ceftriaxone has good activity against viridans group streptococci and HACEK organisms. Empiric treatment of prosthetic valve endocarditis is complex, but one suggested regimen is **vancomycin** plus **cefepime** for optimal coverage of staphylococci as well as gram-negative bacteria. Some experts suggest adding **gentamicin** to this regimen for synergistic killing and **rifampin** to enhance clearance of staphylococci from prosthetic material.

Ideally, blood cultures will eventually yield the bacterium responsible for the infection, allowing more focused treatment of patients with endocarditis. The antibiotic regimens described here not only follow logically from what is known about the

Table 22-2	Examples of Empiric Antimicrobial Regimens for Infective Endocarditis

Native valve endocarditis
Vancomycin
  plus
Ceftriaxone

Prosthetic valve endocarditis
Vancomycin
  plus
Cefepime
  plus
Gentamicin
  plus
Rifampin

Choice of therapy should be guided by the individual's risk factors for specific organisms.

susceptibility of the bacteria that commonly cause infective endocarditis but also have been shown to be efficacious.

Treatment of native valve endocarditis caused by viridans group streptococci depends on the susceptibility of the causative strain to penicillins (Table 22-3; see Figure 22-1). Infections that are caused by highly penicillin-susceptible (minimum inhibitory concentration [MIC] ≤0.12 µg/mL) strains are usually treated with **penicillin G** or **ceftriaxone** for 4 weeks. For viridans group streptococci that have an intermediate level of susceptibility to penicillin (MIC >0.12 and <0.5 µg/mL), **penicillin G** or **ceftriaxone** should be given for 4 weeks along with **gentamicin** for the

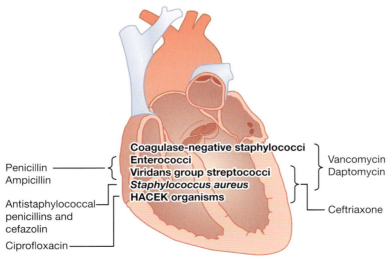

Figure 22-1. Activities of agents used to treat bacterial endocarditis. HACEK, *Haemophilus parainfluenzae*, *Aggregatibacter aphrophilus*, *Aggregatibacter actinomycetemcomitans*, *Cardiobacterium hominis*, *Eikenella corrodens*, and *Kingella kingae*.

Table 22-3. Specific Antimicrobial Therapy for Infective Endocarditis Caused by Viridans Group Streptococci

Antibiotic	Duration (weeks)
Native valve	
Highly penicillin-susceptible strains (MIC ≤0.12 μg/mL)	
Penicillin G or ceftriaxone	4
Intermediate penicillin-resistance strains (MIC >0.12 and <0.5 μg/mL)	
Penicillin G or ceftriaxone	4
+ Gentamicin	2
Highly penicillin-resistant strains (MIC ≥0.5 μg/mL)	
Penicillin G or ampicillin or ceftriaxone	4-6
+ Gentamicin	2-6
Prosthetic valve	
Highly penicillin-susceptible strains (MIC ≤0.12 μg/mL)	
Penicillin G or ceftriaxone	6
± Gentamicin	2
Intermediate or highly penicillin-resistant strains (MIC >0.12 μg/mL)	
Penicillin G or ceftriaxone	6
+ Gentamicin	6

MIC, minimum inhibitory concentration.
In patients who meet specific criteria, intravenous antibiotics may be transitioned to oral antibiotics to complete the course of treatment.

first 2 weeks. Opinions differ on the best antibiotic regimens for infections caused by highly penicillin-resistant (MIC ≥0.5 μg/mL) strains of viridans group streptococci. Some clinicians suggest either **penicillin G** or **ampicillin** for 4 to 6 weeks, in conjunction with **gentamicin** for part or all the duration of therapy. Others recommend **ceftriaxone** in conjunction with **gentamicin**. It is more difficult to eradicate bacteria from prosthetic material than from native valves, so, in prosthetic valve endocarditis, **penicillin G** or **ceftriaxone** is given for 6 weeks instead of 4 weeks. **Gentamicin** is also given for 6 weeks unless the strain is fully susceptible (MIC ≤0.12 μg/mL) to penicillin. In these cases, gentamicin may be given for 2 weeks or not at all. (Note that in patients with endocarditis who meet specific criteria intravenous antibiotics need not be continued for the full duration of therapy. Rather, patients may be transitioned to oral antibiotics to complete the course of treatment.)

Native valve and prosthetic valve endocarditis caused by susceptible enterococci are treated similarly to highly resistant viridans group streptococcal endocarditis (Table 22-4; see Figure 22-1). Either **penicillin G** or **ampicillin** is given for 6 weeks in conjunction with **gentamicin** for 2 to 6 weeks. The gentamicin works synergistically with antibiotics active against the enterococcal cell wall and results in bactericidal activity against this bacterium. Alternatively, **ampicillin** plus **ceftriaxone** can be given

Table 22-4 Specific Antimicrobial Therapy for Infective Endocarditis Caused by Enterococci

Antibiotic	Duration (weeks)
Native valve	
Penicillin- and aminoglycoside-susceptible strains	
Penicillin G or ampicillin	4-6
+ Gentamicin	2-6
Ampicillin	6
+ Ceftriaxone	6
Penicillin-susceptible and aminoglycoside-resistant strains	
Ampicillin	6
+ Ceftriaxone	6
Penicillin-resistant and aminoglycoside-susceptible strains	
Vancomycin	6
+ Gentamicin	2-6
Prosthetic valve	
Penicillin- and aminoglycoside-susceptible strains	
Penicillin G or ampicillin	6
+ Gentamicin	2-6
Ampicillin	6
+ Ceftriaxone	6
Penicillin-susceptible and aminoglycoside-resistant strains	
Ampicillin	6
+ Ceftriaxone	6
Penicillin-resistant and aminoglycoside-susceptible strains	
Vancomycin	6
+ Gentamicin	2-6

Infections caused by highly aminoglycoside-resistant strains should be treated in consultation with an expert. In patients who meet specific criteria, intravenous antibiotics may be transitioned to oral antibiotics to complete the course of treatment.

for 6 weeks. This regimen avoids the toxicity associated with a prolonged course of gentamicin. Infections caused by enterococci resistant to penicillin are treated with **vancomycin** for 6 weeks plus **gentamicin** for 2 to 6 weeks. Treatment of enterococcal endocarditis caused by strains susceptible to penicillin but resistant to aminoglycosides are treated with **ampicillin** plus **ceftriaxone**. Strains resistant to both penicillin and vancomycin are problematic and should be treated in consultation with an expert.

Native valve endocarditis caused by *S. aureus* is treated with **nafcillin, oxacillin,** or **cefazolin** for 6 weeks (Table 22-5; see Figure 22-1). In infections caused by

Table 22-5. Specific Antimicrobial Therapy for Infective Endocarditis Caused by Staphylococci

Antibiotic	Duration (weeks)
Native valve	
Methicillin-susceptible strains	
Nafcillin or oxacillin or cefazolin	6
Methicillin-resistant strains	
Vancomycin	6
Daptomycin	6
Prosthetic valve	
Methicillin-susceptible strains	
Nafcillin or oxacillin or cefazolin	≥6
+ Rifampin	≥6
+ Gentamicin	2
Methicillin-resistant strains	
Vancomycin	≥6
+ Rifampin	≥6
+ Gentamicin	2

In patients who meet specific criteria, intravenous antibiotics may be transitioned to oral antibiotics to complete the course of treatment.

History

Despite appropriate antibiotic therapy, the mortality associated with infective endocarditis remains high (20%-25%). Yet, these statistics are a vast improvement over outcomes in the preantibiotic era, when the diagnosis of infective endocarditis was a death sentence. This was poignantly documented in 1931 by the Harvard medical student Alfred S. Reinhart, who had aortic insufficiency following a bout of rheumatic fever as a child. One night, Reinhart noted the presence of petechiae on his left arm and immediately self-diagnosed infective endocarditis.

"No sooner had I removed the left arm of my coat, than there was on the ventral aspect of my left wrist a sight which I shall never forget until I die. There greeted my eyes about fifteen or twenty bright red, slightly raised, hemorrhagic spots about 1 millimeter in diameter which did not fade on pressure and which stood defiant as if they were challenging the very gods of Olympus.... I took one glance at the pretty little collection of spots and turned to my sister-in-law, who was standing nearby, and calmly said: 'I shall be dead within six months.'"

Used with permission of John Wiley & Sons, from Weiss S. Self-observations and psychological reactions of medical student A. S. R. to the onset and symptoms of subacute bacterial endocarditis. *J Mt Sinai Hosp.* 1942;8:1079-1094; permission conveyed through Copyright Clearance Center, Inc.

Table 22-6. Specific Antimicrobial Therapy for Infective Endocarditis Caused by HACEK Organisms

Antibiotic	Duration (weeks)
Native valve	
Ceftriaxone	4
Ampicillin-sulbactam	4
Ciprofloxacin	4
Prosthetic valve	
Ceftriaxone	6
Ampicillin-sulbactam	6
Ciprofloxacin	6

HACEK, *Haemophilus parainfluenzae*, *Aggregatibacter aphrophilus*, *Aggregatibacter actinomycetemcomitans*, *Cardiobacterium hominis*, *Eikenella corrodens*, and *Kingella kingae*.
In patients who meet specific criteria, intravenous antibiotics may be transitioned to oral antibiotics to complete the course of treatment.

methicillin-resistant *S. aureus* (MRSA), **vancomycin** or **daptomycin** is used in place of antistaphylococcal penicillin. In prosthetic valve endocarditis caused by *S. aureus* or *Staphylococcus epidermidis*, treatment is with **nafcillin**, **oxacillin**, or **cefazolin** in conjunction with **gentamicin** and **rifampin** for methicillin-susceptible strains. Gentamicin acts to synergistically enhance eradication of the bacteria, and rifampin is thought to facilitate clearance of the staphylococci from prosthetic material. In infections caused by strains resistant to antistaphylococcal penicillins, **vancomycin** is substituted for nafcillin, oxacillin, or cefazolin. Nafcillin, oxacillin, cefazolin, or vancomycin is continued for 6 weeks or longer if necessary. Rifampin is continued for 6 weeks, and gentamicin is used for only the first 2 weeks.

Native or prosthetic valve endocarditis caused by one of the HACEK bacteria is treated with **ceftriaxone**, **ampicillin-sulbactam**, or **ciprofloxacin** for 4 to 6 weeks (Table 22-6; see Figure 22-1).

QUESTIONS

1. The three most common bacterial causes of native valve infectious endocarditis are _____, _____, and other _____.
2. The two most common bacterial causes of prosthetic valve infectious endocarditis are _____ and _____.
3. The antibiotics used to treat endocarditis caused by viridans group streptococci with intermediate resistance to penicillin are either _____ or _____ in conjunction with _____.
4. The antibiotics used to treat endocarditis caused by enterococci resistant to penicillin are _____ and _____.

5. The antibiotics used to treat prosthetic valve endocarditis caused by *S. epidermidis* resistant to methicillin are _____ plus _____ plus _____.
6. The antibiotics used to treat native valve endocarditis caused by *S. aureus* susceptible to methicillin are _____, _____, or _____.
7. The antibiotic used to treat endocarditis caused by *E. corrodens* is _____, _____, or _____.

Answers

1. viridans group streptococci, *S. aureus*, enterococci
2. coagulase-negative staphylococci, *S. aureus*
3. penicillin G, ceftriaxone, gentamicin
4. vancomycin, gentamicin
5. vancomycin, rifampin, gentamicin
6. nafcillin, oxacillin, cefazolin
7. ceftriaxone, ampicillin-sulbactam, ciprofloxacin

Additional Readings

Baddour LM, Wilson WR, Bayer AS, et al. Infective endocarditis in adults: diagnosis, antimicrobial therapy, and management of complications: a scientific statement for healthcare professionals from the American Heart Association. *Circulation*. 2015;132:1435-1486.

Delgado V, Marsan NA, de Waha S, et al. 2023 ESC guidelines for the management of endocarditis. *Eur Hear J*. 2023;00:1-95. doi:10.1093/eurheartj/ehad193

Hoen B, Duval X. Clinical practice. Infective endocarditis. *N Engl J Med*. 2013;368:1425-1433.

McDonald EG, Aggrey G, Aslan AT, et al. Guidelines for diagnosis and management of infective endocarditis in adults: a WikiGuidelines group consensus statement. *JAMA Networ Open*. 2023;6(7):e2326366. doi:10.1001/jamanetworkopen.2023.26366

Pannu AK. Optimal empirical antimicrobial therapy in infective endocarditis. *QJM*. 2023;156-157.

CHAPTER 23

Intravascular-Related Catheter Infections

If skin is the human body's equivalent of a castle wall, then intravascular catheters are battering rams that breach this defense, allowing bacteria access to the vulnerable underlying bloodstream. Because intravascular catheters are an essential component of modern hospital care, catheter-related infections are quite common, occurring at a rate of 200,000 per year in the United States. Obviously, recognizing and appropriately treating these infections is crucial.

Diagnosis of intravascular-related catheter infections is problematic in that confirmation usually requires removal and culture of the catheter. Nonetheless, these infections should be suspected in anyone with an intravascular catheter and a fever of unclear etiology. Inflammation or purulence at the exit site of the catheter is specific, but not sensitive, for catheter infections. Growth of bacteria from blood cultures should increase suspicion for these infections.

Most bacterial intravascular-related catheter infections are caused by skin flora that contaminate the catheter during placement or migrate down the catheter after placement. Thus, it is not surprising that coagulase-negative staphylococci (especially *Staphylococcus epidermidis*) and *Staphylococcus aureus* are the pathogens most often associated with catheter infections (Table 23-1). In immunocompromised or severely ill patients, aerobic gram-negative bacilli also cause a significant percentage of these infections.

Empiric treatment of intravascular-related catheter infections is focused on staphylococci. **Vancomycin** has become the agent of choice in many locations (Table 23-2 and Figure 23-1). In regions and hospitals where methicillin-resistant staphylococci are rare, **oxacillin**, **nafcillin**, or **cefazolin** may be used. In severely ill or immunocompromised patients, antibiotics active against aerobic gram-negative bacilli should be added. The choice of these antibiotics should be based on local antibiotic susceptibility data; possible agents include a third- or fourth-generation cephalosporin (**ceftazidime**, **cefepime**), a carbapenem (**meropenem**, **imipenem**), or a penicillin/β-lactamase inhibitor combination (**piperacillin-tazobactam**). Once a causative organism is

Table 23-1. Bacterial Causes of Intravascular-Related Catheter Infections

Bacteria	Incidence (%)
Coagulase-negative staphylococci	32-41
Staphylococcus aureus	5-14
Enteric gram-negative bacilli	5-11
Pseudomonas aeruginosa	4-7

From Haslett TM, Isenberg HD, Hilton E, et al. Microbiology of indwelling central intravascular catheters. *J Clin Microbiol*. 1988;26:696-701; Jarvis WR. Epidemiology and control of Pseudomonas aeruginosa infections in the intensive care unit. In: Hauser AR, Rello J, eds. *Severe Infections Caused by Pseudomonas Aeruginosa*. Kluwer Academic Publishers; 2003:153-168.

Table 23-2. Empiric Antimicrobial Therapy for Intravascular-Related Catheter Infections

Antibiotic Class	Antibiotic
Methicillin resistance uncommon	
Antistaphylococcal penicillin	Nafcillin, oxacillin
Cephalosporin	Cefazolin
Methicillin resistance common	
Glycopeptide	Vancomycin
Immunocompromised or severely ill patient	
Add cephalosporin	Ceftazidime, cefepime
or carbapenem	Meropenem, imipenem
or penicillin/β-lactamase inhibitor	Piperacillin-tazobactam

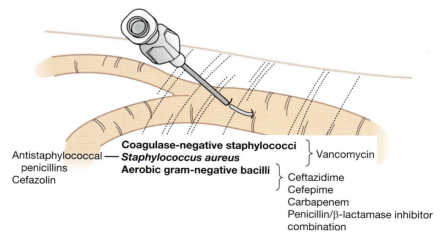

Figure 23-1. Activities of agents used to treat intravascular-related catheter infections.

identified from cultures of blood or the catheter itself, the antibiotic regimen should be focused on the identified bacterium. Antibiotic therapy alone, however, may not be sufficient; catheter removal may be required.

Questions

1. Bacterial pathogens that typically cause intravascular-related catheter infections are _____, _____, and _____.
2. In settings where methicillin-resistant staphylococci are uncommon, _____, _____, and _____ are the empiric antibiotics of choice for these infections.
3. In settings where methicillin-resistant staphylococci are common, _____ is the empiric antibiotic of choice for these infections.
4. In immunocompromised or severely ill patients, an agent with activity against aerobic _____ should be added.

Answers

1. coagulase-negative staphylococci, *S. aureus*, aerobic gram-negative bacilli
2. nafcillin, oxacillin, cefazolin
3. vancomycin
4. gram-negative bacilli

Additional Readings

Fätkenheuer G, Cornely O, Seifert H. Clinical management of catheter-related infections. *Clin Microbiol Infect.* 2002;8:545-550.

Lorente L, Martín MM, Vidal P, et al. Should central venous catheter be systematically removed in patients with suspected catheter related infection? *Crit Care.* 2014;18:564. doi:10.1186/s13054-014-0564-3

Mermel LA, Allon M, Bouza E, et al. Clinical practice guidelines for the diagnosis and management of intravascular catheter-related infection: 2009 update by the Infectious Diseases Society of America. *Clin Infect Dis.* 2009;49:1-45.

Timsit JF, Baleine J, Bernard L, et al. Expert consensus-based clinical practice guidelines management of intravascular catheters in the intensive care unit. *Ann Intensive Care.* 2020;10:118. doi:10.1186/s13613-020-00713-4

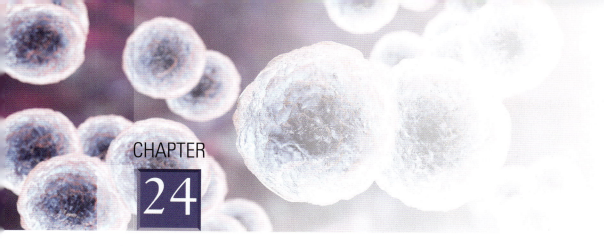

CHAPTER 24

Intra-abdominal Infections

Intra-abdominal infections include peritonitis, biliary tract infections, splenic abscesses, appendicitis, diverticulitis, and infections following loss of bowel integrity from trauma or surgery. Most of these syndromes have in common the contamination of a normally sterile abdominal site with microbial flora of the bowel. Thus, they are often polymicrobial in nature and are caused by aerobic and facultative gram-negative bacilli, anaerobic bacteria, and gram-positive aerobic cocci (Table 24-1). These infections can be quite severe and frequently lead to sepsis and death.

The presentations of patients with intra-abdominal infections vary depending on the site and type of the infection but often include abdominal pain with tenderness, rebound, and guarding on examination, fever, chills, nausea, and vomiting. Laboratory examination is often remarkable for peripheral blood leukocytosis. Abdominal imaging studies may show evidence of ileus, obstruction, or abdominal abscesses or fluid collections.

As mentioned, the bacteria most often responsible for intra-abdominal infections are the flora of the bowel. This flora can vary markedly depending on whether the illness is community acquired or health care associated. In community-acquired infections, enteric gram-negative facultative and aerobic bacilli, gram-positive cocci, and anaerobic bacilli are most frequently isolated. Recommended treatment depends on the severity of the infection and may include a single agent or a combination of agents (Figure 24-1 and Table 24-2). Antibiotics used in these regimens include carbapenems (**imipenem, meropenem**), penicillin/β-lactamase inhibitor combinations (**piperacillin/tazobactam**), cephalosporins (**cefuroxime, ceftriaxone, cefotaxime, ceftazidime, cefepime**), quinolones (**ciprofloxacin, levofloxacin**), and **metronidazole**.

In health care–associated infections, antibiotic-resistant bacteria are more common, including *Pseudomonas aeruginosa*, penicillin- or vancomycin-resistant enterococci, and methicillin-resistant *Staphylococcus aureus*. Recommended regimens include the following: **piperacillin/tazobactam** alone, carbapenem alone (**imipenem, meropenem**), or cephalosporin (**ceftazidime, cefepime**) plus **metronidazole** (Table 24-2). When risk factors for methicillin-resistant *S. aureus* are present, **vancomycin** should be added.

Table 24-1. Bacterial Causes of Complicated Intra-Abdominal Infection

Bacterium	Percentage of Patients
Gram-negative facultative and aerobic bacilli	
Escherichia coli	48-71
Klebsiella spp.	8-14
Pseudomonas aeruginosa	7-14
Anaerobic bacteria	
Bacteroides fragilis	16-35
Other *Bacteroides* spp.	15-71
Clostridium spp.	29
Gram-positive aerobic cocci	
Streptococcus spp.	24-38
Enterococcus faecalis	7-12
Enterococcus faecium	3-9

From Solomkin JS, Mazuski JE, Bradley JS, et al. Diagnosis and management of complicated intra-abdominal infection in adults and children: guidelines by the Surgical Infection Society and the Infectious Diseases Society of America. *Clin Infect Dis*. 2010;50:133-164; Solomkin J, Evans D, Slepavicius A, et al. Assessing the efficacy and safety of eravacycline vs. ertapenem in complicated intra-abdominal infections in the Investigating Gram-Negative Infections Treated with Eravacycline (IGNITE 1) trial: a randomized clinical trial. *JAMA Surg*. 2017;152:224-232.

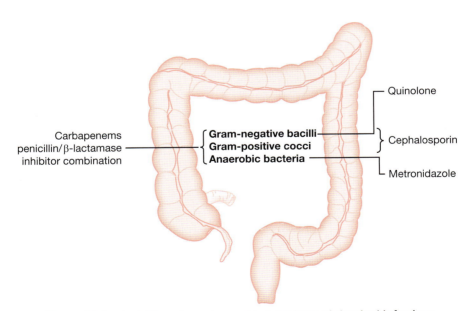

Figure 24-1. Activities of agents used to treat intra-abdominal infections.

Table 24-2. Empiric Antimicrobial Therapy for Intra-Abdominal Infections

Antibiotic Class	Antibiotic
Community acquired	
For mild-to-moderate infections	
Single agent: piperacillin/tazobactam Combination therapy: (cefuroxime, ceftriaxone, cefotaxime, ciprofloxacin, or levofloxacin) plus metronidazole	
For severe infections	
Single agent: imipenem, meropenem, piperacillin/tazobactam Combination therapy: (cefepime, ceftazidime, ciprofloxacin, or levofloxacin) plus metronidazole	
Health care associated	
Penicillin/β-lactamase inhibitor	Piperacillin/tazobactam
or	
Carbapenem	Imipenem, meropenem
or	
Third- or fourth-generation cephalosporin	Ceftazidime, cefepime
plus	
Metronidazole	

QUESTIONS

1. Intra-abdominal infections are usually polymicrobial and are caused by the three main groups of bacteria found in the bowel: _____, _____, and _____.
2. The facultative gram-negative bacillus most commonly isolated from intra-abdominal infections is _____.
3. The following classes of antibiotics can be used as single agents to treat severe community-acquired intra-abdominal infections because they have broad activity against the three different groups of bacteria that cause these infections: _____ and _____.
4. Intra-abdominal infections acquired in a health care setting can be treated with ceftazidime or cefepime, but because these agents lack activity against anaerobes, it is recommended that they be used in conjunction with _____.

ANSWERS

1. facultative and aerobic gram-negative bacilli, gram-positive cocci, anaerobic bacilli
2. *Escherichia coli*
3. penicillin/β-lactamase inhibitor combinations, carbapenems
4. metronidazole

ADDITIONAL READINGS

Blot S, De Waele JJ. Critical issues in the clinical management of complicated intra-abdominal infections. *Drugs.* 2005;65:1611-1620.

Montravers P, Gauzit R, Muller C, et al. Emergence of antibiotic-resistant bacteria in cases of peritonitis after intraabdominal surgery affects the efficacy of empirical antimicrobial therapy. *Clin Infect Dis.* 1996;23:486-494.

Sartelli M, Chichom-Mefire A, Labricciosa FM, et al. The management of intra-abdominal infections from a global perspective: 2017 WSES guidelines for management of intra-abdominal infections. *World J Emerg Surg.* 2017;12:29. doi:10.1186/s13017-017-0141-6

Solomkin JS, Mazuski JE, Bradley JS, et al. Diagnosis and management of complicated intra-abdominal infection in adults and children: guidelines by the Surgical Infection Society and the Infectious Diseases Society of America. *Clin Infect Dis.* 2010;50:133-164.

PART 5

Clinical Cases

"All things, at first try, are difficult to handle. The bow is difficult to draw and the halberd is difficult to wield. When you grow accustomed to a weapon it gets to be easy to handle."
—**The Book of Five Rings, Miyamoto Musashi**

The acquisition of any skill requires practice, and prescribing appropriate antibiotics is no exception. In this section, a series of clinical cases is presented to help you assimilate the information from the previous sections. The answers to the clinical case questions are at the end of this section.

CASE 1

A 62-year-old man presents with a 4-day history of fevers, chills, malaise, and a cough productive of purulent sputum. He also states that his right chest hurts when he coughs or takes a deep breath. Although he feels ill, his oral intake has been near his normal level. His past medical and surgical history is remarkable for hypertension and arthroscopic surgery on the left knee 10 years prior to admission. He has not been hospitalized since his knee surgery. His only medication is lisinopril. He has not taken any antibiotics over the past 3 months. He works as an accountant and drinks socially and does not smoke. He denies any recent travel or exposure to birds or animals other than his pet dog.

The patient has a temperature of 38.5°C, blood pressure of 152/84, pulse of 74, respiratory rate of 16, and oxygen saturation of 98% on room air. Examination is otherwise remarkable for dullness to percussion of the chest wall, bronchial breath sounds, and splinting on the right side of the chest. His neck is supple, and no heart murmurs are heard.

Laboratory analysis is remarkable for a peripheral blood leukocyte count of 16,600 cells/mm^3 with 75% neutrophils and 10% band forms. Electrolytes are within normal limits, and glucose is 155 mg/dL. A chest radiograph shows lobar consolidation with a questionable effusion on the right side.

QUESTIONS

1. What is your diagnosis?
2. What are the bacteria that most commonly cause this syndrome?
3. Which antibiotic(s) would you use to empirically treat this patient?
4. Which antibiotic(s) would you use to empirically treat this patient if he became hypoxemic and required admission to a medical ward?
5. Which antibiotic(s) would you use to empirically treat this patient if he became hypotensive, required vasopressor support, and was admitted to the intensive care unit?
6. If a blood culture later grows *Streptococcus pneumoniae*, which antibiotic(s) would you then use to treat this patient?
7. If instead a urinary antigen test result for *Legionella pneumophila* was reported as positive, which antibiotic(s) would you use to treat this patient?

CASE 2

A 68-year-old woman is admitted to the surgical service for colectomy following the diagnosis of nonmetastatic colon cancer. The colectomy is performed on the second day of hospitalization. Her postoperative course is complicated by poor respiratory function due to underlying chronic obstructive pulmonary disease, which has recently been treated with multiple courses of antibiotics. As a result, she remains mechanically ventilated. On postoperative day 6, she is noted to have a fever and a marked increase in the purulence and quantity of her respiratory secretions. Her pulmonary examination is remarkable for bilateral rhonchi. Her peripheral leukocyte count has risen to 18,200 cells/mm^3 with 81% neutrophils. A chest radiograph shows the development of bilateral patchy infiltrates. Preliminary examination of a tracheal aspirate sample shows many neutrophils and gram-negative bacilli.

QUESTIONS

1. What is your diagnosis?
2. What are the bacteria that most commonly cause this syndrome?
3. Which antibiotic(s) would you use to empirically treat this patient?
4. If a tracheal aspirate subsequently grows many colonies of *P. aeruginosa*, which antibiotic(s) would you use?
5. If a tracheal aspirate subsequently grows many colonies of *Staphylococcus aureus*, which antibiotic(s) would you use?

CASE 3

A 23-year-old sexually active woman presents with a 3-day history of dysuria, frequency, and hematuria. She denies fever, chills, nausea, vomiting, or flank pain and states that she is not pregnant. Her past medical history is remarkable for a "bladder infection" 1 year ago. Examination reveals no fevers or costovertebral angle tenderness. A urine dipstick is positive for leukocyte esterase.

QUESTIONS

1. What is your diagnosis?
2. Is this a "complicated" or "uncomplicated" infection?
3. Which antibiotic(s) would you use to empirically treat this patient?
4. Which antibiotic(s) would you use to empirically treat this patient if she resided in a region where 40% of community-acquired *Escherichia coli* are resistant to trimethoprim-sulfamethoxazole?
5. Which antibiotic(s) would you use to empirically treat this patient if she were diabetic and a urine Gram stain showed many gram-negative bacilli?

CASE 4

A 26-year-old sexually active woman presents with a 6-day history of fevers, chills, dysuria, frequency, and flank pain. She also reports nausea and has repeatedly vomited and has been unable to maintain oral intake. Her past medical history is remarkable only for the normal vaginal delivery of a daughter 3 years ago. Vital signs are as follows: a temperature of 38.7°C, a recumbent blood pressure of 98/66 mm Hg and pulse of 88 beats per minute, a standing blood pressure of 88/55 mm Hg and pulse of 101 beats per minute, and a respiratory rate of 13 breaths per minute. Physical examination is otherwise remarkable for costovertebral angle tenderness to palpation on the left side. Laboratory analysis shows a peripheral blood leukocyte count of 26,200 cells/mm^3 with 82% neutrophils and 15% band forms. Electrolytes are within normal limits, and glucose is 93 mg/dL. A pregnancy test is negative. A urine sample shows pyuria and greater than 100,000 bacteria.

Questions

1. What is your diagnosis?
2. Is this a "complicated" or "uncomplicated" infection?
3. Which antibiotic(s) would you use to empirically treat this patient?

CASE 5

A 17-year-old sexually active woman presents with a 1-week history of fevers, chills, lower abdominal pain, and vaginal discharge. She denies nausea, vomiting, and diarrhea. Her past medical history is remarkable for two episodes of *Chlamydia* infections during the past 2 years. Vital signs are as follows: temperature of 37.4°C, blood pressure of 126/78 mm Hg, pulse of 72 beats per minute, and respiratory rate of 11 breaths per minute. Physical examination is otherwise remarkable for bilateral lower abdominal tenderness without evidence of a mass. On pelvic examination, cervical motion tenderness, bilateral adnexal tenderness, and mucopurulent cervical discharge are noted. Laboratory analysis shows a peripheral blood leukocyte count of 8,300 cells/mm^3 with 60% neutrophils and no band forms. Electrolytes and glucose are within normal limits.

QUESTIONS

1. What is your diagnosis?
2. What are the likely causes of this patient's infection?
3. Which antibiotic(s) would you use to empirically treat this patient?
4. If her sexual partner is subsequently found to be infected with *Chlamydia trachomatis*, which antibiotic(s) would you use to treat the sexual partner?
5. If her sexual partner is subsequently found to be infected with *Neisseria gonorrhoeae*, which antibiotic(s) would you use to treat the sexual partner?

CASE 6

A 62-year-old man complains of fever, chills, nausea, vomiting, headache, confusion, and a stiff neck for the past 24 hours. He states that he has had nasal congestion and a cough for the past week but has otherwise been healthy. His past medical history is remarkable for hypertension and alcohol abuse. His examination is remarkable for a temperature of 38.7°C, pain on flexion of the neck, questionable papilledema, and orientation to self and place, but not year. Because of concerns about the presence of a central nervous system mass, a head computed tomography (CT) scan is ordered prior to performing a lumbar puncture.

QUESTIONS

1. What infection should you be concerned about?
2. Which bacteria frequently cause this infection?
3. Should this patient receive antibiotics prior to being sent for his head CT scan?
4. If it is decided that antibiotics are appropriate, which agents should be given?

A head CT is performed and shows no evidence of a central nervous system mass lesion. A lumbar puncture is performed, which yields cerebrospinal fluid (CSF) with the following parameters: white cells, 412 cells/mm^3 (96% neutrophils); protein, 110 mg/dL; and glucose, 23 mg/dL (simultaneous serum glucose of 98 mg/dL). Gram stain examination reveals gram-positive cocci in pairs.

QUESTIONS

5. Which organism is the likely cause of this patient's illness?
6. What changes would you now make to this patient's antibiotic regimen?

Several days later, the microbiology laboratory reports that *S. pneumoniae* susceptible to penicillin is growing from the CSF.

QUESTIONS

7. What changes would you now make to this patient's antibiotic regimen?
8. Which antibiotics would you choose if the Gram stain results show gram-negative cocci in pairs?
9. Which antibiotics would you choose if the Gram stain results show gram-positive bacilli?

CASE 7

A 56-year-old woman complains of a painful rash on her right foot. Five days ago, she developed a blister on her foot after wearing a new pair of shoes. Three days ago, the skin around the blister became red and tender. Over the following days, the redness spread and now involves most of her foot and ankle, and she now has difficulty putting weight on the foot because of pain. She has also noted fever, chills, and rigors over the past 24 hours. Her past medical history is remarkable for hypertension, hyperlipidemia, and hypothyroidism. Her medications are hydrochlorothiazide, lovastatin, and levothyroxine. Two years earlier, she had a small skin abscess drained, and the culture grew MRSA. Her vital signs are as follows: temperature, 39.1°C; pulse, 96 beats per minute; respiratory rate, 16 breaths per minute; and blood pressure, 123/74 mm Hg. On physical examination, an erythematous, warm, somewhat tender, swollen region is noted over her right foot and extending halfway up her calf. No bullae are noted. Pedal pulses are intact, as is sensation over the region of the rash. She is able to move her foot with minimal pain.

QUESTIONS

1. What is your diagnosis?
2. Which bacteria frequently cause this infection?
3. Which antibiotic(s) would you use to empirically treat this patient?
4. If a blood culture later grows *Streptococcus pyogenes*, which antibiotic(s) would you then use to treat this patient?
5. If a blood culture later grows *Staphylococcus aureus* susceptible to methicillin, which antibiotic(s) would you then use to treat this patient?

A mother brings her 5-year-old daughter to be seen for complaints of right ear pain for the last 72 hours. One of your partners saw the patient 2 days ago and diagnosed acute otitis media at that time. He had told the patient's mother to watch her carefully and to return if her symptoms did not resolve over the next 2 days. Since that time, her ear pain has persisted, and she now has a fever. Her past medical history is remarkable for one prior ear infection, which occurred 24 months earlier. On examination, her temperature is 38.8°C; her other vital signs are within normal limits. The right tympanic membrane is bulging and inflamed. There is no evidence of conjunctivitis.

Questions

1. What is your diagnosis?
2. Which bacteria frequently cause this infection?
3. Which antibiotic would you use to empirically treat this patient?

Upon further questioning, the mother informs you that the patient received amoxicillin for her last ear infection but developed a rash shortly after starting the medication. She states that the rash did not itch, and she was told by her physician, who saw the rash, that it was not hives.

Questions

4. Which antibiotic would you use to treat this patient?
5. Which antibiotic would you use if the patient did have a history of hives (urticaria) associated with amoxicillin?

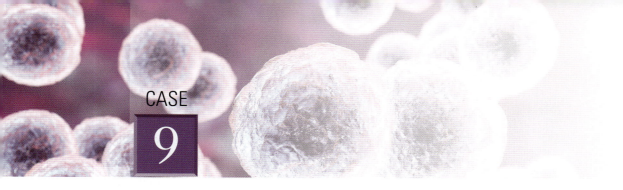

CASE 9

A 38-year-old woman presents with a 2-week history of fevers, chills, and malaise. Her past medical history is remarkable for poor dentition, which resulted in the extraction of several teeth 6 weeks prior to admission, and for rheumatic fever as a child, although she has neglected to take antibiotic prophylaxis before procedures. She works as an accountant and drinks socially and does not smoke or use recreational drugs.

The patient is a thin woman with a temperature of 38.2°C, blood pressure of 122/54 mm Hg, pulse of 83 beats per minute and bounding, and respiratory rate of 12 breaths per minute. Examination is otherwise remarkable for a III/VI early high-pitched diastolic murmur heard at the upper right sternal border that was not present at her last visit. Conjunctival petechiae are also noted. Laboratory evaluation is remarkable for a peripheral blood leukocyte count of 10,600 cells/mm^3 with 65% neutrophils and a hemoglobin content of 12 g/dL. Electrolytes are within normal limits, and glucose is 95 mg/dL. Urinalysis is remarkable for hematuria. Echocardiography shows aortic regurgitation with a vegetation on a leaflet of the aortic valve.

QUESTIONS

1. What is your diagnosis?
2. What are the bacteria that most commonly cause this syndrome?
3. Blood cultures are drawn, and a decision is made to empirically treat the patient while awaiting their results. Which antibiotic(s) would you use to empirically treat this patient?
4. If blood cultures subsequently grow viridans group streptococci fully susceptible to penicillin (minimum inhibitory concentration ≤0.12 μg/mL), which antibiotic(s) would you use to treat this patient?
5. If blood cultures subsequently grow *S. aureus* resistant to methicillin, which antibiotic(s) would you use to treat this patient?
6. If blood cultures subsequently grow enterococci susceptible to penicillin and aminoglycosides, which antibiotic(s) would you use to treat this patient?

CASE 10

A 74-year-old man presents with a 1-week history of fevers, chills, and increasing shortness of breath. His past medical history is remarkable for placement of a prosthetic mitral valve 5 months prior to admission. He is a retired banking executive. He reports moderate alcohol consumption and smokes one pack of cigarettes per day.

Vital signs are as follows: temperature of 38.4°C, blood pressure of 112/75 mm Hg, pulse of 92 beats per minute, and respiratory rate of 19 breaths per minute. Examination is otherwise remarkable for venous jugular distention, crackles at the bases of both lungs, and a low-pitched early diastolic murmur. Laboratory evaluation is remarkable for a peripheral blood leukocyte count of 12,400 cells/mm^3 with 70% neutrophils and a hemoglobin content of 13.2 g/dL. Electrolytes are within normal limits, and glucose is 89 mg/dL. Echocardiography shows a malfunctioning prosthetic valve with vegetations.

QUESTIONS

1. What is your diagnosis?
2. What are the bacteria that most commonly cause this syndrome?
3. Blood cultures are drawn, and a decision is made to empirically treat the patient while awaiting their results. Which antibiotic(s) would you use to empirically treat this patient?
4. If blood cultures subsequently grow *Staphylococcus epidermidis* resistant to methicillin, which antibiotic(s) would you use to treat this patient?
5. If blood cultures subsequently grow *Staphylococcus aureus* susceptible to methicillin, which antibiotic(s) would you use to treat this patient?
6. If blood cultures subsequently grow *Haemophilus aphrophilus*, which antibiotic(s) would you use to treat this patient?

CASE 11

A 75-year-old woman is in the intensive care unit following resection of her colon for colon cancer. On postoperative day 3, you are asked to see her because she has developed a fever.

The patient is mechanically ventilated and sedated. Her temperature is 38.6°C, blood pressure is 128/75 mm Hg, and pulse is 96 beats per minute. She is receiving minimal respiratory support, and the nurse reports scant respiratory secretions on suctioning. On examination, her lungs are clear, and her abdomen is soft. The surgical wound is only minimally erythematous without purulence or drainage, and stool is present in the colostomy bag. A Foley catheter is in place. She has no rash, but there is purulent drainage from the exit site of her femoral triple-lumen catheter. Laboratory evaluation is remarkable for a peripheral blood leukocyte count of 13,400 cells/mm^3 with 85% neutrophils. Electrolytes, glucose, and urinalysis are within normal limits. Chest radiograph shows no evidence of an infiltrate.

QUESTIONS

1. What diagnosis do you suspect?
2. What are the bacteria that most commonly cause this infection?
3. You ask that blood cultures be obtained, the catheter be removed, and the catheter tip sent for culture. While awaiting culture results, you wish to empirically start antibiotics. Which antibiotic(s) would you use to empirically treat this patient?
4. Upon further review of the patient's chart, you find that she has a history of systemic lupus erythematosus and has been on high doses of steroids for some time. Which antibiotic(s) would you use to empirically treat this patient?
5. If blood cultures subsequently grow *Staphylococcus aureus* susceptible to methicillin, which antibiotic(s) would you use to treat this patient?
6. If blood cultures subsequently grow *S. aureus* susceptible to methicillin but the patient has a history of an anaphylactic reaction to amoxicillin, which antibiotic(s) would you use?

CASE 12

A 21-year-old man presents with a 4-day history of severe abdominal pain that initially was centered in his right lower quadrant but is now more diffuse. He also reports fevers, chills, nausea, and vomiting. His past medical history is unremarkable, and he is not taking any medications.

The patient's temperature is 38.5°C, blood pressure is 90/53 mm Hg, and pulse is 121 beats per minute. His physical examination is remarkable for diffuse abdominal tenderness with rigidity, rebound, and guarding. Bowel sounds are absent. Laboratory evaluation shows a peripheral blood leukocyte count of 23,100 cells/mm^3 with 95% neutrophils. Electrolytes, glucose, and urinalysis are within normal limits. Abdominal radiograph shows an ileus with air-fluid levels and free air. Ultrasound examination is consistent with appendicitis with rupture. The patient is immediately prepared for surgery.

QUESTIONS

1. The patient has secondary peritonitis and a ruptured appendix. What are the bacteria that most commonly cause this syndrome?
2. Which antibiotic(s) would you use to empirically treat this patient?
3. If this patient had cystic fibrosis and had recently been hospitalized and had in the past received multiple courses of antibiotics for respiratory infections, which antibiotic(s) would you use to empirically treat him?

ANSWERS TO CLINICAL CASES

Case 1

1. This patient has pneumonia, as evidenced by the recent onset of fevers, chills, a productive cough, an elevated peripheral blood leukocyte count, and an infiltrate on his chest radiograph. The pneumonia is classified as community acquired because the patient has not recently been hospitalized or otherwise exposed to the health care environment or taken antibiotics.

2. The most common bacterial causes of community-acquired pneumonia in adults are *Streptococcus pneumoniae*, *Haemophilus influenzae*, *Legionella* spp., *Mycoplasma pneumoniae*, other aerobic gram-negative bacteria, and *Chlamydia pneumoniae*. The age of the patient, the productive cough, and the lobar consolidation would make one suspicious of a "typical" organism, as opposed to an "atypical" organism. However, these clinical distinctions have been shown to be unreliable, and the choice of therapy should not be based on them.

3. This patient's pneumonia is mild and can be treated in the outpatient setting. He has no significant comorbidities. Appropriate antibiotic choices include high-dose amoxicillin or doxycycline.

4. If the patient's pneumonia was severe enough to require admission to a medical ward, treatment should be given intravenously and include a combination of a macrolide (azithromycin, clarithromycin) and a β-lactam (cefotaxime, ceftriaxone, ceftaroline, ampicillin/sulbactam). An intravenous quinolone with antistreptococcal activity (moxifloxacin, levofloxacin) would also be appropriate.

5. If the patient's illness was severe and required admission to an intensive care unit, treatment should be given intravenously using a β-lactam (cefotaxime, ceftriaxone, ceftaroline, ampicillin/sulbactam) in combination with either a macrolide (azithromycin) or a quinolone with antistreptococcal activity (moxifloxacin, levofloxacin). Note that this patient does not have risk factors for *Pseudomonas aeruginosa* or methicillin-resistant *S. aureus* (MRSA) infection, so antipseudomonal or anti-MRSA antibiotics are not indicated.

6. The presence of *S. pneumoniae* in the patient's blood indicates that his pneumonia is caused by this bacterium. The treatment regimen should be narrowed and focused on this pathogen. Appropriate antibiotic therapy would be high-dose penicillin G or ampicillin. A second- or third-generation cephalosporin would also be appropriate. Note that there have been several reports suggesting that patients with bacteremic pneumococcal pneumonia have better outcomes with combination therapy consisting of a β-lactam plus a macrolide (azithromycin) compared to β-lactams alone, so combination therapy should be considered.

7. If diagnostic testing indicated that this patient's pneumonia is caused by *Legionella* spp., therapy should be targeted against this bacterium. Appropriate antibiotics would be either levofloxacin or azithromycin.

Case 2

1. This patient has pneumonia, as evidenced by the new onset of fever, increased production of purulent respiratory secretions, an elevated peripheral blood leukocyte

count, and an infiltrate on her chest radiograph. The pneumonia is classified as hospital acquired because it developed after the patient was in the hospital.

2. This patient's pneumonia developed after she had been in the hospital for 8 days. She has also received recent courses of antibiotics for her chronic obstructive pulmonary disease. In such a patient, one must be especially concerned about *Pseudomonas aeruginosa*, *Acinetobacter* spp., antibiotic-resistant Enterobacterales, and MRSA. The presence of many gram-negative bacilli in the endotracheal aspirate suggests *P. aeruginosa* or antibiotic-resistant Enterobacterales.

3. Appropriate therapy would include one agent from each of the two groups of antipseudomonal antibiotics. Group 1 includes antipseudomonal cephalosporins (ceftazidime, cefepime), carbapenems (imipenem, meropenem), antipseudomonal penicillin/β-lactamase inhibitor combinations (piperacillin/tazobactam), and a monobactam (aztreonam). Group 2 includes quinolones (ciprofloxacin, levofloxacin) and polymyxin (colistin, polymyxin B). It would also be appropriate to add *Staphylococcus aureus* coverage, which would be vancomycin or linezolid.

4. Growth of *P. aeruginosa* from the tracheal aspirate suggests that this bacterium is the cause of pneumonia. Appropriate therapy would include two agents with antipseudomonal activity. For example, a typical regimen might include an antipseudomonal cephalosporin (ceftazidime, cefepime) or piperacillin-tazobactam in combination with ciprofloxacin. Actual choices should be guided by local resistance patterns and the previous antibiotic exposure of this patient. Recall that ciprofloxacin has the best antipseudomonal activity of the quinolones.

5. Growth of *S. aureus* from the tracheal aspirate suggests that this bacterium is the cause of pneumonia. Appropriate therapy would be linezolid or vancomycin. If the isolate is subsequently shown to be susceptible to β-lactams, nafcillin, oxacillin, or cefazolin could be used.

Case 3

1. This patient has acute cystitis, as evidenced by the symptoms of dysuria, frequency, and a positive urine dipstick. The absence of fever, chills, nausea, vomiting, or flank pain makes pyelonephritis unlikely.

2. This urinary tract infection would be classified as "uncomplicated" acute cystitis because the patient is young, healthy, not pregnant, not hospitalized, and without evidence of structural abnormalities of her urinary tract.

3. Appropriate therapy for this patient would be a 5-day course of nitrofurantoin or a single dose of fosfomycin or possibly a 3-day course of oral trimethoprim-sulfamethoxazole if she lives in a region in which the prevalence of uropathogens resistant to this agent is less than 20%.

4. If this patient resided in a region in which resistance to trimethoprim-sulfamethoxazole was common, nitrofurantoin or fosfomycin would be appropriate therapies.

5. A past diagnosis of diabetes would predispose this patient to infection by a broader range of bacteria and would cause her urinary tract infection to be classified as a "complicated" acute cystitis. Because her infection is mild, she could be treated with oral antibiotics. Ciprofloxacin would be a good choice because it is effective

against many of the gram-negative bacilli that might cause this infection, including *Pseudomonas aeruginosa* and many members of the Enterobacterales.

Case 4

1. This patient has acute pyelonephritis, as evidenced by symptoms of fever, chills, dysuria, frequency, and flank pain.
2. This case of acute pyelonephritis would be classified as uncomplicated because the patient is young, healthy, not pregnant, not hospitalized, and without evidence of structural abnormalities of her urinary tract.
3. Because this patient is dehydrated and unable to tolerate oral intake, she should be hospitalized and receive intravenous antibiotics as well as hydration. Appropriate empiric antibiotic therapy would be a quinolone (ciprofloxacin, levofloxacin), a penicillin/β-lactamase inhibitor combination (piperacillin-tazobactam), a fourth-generation cephalosporin (cefepime), or a carbapenem (imipenem, meropenem).

Case 5

1. This patient has pelvic inflammatory disease (PID), as evidenced by symptoms of fever, chills, lower abdominal pain, and findings of cervical motion tenderness, bilateral adnexal tenderness, and mucopurulent cervical discharge.
2. The sexually transmitted bacteria that are most often implicated are *Neisseria gonorrhoeae* and *Chlamydia trachomatis*. Many other bacteria are frequently isolated from PID lesions, including *Bacteroides* and *Peptostreptococcus* spp. as well as *Escherichia coli*, *Gardnerella vaginalis*, *Haemophilus influenzae*, and group B streptococci. Of these, anaerobic bacteria most likely play a significant role in the pathogenesis of PID, and many experts feel that antibiotics effective against anaerobic bacteria should be included in PID treatment regimens.
3. Because this patient's illness is relatively mild, she is a candidate for outpatient therapy. An appropriate antibiotic regimen would be a single intramuscular dose of cephalosporin (ceftriaxone, cefotaxime, cefoxitin plus probenecid) plus oral doxycycline. The addition of oral metronidazole would also be reasonable.
4. Uncomplicated *C. trachomatis* urethritis is treated with doxycycline. Azithromycin is an alternative.
5. Gonorrhea is treated with ceftriaxone. Doxycycline is also given for the possibility of a coexisting *C. trachomatis* infection.

Case 6

1. This patient may have acute bacterial meningitis, as evidenced by the acute onset of fever, chills, nausea, vomiting, headache, confusion, and a stiff neck. Examination of the CSF is necessary to definitively make the diagnosis.
2. In an adult patient, acute bacterial meningitis is most frequently caused by *Streptococcus pneumoniae* or *Neisseria meningitidis*. In an older individual such as this patient, *Listeria monocytogenes* and aerobic gram-negative bacilli are also a concern.

3. Even a delay of several hours can have a detrimental effect on the outcomes of patients with acute bacterial meningitis. For this reason, antibiotic therapy should not be withheld while awaiting the results of neuroimaging studies. Note that most experts would also initiate steroid therapy prior to or at the same time as starting antibiotics.

4. Empiric therapy in this patient would include a third-generation cephalosporin (ceftriaxone or cefotaxime) to cover *N. meningitidis* and most strains of *S. pneumoniae*. Vancomycin should be added to cover highly penicillin-resistant strains of *S. pneumoniae*. Because this patient is older than 50 years, ampicillin should also be added to cover *L. monocytogenes*.

5. The lumbar puncture results confirm the diagnosis of acute bacterial meningitis. The gram-positive cocci in pairs seen on Gram stain of the CSF indicate that *S. pneumoniae* is the likely cause. If the patient were an infant, one would also be concerned about *Streptococcus agalactiae*, but meningitis caused by this bacterium is rare in adults.

6. Acute bacterial meningitis caused by *S. pneumoniae* is treated with a third-generation cephalosporin plus vancomycin, so ampicillin should be discontinued.

7. Meningitis caused by penicillin-susceptible *S. pneumoniae* can be treated with either a penicillin or a third-generation cephalosporin.

8. CSF containing gram-negative cocci in pairs indicates that *N. meningitidis* is the cause of the meningitis. The patient should be treated with a third-generation cephalosporin (ceftriaxone, cefotaxime).

9. CSF containing gram-positive bacilli indicates that *L. monocytogenes* is the cause of meningitis. The patient should be treated with ampicillin plus gentamicin.

Case 7

1. This patient has cellulitis, as evidenced by an erythematous and tender skin rash, fevers, chills, and rigors. One would also be concerned about deeper infections, such as necrotizing fasciitis, but she does not have bullae, violaceous skin discoloration, paresthesia, or intense pain with movement of the foot, making these more serious infections less likely.

2. This patient is not immunocompromised, and the infection did not result from an unusual exposure, such as to seawater. Therefore, her cellulitis is most likely caused by skin bacteria, such as *Staphylococcus aureus*, *Streptococcus pyogenes*, or other streptococci.

3. Given her high fever and decreased mobility, this patient should be admitted to the hospital and treated with intravenous antibiotics. Because she previously had an MRSA infection, agents should be chosen that are effective against this organism as well as streptococci. Vancomycin or daptomycin would be appropriate.

4. The presence of *S. pyogenes* in the blood indicates that this bacterium is the cause of cellulitis. The antibiotic regimen can, therefore, be changed to penicillin G, which has excellent activity against this organism.

5. The presence of methicillin-susceptible *S. aureus* in the blood indicates that this bacterium is the cause of cellulitis. The antibiotic regimen can, therefore, be

changed to an antistaphylococcal penicillin, such as nafcillin, oxacillin, or a cephalosporin such as cefazolin because MRSA is no longer a concern.

Case 8

1. This patient has acute otitis media, as evidenced by ear pain, fever, and an inflamed tympanic membrane.
2. Acute otitis media is most commonly caused by *Streptococcus pneumoniae*, *Haemophilus influenzae*, or *Moraxella catarrhalis*.
3. This patient's ear infection has not resolved over 72 hours, and she now has a fever, so antibiotic therapy is definitely indicated. There are no risk factors for β-lactamase–producing bacteria, so high-dose amoxicillin is the treatment of choice.
4. The patient has a mild allergy to penicillin, so an oral cephalosporin (cefdinir, cefpodoxime, cefuroxime) should be used to treat the ear infection.
5. When there is a history of a type I hypersensitivity allergic reaction to penicillin, a macrolide (azithromycin, clarithromycin) or clindamycin should be used to treat otitis media.

Case 9

1. This patient has infective endocarditis, as evidenced by a fever and a new murmur in a patient with a history of rheumatic fever and a recent dental procedure during which she did not receive antibiotic prophylaxis. Other supporting features include conjunctival petechiae, mild anemia, and hematuria. The finding of a vegetation by echocardiography confirms the diagnosis.
2. Native valve endocarditis is most frequently caused by viridans group streptococci, *Staphylococcus aureus*, enterococci, and the HACEK organisms.
3. Vancomycin plus ceftriaxone is appropriate empiric therapy. This regimen will cover most viridans group streptococci, staphylococci, enterococci, and HACEK organisms.
4. Appropriate antimicrobial therapy for endocarditis caused by penicillin-susceptible viridans group streptococci is penicillin G or ceftriaxone for 4 weeks.
5. Appropriate antimicrobial therapy for endocarditis caused by MRSA is vancomycin or daptomycin for 6 weeks.
6. Appropriate antimicrobial therapy for endocarditis caused by penicillin- and gentamicin-susceptible enterococci is penicillin G or ampicillin for 4 to 6 weeks plus gentamicin for 2 to 6 weeks to allow for synergistic bactericidal killing of the enterococci. Ampicillin plus ceftriaxone for 6 weeks would also be appropriate.

Case 10

1. This patient has prosthetic valve endocarditis, as evidenced by a fever and a new murmur in an individual with a history of mitral valve replacement. Infection of the prosthetic valve has caused it to malfunction, resulting in the signs and symptoms of congestive heart failure. The finding of a vegetation and malfunctioning prosthetic valve by echocardiography confirms the diagnosis.

2. Prosthetic valve endocarditis is most frequently caused by coagulase-negative staphylococci and *Staphylococcus aureus*.
3. Vancomycin plus cefepime plus gentamicin plus rifampin is appropriate empiric therapy. This regimen will cover staphylococci as well as other gram-positive and gram-negative bacteria that cause prosthetic valve endocarditis.
4. Appropriate antimicrobial therapy for prosthetic valve endocarditis caused by methicillin-resistant *Staphylococcus epidermidis* is vancomycin plus rifampin for 6 weeks or more. Gentamicin should be given for the first 2 weeks.
5. Appropriate antimicrobial therapy for prosthetic valve endocarditis caused by methicillin-susceptible *S. aureus* is nafcillin, oxacillin, or cefazolin for 6 weeks or more. Rifampin should also be given for 6 weeks or more, and gentamicin should be added for the first 2 weeks.
6. Appropriate antimicrobial therapy for prosthetic valve endocarditis caused by one of the HACEK organisms is ceftriaxone, ampicillin-sulbactam, or ciprofloxacin for 6 weeks.

Case 11

1. This patient likely has an intravascular catheter infection, as evidenced by fever, purulent drainage from the catheter exit site, and lack of evidence to support an alternative diagnosis.
2. Intravascular-related catheter infections are most commonly caused by coagulase-negative staphylococci and *Staphylococcus aureus*.
3. If methicillin-resistant staphylococci are rarely isolated in this hospital, one could use nafcillin, oxacillin, or cefazolin. Otherwise, vancomycin would be the antibiotic of choice.
4. In an immunocompromised host, one would add coverage for aerobic gram-negative bacilli such as ceftazidime, cefepime, carbapenem, or penicillin/β-lactamase inhibitor combination.
5. Nafcillin, oxacillin, or cefazolin would be appropriate antimicrobial therapy for an intravascular catheter infection caused by methicillin-susceptible *S. aureus*.
6. Antistaphylococcal penicillins should not be given to a patient with a history of an anaphylactic reaction to penicillins. Likewise, cephalosporins should be avoided. Vancomycin would be the agent of choice in this situation.

Case 12

1. The bacteria that most commonly cause secondary peritonitis are enteric gram-negative bacilli, such as *Escherichia coli*; gram-positive cocci, such as enterococci and streptococci; and anaerobic bacteria, such as *Bacteroides* spp.
2. This patient has a community-acquired infection and is severely ill, so appropriate single-agent antimicrobial therapy would be a carbapenem (imipenem, meropenem) or piperacillin/tazobactam. Combination regimens would include metronidazole together with one of the following: cefepime, ceftazidime, ciprofloxacin, or levofloxacin.
3. If this patient's intra-abdominal infection was health care–associated, antibiotics with activity against resistant bacteria, including *Pseudomonas aeruginosa* and

resistant Enterobacterales, would be preferred. Such regimens would be piperacillin/tazobactam, imipenem, meropenem, cefepime plus metronidazole, or ceftazidime plus metronidazole. The actual regimen chosen would depend on the antibiotics to which this patient had been previously exposed, the bacteria with which he is colonized, and regional antibiotic resistance patterns.

PART 6

Review Questions and Answers

1. Which of the following antibiotics is NOT a β-lactam?
   a. ampicillin
   b. meropenem
   c. ceftriaxone
   d. vancomycin
   e. aztreonam

2. Which of the following antibiotics has little activity against anaerobic bacteria?
   a. imipenem
   b. metronidazole
   c. ceftriaxone
   d. clindamycin
   e. amoxicillin/clavulanate

3. Which of the following antibiotics could be used in someone who has a history of developing anaphylaxis after taking penicillin?
   a. aztreonam
   b. ampicillin
   c. cefazolin
   d. piperacillin/tazobactam
   e. cefotetan

4. Which of the following agents is NOT useful in the treatment of enterococcal infections?
   a. penicillin
   b. cefazolin
   c. ampicillin
   d. gentamicin
   e. vancomycin

5. Which of the following quinolones has the greatest activity against *Pseudomonas aeruginosa*?
   a. levofloxacin
   b. moxifloxacin
   c. delafloxacin
   d. gemifloxacin
   e. ciprofloxacin

6. Rifampin is useful in treatment or prophylaxis against all of the following bacteria EXCEPT:
   a. *Staphylococcus aureus*
   b. *Staphylococcus epidermidis*
   c. *Bacteroides fragilis*
   d. *Neisseria meningitidis*
   e. *Mycobacterium tuberculosis*

7. Severe infections caused by which of the following bacteria are routinely treated with a single antibiotic?
   a. *Treponema pallidum*
   b. *Brucella melitensis*
   c. *Mycobacterium leprae*
   d. *M. tuberculosis*
   e. *Helicobacter pylori*

8. Which of the following agents is NOT useful in treating infections caused by *Mycobacterium avium* complex?
   a. clarithromycin
   b. isoniazid
   c. ethambutol
   d. rifabutin
   e. ciprofloxacin

9. Which of the following agents is useful in the treatment of infections caused by *Clostridioides difficile*?
   a. clindamycin
   b. imipenem
   c. penicillin
   d. vancomycin
   e. piperacillin/tazobactam

10. Which of the following agents would be useful in the treatment of an infection caused by an *Escherichia coli* strain that produces an extended-spectrum β-lactamase?
    a. ceftriaxone
    b. ceftazidime
    c. meropenem
    d. aztreonam
    e. piperacillin

11. Which of the following agents does NOT inhibit bacterial cell wall synthesis?
    a. gentamicin
    b. aztreonam
    c. imipenem
    d. vancomycin
    e. ampicillin

12. Penicillin is still commonly used to treat all of the following bacteria EXCEPT:
    a. *T. pallidum*
    b. *Streptococcus pyogenes*
    c. *Clostridium perfringens*

d. *N. meningitidis*
   e. *S. aureus*

13. Which of the following bacteria is susceptible to vancomycin?
   a. *Bordetella pertussis*
   b. *C. difficile*
   c. *P. aeruginosa*
   d. *Haemophilus influenzae*
   e. *Enterobacter cloacae*

14. All of the following would be appropriate treatment for an infection caused by *H. influenzae* EXCEPT:
   a. amoxicillin/clavulanate
   b. cefuroxime
   c. ampicillin
   d. doxycycline
   e. cefotaxime

15. Which of the following antibiotics can be safely used in small children?
   a. ciprofloxacin
   b. azithromycin
   c. tetracycline
   d. gemifloxacin
   e. doxycycline

16. All of the following are relatively common adverse reactions to aminoglycosides EXCEPT:
   a. auditory impairment
   b. nephrotoxicity
   c. vestibular toxicity
   d. biliary sludging
   e. decreased renal function

17. Pyrazinamide is used to treat infections caused by which of the following?
   a. *M. tuberculosis*
   b. *M. avium* complex
   c. *M. leprae*
   d. *Rickettsia rickettsii*
   e. *Legionella pneumophila*

18. The sexually transmitted disease chlamydia may be treated with which of the following agents:
   a. doxycycline
   b. penicillin
   c. cefazolin
   d. vancomycin
   e. ceftriaxone

19. Empiric use of vancomycin in a patient with infective endocarditis would fail to cover which of the following organisms?
   a. *S. aureus*
   b. *S. epidermidis*
   c. viridans group streptococci
   d. enterococci
   e. HACEK organisms

20. Which of the following antibiotics targets the bacterial ribosome?
   a. isoniazid
   b. vancomycin
   c. tetracycline
   d. levofloxacin
   e. trimethoprim-sulfamethoxazole

21. Which of the following antibiotics would NOT be used to treat a patient infected with *Borrelia burgdorferi*?
   a. doxycycline
   b. clindamycin
   c. amoxicillin
   d. cefuroxime
   e. ceftriaxone

22. Doxycycline is useful in treating infections caused by all of the following bacteria EXCEPT:
   a. *Leptospira interrogans*
   b. *Brucella abortus*
   c. *Chlamydia trachomatis*
   d. *P. aeruginosa*
   e. *R. rickettsii*

23. Which of the following antibiotics targets bacterial RNA polymerase?
   a. cefotetan
   b. amikacin
   c. rifampin
   d. azithromycin
   e. daptomycin

24. Which of the following agents does NOT have activity against vancomycin-resistant *Enterococcus faecium*?
   a. tedizolid
   b. linezolid
   c. daptomycin
   d. tigecycline
   e. vancomycin

25. Which of the following antibiotic regimens would be appropriate for a patient with a severe infection caused by P. aeruginosa prior to knowledge of the isolate's susceptibilities?
    a. ceftazidime plus ciprofloxacin
    b. ceftriaxone plus gentamicin
    c. piperacillin/tazobactam plus rifampin
    d. ertapenem plus ciprofloxacin
    e. ampicillin plus tobramycin

26. Vancomycin is added to ceftriaxone in the empiric treatment of community-acquired acute bacterial meningitis to allow for effective treatment of which organism?
    a. N. meningitidis
    b. Streptococcus pneumoniae
    c. S. aureus
    d. H. influenzae
    e. E. faecium

27. Which of the following types of bacteria have acquired resistance to all β-lactam antibiotics by producing a special penicillin-binding protein that is NOT bound by these agents?
    a. Klebsiella pneumoniae that produce a carbapenemase
    b. E. coli strains that produce extended-spectrum β-lactamases
    c. E. cloacae strains that constitutively express AmpC β-lactamases
    d. methicillin-resistant S. aureus (MRSA)
    e. multidrug-resistant P. aeruginosa

28. The β-lactamase inhibitors clavulanate, sulbactam, and tazobactam effectively inhibit many of the β-lactamases of the following groups of bacteria EXCEPT:
    a. P. aeruginosa
    b. B. fragilis
    c. S. aureus
    d. H. influenzae
    e. Proteus mirabilis

29. Accepted regimens for the treatment of H. pylori may contain each of the following agents EXCEPT:
    a. amoxicillin
    b. clarithromycin
    c. cefotaxime
    d. metronidazole
    e. bismuth subsalicylate

30. Which of the following antibiotics is effective against bacteria that cause an atypical pneumonia?
    a. amoxicillin
    b. amoxicillin/clavulanate
    c. cefotaxime
    d. vancomycin
    e. azithromycin

31. Which of the following bacteria frequently alters the composition of the peptide side chain of peptidoglycan to cause resistance to vancomycin?
    a. S. aureus
    b. S. epidermidis
    c. E. faecium
    d. S. pneumoniae
    e. E. cloacae

32. Azithromycin may be used to treat infections caused by all of the following bacteria EXCEPT:
    a. C. trachomatis
    b. Mycoplasma pneumoniae
    c. Campylobacter jejuni
    d. M. tuberculosis
    e. M. avium complex

33. All of the following agents are used to treat patients with tuberculosis EXCEPT:
    a. pyrazinamide
    b. isoniazid
    c. rifampin
    d. dapsone
    e. ethambutol

34. Which of the following would be considered appropriate therapy for an acute uncomplicated urinary tract infection?
    a. nitrofurantoin
    b. amoxicillin
    c. ampicillin
    d. ceftriaxone
    e. meropenem

35. Which of the following antibiotics is effective against *H. pylori*, *M. avium* complex, *B. pertussis*, and some strains of *S. aureus* and *S. pneumoniae*?
   a. amoxicillin
   b. amoxicillin/clavulanate
   c. ceftriaxone
   d. doxycycline
   e. clarithromycin

36. Which of the following is NOT an aminoglycoside?
   a. plazomicin
   b. gentamicin
   c. tobramycin
   d. erythromycin
   e. amikacin

37. All of the following are appropriate antimicrobial regimens for hospital-acquired pneumonia in a patient with septic shock and risk factors for infection with a multidrug-resistant bacterium EXCEPT:
   a. cefepime plus levofloxacin plus vancomycin
   b. piperacillin/tazobactam plus ceftazidime plus vancomycin
   c. imipenem plus ciprofloxacin plus linezolid
   d. ceftazidime plus polymyxin plus vancomycin
   e. piperacillin/tazobactam plus ciprofloxacin plus linezolid

38. Which of the following is appropriate therapy for infections caused by *L. interrogans*?
   a. amoxicillin
   b. vancomycin
   c. linezolid
   d. amikacin
   e. metronidazole

39. Relatively common adverse reactions to penicillin include all of the following EXCEPT:
   a. diarrhea
   b. rash
   c. anaphylaxis
   d. cartilage damage
   e. serum sickness

40. Clindamycin predisposes to infection by which of the following bacteria?
   a. *C. perfringens*
   b. *C. difficile*
   c. *Clostridium tetani*
   d. *Clostridium botulinum*
   e. *Clostridium septicum*

41. Third-generation cephalosporins should be used with caution in infections caused by certain bacteria that produce inducible chromosomal AmpC β-lactamases because resistance may develop during treatment. Each of the following is an example of such a bacterium EXCEPT:
   a. *Klebsiella aerogenes*
   b. *Haemophilus* spp.
   c. *Enterobacter* spp.
   d. *Citrobacter* spp.

42. Which of the following antibiotics has clinically useful activity against anaerobic bacteria?
   a. cefotetan
   b. cefotaxime
   c. cefuroxime
   d. cefazolin
   e. ceftazidime

43. Which of the following antibiotics has the least activity against *P. aeruginosa*?
   a. imipenem
   b. meropenem
   c. ertapenem
   d. ceftazidime
   e. piperacillin

44. Which of the following antibiotics does NOT have activity against *L. pneumophila*?
   a. azithromycin
   b. levofloxacin
   c. moxifloxacin
   d. ciprofloxacin
   e. piperacillin/tazobactam

45. Which of the following antibiotics is used to treat leprosy?
   a. isoniazid
   b. ethambutol
   c. clofazimine
   d. streptomycin

e. amoxicillin/clavulanate

46. Which of the following would be appropriate antibiotic therapy for a patient with native valve infective endocarditis caused by a highly penicillin-resistant (minimum inhibitory concentration >0.5 μg/mL) strain of viridans group streptococci?
  a. penicillin G
  b. ampicillin plus amikacin
  c. ceftriaxone
  d. ampicillin plus gentamicin
  e. oxacillin plus gentamicin

47. All of the following antibiotics are active against *C. jejuni* EXCEPT:
  a. clarithromycin
  b. cefazolin
  c. azithromycin
  d. ciprofloxacin
  e. doxycycline

48. Each of the following might be appropriate empiric monotherapy for cellulitis EXCEPT:
  a. ceftazidime
  b. vancomycin
  c. oxacillin
  d. cefazolin
  e. clindamycin

49. Which of the following is a major toxicity of the antimycobacterial drug ethambutol?
  a. rash
  b. hepatotoxicity
  c. gout
  d. serum sickness
  e. optic neuritis

50. Optimal initial antibiotic therapy for a patient with prosthetic valve endocarditis caused by *S. aureus* might include each of the following agents EXCEPT:
  a. nafcillin
  b. rifampin
  c. linezolid
  d. vancomycin
  e. gentamicin

ANSWERS TO REVIEW QUESTIONS

1. d. vancomycin. Like the β-lactams, vancomycin works by inhibiting cell wall synthesis. However, its structure lacks the β-lactam ring that is characteristic of β-lactam antibiotics, and it is, therefore, not included in this group. β-Lactam antibiotics include penicillins (eg, ampicillin), cephalosporins (eg, ceftriaxone), carbapenems (eg, meropenem), and monobactams (eg, aztreonam).

2. c. ceftriaxone. Whereas imipenem, metronidazole, clindamycin, and amoxicillin/clavulanate all have good or excellent activity against anaerobic bacteria, ceftriaxone has limited activity against them.

3. a. aztreonam. Most β-lactam antibiotics should be avoided in someone with a history of an immediate hypersensitivity response (eg, urticaria or anaphylaxis) to penicillin, with the exception of the monobactam aztreonam. There are few allergic cross-reactions between aztreonam and other β-lactam agents.

4. b. cefazolin. Enterococcal infections are usually treated with penicillin (eg, penicillin, ampicillin, or piperacillin) in conjunction with an aminoglycoside (gentamicin or streptomycin). Vancomycin is often used for penicillin-resistant strains. All enterococci are resistant to cephalosporins when used as single agents, although ceftriaxone may be used in combination therapy.

5. e. ciprofloxacin. Of the commercially available quinolones, ciprofloxacin has the greatest activity against *P. aeruginosa*.

6. c. *B. fragilis*. Rifampin is used in conjunction with an antistaphylococcal penicillin or vancomycin to treat infections involving prosthetic material caused by staphylococci. It is used as prophylaxis in individuals exposed to *N. meningitidis* and is one of the major reagents used to treat *M. tuberculosis* infections. It is not used in the treatment of anaerobic infections, such as those caused by *B. fragilis*.

7. a. *T. pallidum*. Infections caused by *T. pallidum*, the etiologic agent of syphilis, are usually treated with penicillin alone. *Brucella* infections are usually treated with doxycycline plus rifampin, gentamicin, or streptomycin. Active infections caused by *M. tuberculosis*, *M. leprae*, and *H. pylori* are routinely treated with multiple drug regimens.

8. b. isoniazid. Although isoniazid is part of the core antibiotic regimen used to treat *M. tuberculosis*, it is not active against *M. avium* complex. Clarithromycin, ethambutol, rifabutin, and ciprofloxacin are active against *M. avium* complex.

9. d. vancomycin. *C. difficile* infections are treated with oral vancomycin. Clindamycin, imipenem, penicillin, and piperacillin/tazobactam have no activity against this organism. Clindamycin, in particular, predisposes to disease by *C. difficile*.

10. c. meropenem. Extended-spectrum β-lactamase–producing bacteria are frequently resistant to all classes of antibiotics, except the carbapenems. Thus, of the agents listed, only meropenem would reliably have activity against these bacteria.

11. a. gentamicin. Aztreonam, imipenem, and ampicillin are all β-lactam antibiotics that act by inhibiting penicillin-binding proteins, which are essential for cell wall synthesis. Likewise, vancomycin prevents incorporation of new peptidoglycan subunits into the cell wall. Gentamicin, on the other hand, is an aminoglycoside and acts by inhibiting the bacterial ribosome.

12. e. *S. aureus*. Penicillin is still commonly used to treat infections caused by *T. pallidum* (syphilis), *S. pyogenes* (streptococcal pharyngitis), and *C. perfringens* (gas gangrene). In addition, many strains of *N. meningitidis* (meningococcemia) remain susceptible to this agent. Penicillin, however, is not active against most strains of *S. aureus*.

13. b. *C. difficile*. Vancomycin has activity against only gram-positive bacteria. *B. pertussis*, *P. aeruginosa*, *H. influenzae*, and *E. cloacae* are all gram-negative bacteria.

14. c. ampicillin. A significant proportion of *H. influenzae* strains now produce β-lactamases that destroy ampicillin and amoxicillin. These β-lactamases, however, are inhibited by commercially available β-lactamase inhibitors, so amoxicillin/clavulanate is effective against strains that produce them. Cefuroxime and cefotaxime are resistant to degradation by these β-lactamases and are, therefore, also effective against these strains. Doxycycline is also active against most *H. influenzae* strains.

15. b. azithromycin. Quinolones, such as ciprofloxacin and gemifloxacin, should be used with caution in infants and children younger than 18 years of age because they have been associated with cartilage damage in juvenile animals. Tetracycline and doxycycline should usually be avoided in children younger than 8 years of age. Azithromycin is safe for use in children.

16. d. biliary sludging. Relatively common adverse effects associated with the use of aminoglycosides include nephrotoxicity (which results in decreased renal function), auditory impairment, and vestibular toxicity. Biliary sludging is associated with the use of ceftriaxone.

17. a. *M. tuberculosis*. Pyrazinamide is a core component of the basic four-drug regimen used to treat tuberculosis: isoniazid, rifampin, pyrazinamide, and ethambutol. It does not have significant activity against *M. avium* complex, *M. leprae*, or nonmycobacterial organisms.

18. a. doxycycline. *C. trachomatis*, which causes chlamydia, is susceptible to doxycycline, but not to ceftriaxone, cefazolin, vancomycin, or penicillin.

19. e. HACEK organisms. The HACEK organisms (*Haemophilus parainfluenzae*, *Aggregatibacter aphrophilus*, *Aggregatibacter actinomycetemcomitans*, *Cardiobacterium hominis*, *Eikenella corrodens*, and *Kingella kingae*) are gram-negative bacteria and, therefore, not susceptible to vancomycin.

20. c. tetracycline. Tetracycline binds to the 30S subunit of the bacterial ribosome and prevents the binding of transfer RNA (tRNA) loaded with an amino acid. Isoniazid inhibits the synthesis of mycolic acid. Vancomycin inhibits cell wall synthesis. Levofloxacin inhibits topoisomerases. Trimethoprim-sulfamethoxazole inhibits the synthesis of tetrahydrofolate, a precursor necessary for the production of DNA.

21. b. clindamycin. Clindamycin is active against many gram-positive bacteria and anaerobic bacteria, but not spirochetes such as *B. burgdorferi*. This bacterium, which causes Lyme disease, is susceptible to doxycycline, amoxicillin, cefuroxime, and ceftriaxone.

22. d. *P. aeruginosa*. Doxycycline has excellent activity against *L. interrogans*, *B. abortus*, *C. trachomatis*, and *R. rickettsii*, but not against *P. aeruginosa*.

23. c. rifampin. Rifampin targets bacterial RNA polymerase, whereas cefotetan prevents cell wall synthesis, amikacin and azithromycin target the bacterial ribosome, and daptomycin forms an ion-conducting channel in the bacterial cytoplasmic membrane.

24. e. vancomycin. Just checking if you were paying attention. The point is that tedizolid, linezolid, daptomycin, and tigecycline each are effective against many strains of vancomycin-resistant *E. faecium*.

25. a. ceftazidime plus ciprofloxacin. Both ceftazidime and ciprofloxacin have antipseudomonal activity and would allow two agents to be targeted against *P. aeruginosa*. In contrast, each of the remaining regimens contains at least one agent lacking activity against this bacterium. Ceftriaxone, rifampin, ertapenem, and ampicillin have poor or no antipseudomonal activity. The use of gentamicin to treat *P. aeruginosa* infections is controversial.

26. b. *S. pneumoniae*. Some strains of *S. pneumoniae* are resistant to ceftriaxone, so vancomycin is added to empirically cover for this possibility. *N. meningitidis* and *H. influenzae* would be adequately covered with ceftriaxone alone. Vancomycin would be appropriate empiric therapy for *S. aureus* and *S. epidermidis*, but these bacteria rarely cause community-acquired acute bacterial meningitis.

27. d. MRSA. MRSA produce PBP2, a penicillin-binding protein (PBP) that is not recognized by any β-lactam antibiotics. For this reason, MRSA cannot be treated with these agents.

28. a. *P. aeruginosa*. The addition of clavulanate, sulbactam, or tazobactam to penicillin increases activity against anaerobes such as *B. fragilis*; many gram-negative bacteria such as *H. influenzae* and *P. mirabilis*; and some staphylococci such as *S. aureus*. These inhibitors, however, do not appreciably increase activity against *P. aeruginosa*.

29. c. cefotaxime. Regimens used to treat *H. pylori* infections include amoxicillin plus clarithromycin plus a proton pump inhibitor; metronidazole plus clarithromycin plus a proton pump inhibitor; and bismuth subsalicylate plus metronidazole plus tetracycline plus a proton pump inhibitor. Cefotaxime has not been used to treat this bacterium.

30. e. azithromycin. The common bacterial causes of atypical pneumonia are *M. pneumoniae*, *Chlamydia pneumoniae*, and *L. pneumophila*. Antibiotics that target the cell wall, such as β-lactams (amoxicillin, amoxicillin/clavulanate, and cefotaxime) and vancomycin, are not effective against these bacteria. They are, however, susceptible to the macrolides, such as azithromycin.

31. c. *E. faecium*. Some *E. faecium* strains substitute D-alanine-D-lactate for the terminal D-alanine-D-alanine residues of the peptide side chain of peptidoglycan. This prevents binding of vancomycin, resulting in resistance. Although some *S. aureus* strains that also have this capability have been identified, this mode of resistance to vancomycin is most common among the enterococci.

32. d. *M. tuberculosis* Azithromycin is used to treat *C. trachomatis* (sexually transmitted infection), *M. pneumoniae* (community-acquired pneumonia), *Campylobacter pneumoniae* (gastroenteritis), and *M. avium* complex infections. It is not active against *M. tuberculosis*, the cause of tuberculosis.

33. d. dapsone. Isoniazid, rifampin, pyrazinamide, and ethambutol are commonly used to treat tuberculosis. Dapsone is used to treat leprosy.

34. a. nitrofurantoin. Nitrofurantoin, fosfomycin, or trimethoprim-sulfamethoxazole is the recommended antibiotic for acute uncomplicated urinary tract infections.

35. e. clarithromycin. Clarithromycin is routinely used to treat infections caused by *H. pylori*, *M. avium* complex, and *B. pertussis*. In addition, some strains of *S. aureus* and *S. pneumoniae* remain susceptible to it. Amoxicillin is not active against *S. aureus*, *M. avium* complex, or *B. pertussis*. Amoxicillin/clavulanate is not used to treat infections caused by *M. avium* complex or *B. pertussis*. Ceftriaxone is not used to treat infections caused by *H. pylori*, *M. avium* complex, or *B. pertussis*. Doxycycline is not routinely used to treat infections caused by *M. avium* complex or *S. aureus*.

36. d. erythromycin. Erythromycin is a macrolide, whereas plazomicin, gentamicin, tobramycin, and amikacin are all aminoglycosides.

37. b. piperacillin/tazobactam plus ceftazidime plus vancomycin. Recommended therapy for hospital-acquired pneumonia with risk factors for multidrug resistance includes two agents with activity against resistant gram-negative bacteria. The first agent should be an antipseudomonal cephalosporin, antipseudomonal carbapenem, piperacillin/tazobactam, or aztreonam. The second agent should be an antipseudomonal quinolone or a polymyxin. Linezolid or vancomycin should be added to cover MRSA.

38. a. amoxicillin. Amoxicillin is appropriate therapy for mild leptospirosis. Vancomycin, linezolid, amikacin, and metronidazole are not recommended for these infections.

39. d. cartilage damage. Penicillins have been associated with diarrhea, rash, anaphylaxis, and serum sickness. Cartilage damage, however, has occurred in juvenile animals exposed to quinolones.

40. b. *C. difficile*. Use of clindamycin is associated with the development of diarrhea and pseudomembranous colitis caused by *C. difficile*.

41. b. *Haemophilus* spp. Whereas *Enterobacter* spp., *Citrobacter* spp., and *K. aerogenes* each produce an inducible chromosomally encoded AmpC β-lactamase that may lead to treatment failures with third-generation cephalosporins, *Haemophilus* spp. do not produce these β-lactamases.

42. a. cefotetan. Of the listed cephalosporins, only cefotetan and cefoxitin have appreciable activity against anaerobic bacteria.

43. c. ertapenem. Unlike the carbapenems imipenem and meropenem, ertapenem has relatively weak antipseudomonal activity. Ceftazidime and piperacillin have potent antipseudomonal activity.

44. e. piperacillin/tazobactam. Antibiotics for infections caused by *L. pneumophila* include azithromycin, levofloxacin, ciprofloxacin, and moxifloxacin. Piperacillin/tazobactam does not have activity against this bacterium, presumably because it does not penetrate as well into macrophages, where the *Legionella* bacteria reside.

45. c. clofazimine. The recommended antibiotic regimen for the treatment of leprosy is dapsone plus rifampin plus clofazimine. Isoniazid, ethambutol, and streptomycin are used to treat tuberculosis but do not have activity against *M. leprae*. Amoxicillin/clavulanate also does not have activity against this bacterium.

46. d. ampicillin plus gentamicin. Ampicillin plus gentamicin or penicillin G plus gentamicin is the recommended antibiotic regimen for patients with native valve endocarditis caused by highly penicillin-resistant strains of viridans group streptococci. Penicillin G or ceftriaxone would be appropriate for infections caused by penicillin-susceptible strains. Oxacillin would be used for infective endocarditis caused by susceptible strains of *S. aureus*. Ampicillin plus amikacin would not be appropriate therapy for endocarditis.

47. b. cefazolin. Cefazolin is not effective in the treatment of patients with *C. jejuni* diarrhea. Clarithromycin, azithromycin, doxycycline, and ciprofloxacin each have activity against this organism.

48. a. ceftazidime. Appropriate empiric therapy for cellulitis should include agents with potent activity against gram-positive cocci, which cause most of these infections. Vancomycin, oxacillin, cefazolin, and clindamycin are highly active against gram-positive cocci, but ceftazidime has poor activity against these bacteria.

49. e. optic neuritis. Use of ethambutol is associated with the development of optic neuritis, which may lead to decreased visual acuity and loss of red-green discrimination.

50. c. linezolid. Recommended initial antimicrobial therapy for patients with prosthetic valve endocarditis caused by methicillin-susceptible *S. aureus* is antistaphylococcal penicillin (nafcillin or oxacillin) plus rifampin plus gentamicin. Recommended initial therapy for methicillin-resistant *S. aureus* infections is vancomycin plus rifampin plus gentamicin. Linezolid would not be optimal as initial treatment for staphylococcal infective endocarditis.

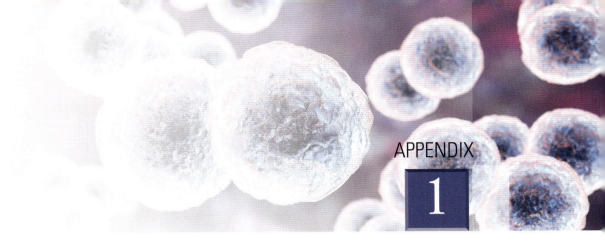

APPENDIX 1

Dosing of Antibacterial Agents in Adults

Agent	Usual Adult Dosage With Normal Renal Function
Natural penicillins	
Penicillin G	2-30 million units/day in divided doses IV/IM q4-6h (Note: IM route should not be used for concentrations >10 million units/mL.)
Penicillin V	125-500 mg PO q6-8h
Antistaphylococcal penicillins	
Nafcillin	0.5-2 g IV/IM q4-6h
Oxacillin	Mild-to-moderate infections: 250-500 mg IV/IM q4-6h Severe infections: 1-2 g IV q4-6h
Dicloxacillin	125-500 mg PO q6h
Aminopenicillins	
Ampicillin	Mild-to-moderate infections: 250-1,000 mg PO, IM, or IV q6h Severe infections: 150-200 mg/kg/day IV/IM in divided doses q3-4h (usual dose: 2 g IV q4h)
Amoxicillin	250-500 mg PO q8h or 500-875 mg PO q12h (1 g PO q8h for *Streptococcus pneumoniae* pneumonia)
Extended-spectrum penicillin	
Piperacillin (not available in the United States)	3-4 g IV/IM q4-6h (maximum: 24 g/day) (IM route should not be used for doses exceeding 3 g.)
Penicillin plus β-lactamase inhibitor combinations	
Ampicillin-sulbactam	1.5-3 g IV/IM q6h (maximum: 12 g/day)

(continued)

APPENDIX 1 — Dosing of Antibacterial Agents in Adults

Agent	Usual Adult Dosage With Normal Renal Function
Amoxicillin-clavulanate	250 mg amoxicillin/125 mg clavulanate, 1 tab PO q8h 500 mg amoxicillin/125 mg clavulanate, 1 tab PO q8-12h or 875 mg amoxicillin/125 mg clavulanate, 1 tab PO q12h
Amoxicillin-clavulanate extended release	1,000 mg amoxicillin/62.5 mg clavulanate, 2 tabs PO q12h (Use extended-release formulation for *S. pneumoniae* pneumonia.)
Piperacillin-tazobactam	3.375 g q6h or 4.5 g IV q8h (4.5 g IV q6h for *Pseudomonas aeruginosa*)
First-generation cephalosporins	
Cefazolin	0.5-2 g IV/IM q6-8h (maximum: 12 g/day)
Cefadroxil	1-2 g PO in divided doses q12-24h
Cephalexin	0.25-1 g PO q6h (maximum: 4 g/day)
Second-generation cephalosporins	
Cefotetan	1-3 g IV/IM q12h (maximum: 6 g/day)
Cefoxitin	1-2 g IV/IM q4-8h or 1-2 g IV q4h (maximum: 12 g/day)
Cefuroxime	0.75-1.5 g IV/IM q8h; meningitis: 3 g IV q8h
Cefuroxime axetil	250-500 mg PO q12h
Cefprozil	250 mg PO q12h or 500 mg PO q12-24h
Cefaclor	250-500 mg PO q8h
Third-generation cephalosporins	
Cefotaxime	1 g IV q8-12h to 2 g IV q4h
Ceftazidime	1-2 g IV q8-12h
Ceftriaxone	1-2 g IV q12-24h
Cefdinir	300 mg PO q12h or 600 mg PO q24h
Cefpodoxime	100-400 mg PO q12h
Cefixime	400 mg/day PO in divided doses q12-24h
Fourth-generation cephalosporin	
Cefepime	1-2 g IV q8-12h
Fifth-generation cephalosporin	
Ceftaroline	600 mg IV q12h
Cephalosporins plus β-lactamase inhibitors	
Ceftazidime-avibactam	2.5 g IV q8h
Ceftolozane-tazobactam	1.5 g IV q8h
Siderophore cephalosporins	
Cefiderocol	2 g IV q8h

Agent	Usual Adult Dosage With Normal Renal Function
Carbapenems	
Imipenem/cilastatin	0.5-1 g (imipenem component) IV q6-8h (maximum: 50 mg [imipenem component]/kg or 4 g [imipenem component]/day, whichever is lower) or 500-750 mg IM q12h
Meropenem	0.5-2 g IV q8h
Ertapenem	1 g IV/IM q24h
Imipenem-relebactam	1.25 g IV q6h
Meropenem-vaborbactam	4 g IV q8h
Monobactam	
Aztreonam	1-2 g IV/IM q8-12h up to 2 g q6-8h (maximum: 8 g/day)
Glycopeptides	
Vancomycin	15 mg/kg IV q12h 0.5-2 g/day PO in divided doses q6-8h (PO should not be used for systemic infections; dose should be adjusted based on serum levels when appropriate.)
Telavancin	10 mg/kg IV q24h
Dalbavancin	1.5 g IV single dose or 1 g IV followed by 0.5 g IV 1 wk later
Oritavancin	1.2 g IV single dose
Daptomycin	4-10 mg/kg IV q24h
Polymyxins	
Colistin (colistimethate)	2.5-5 mg/kg/day IM/IV in 2-4 divided doses
Polymyxin B	20,000-25,000 units/kg loading dose; then 12,500-15,000 units/kg q12h
Rifamycins	
Rifampin	Tuberculosis therapy: 10 mg/kg PO/IV q24h (maximum: 600 mg/day) Synergy for staphylococcal infections: 300-600 mg PO/IV q8-12h with other antibiotics
Rifabutin	*Mycobacterium avium* intracellulare complex therapy: initial phase: 5 mg/kg PO q24h (maximum: 300 mg/day); second phase: 5 mg/kg PO daily or twice weekly; may need to adjust dose in patients receiving concomitant protease inhibitor therapy
Rifapentine	Tuberculosis therapy: 600 mg PO given twice weekly (q72h) during the first 2 mo of treatment, once weekly thereafter
Rifaximin	200 mg PO q8h

(*continued*)

APPENDIX 1 — Dosing of Antibacterial Agents in Adults

Agent	Usual Adult Dosage With Normal Renal Function
Aminoglycosides	(Doses should be adjusted based on body weight and on peak and trough concentrations.)
Streptomycin	1-2 g/day IM in divided doses q6-12h Tuberculosis therapy: 15 mg/kg IM q24h (maximum: 1 g/day)
Gentamicin	2 mg/kg IV/IM load and then 5.1 mg/kg/day IV/IM in divided doses q8h; once-per-day dosing: 4-7 mg/kg IV q24h
Tobramycin	2 mg/kg IV load and then 5.1 mg/kg/day IV in divided doses q8h; once-per-day dosing: 4-7 mg/kg IV q24h
Amikacin	15 mg/kg IV in divided doses q8-12h; once-per-day dosing: 15 mg/kg IV q24h
Plazomicin	15 mg/kg IV q24h
Macrolides	
Erythromycin	Base, estolate, stearate preparations: 250-500 mg PO q6-12h (maximum: 4 g/day) Ethylsuccinate preparation: 400-800 mg PO q6h (maximum: 3.2 g/day) Lactobionate preparation: 15-20 mg/kg/day IV in divided doses q6h or 0.5-1 g IV q6h (maximum: 4 g/day)
Azithromycin	500 mg in a single loading dose PO on day 1, followed by 250 mg/day as a single dose on days 2-5 or 500 mg/day PO for a total of 3 d Extended-release suspension: 2 g PO as a single dose 500 mg IV q24h
Clarithromycin	250-500 mg PO q12h Extended-release formulation: 1 g PO q24h
Tetracyclines	
Tetracycline	250-500 mg PO q6h
Doxycycline	100-200 mg/day PO/IV in divided doses q12-24h
Minocycline	200 mg PO first dose and then 100 mg PO q12h
Tigecycline	100 mg IV first dose, followed by 50 mg IV q12h
Eravacycline	1 mg/kg IV q12h
Omadacycline	200 mg IV as a single dose or 100 mg IV q12h on day 1, followed by 100 mg IV q24h 300 mg PO q12h on day 1 or 450 mg PO q24h on days 1 and 2, followed by 300 mg PO q24h
Clindamycin	150-450 mg PO q6-8h (maximum: 1.8 g/day) 0.6-2.7 g IV/IM in divided doses q6-12h
Oxazolidinones	
Linezolid	600 mg PO/IV q12h
Tedizolid	200 mg PO/IV q24h

APPENDIX 1 — Dosing of Antibacterial Agents in Adults

Agent	Usual Adult Dosage With Normal Renal Function
Nitrofurantoin	Furadantin, Macrodantin: 50-100 mg PO q6h Macrobid: 100 mg q12h
Trimethoprim-sulfamethoxazole	1 DS tablet PO q12h 8-10 mg (trimethoprim component)/kg/day IV in divided doses q6-12h up to 15-20 mg (trimethoprim component)/kg/day in divided doses q6-8h
Quinolones	
Ofloxacin	200-400 mg PO q12h
Ciprofloxacin	250-750 mg PO q12h Cipro XR 500-1,000 mg PO q24h 200-400 mg IV q8-12h
Levofloxacin	250-750 mg PO/IV q24h
Moxifloxacin	400 mg PO/IV q24h
Delafloxacin	300 mg IV q12h 450 mg PO q12h
Gemifloxacin (not available in the United States)	320 mg PO q24h
Metronidazole	250-750 mg PO/IV q6-8h
Antimycobacterial agents	(Doses are those recommended for once-daily regimens.)
Isoniazid	5 mg/kg PO/IM q24h (maximum: 300 mg/day)
Rifampin	Tuberculosis therapy: 10 mg/kg PO/IV q24h (maximum: 600 mg/day)
Pyrazinamide	25-30 mg/kg/day PO q24h (maximum: 2 g/day)
Ethambutol	15-25 mg/kg/day PO q24h

Adapted from Gilbert DN, Moellering RC Jr, Eliopoulos GM, et al. *The Sanford Guide to Antimicrobial Therapy, 2011*. 41st ed. Antimicrobial Therapy, Inc.; 2011; UpToDate. Drug Information. In: Connor RF, ed. Wolters Kluwer. Accessed June 1, 2017 and December 29, 2023. http://www.uptodate.com; Thomson M. *Micromedex Healthcare Series*. Thomson Micromedex; 2006. Accessed September 1, 2006. http://www.micromedex.com; *Clinical Pharmacology*. Gold Standard, Inc.; 2006. Accessed September 1, 2006. http://www.clinicalpharmacology.com; https://www.clinicalkey.com/pharmacology/login; and American Society of Health-System Pharmacists. *AHFS Drug Information 2011*. American Society of Health-System Pharmacists; 2011.

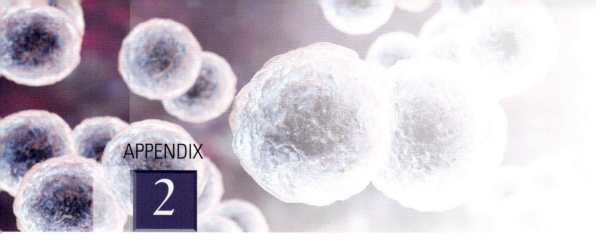

APPENDIX 2

Dosing of Antibacterial Agents in Children

Agent	Usual Pediatric Dosage With Normal Renal Function[a]
Natural penicillins	
Penicillin G	Infants and children: Mild-to-moderate infections: 25,000-50,000 units/kg/day IV/IM in divided doses q4h Severe infections: 250,000-400,000 units/kg/day IV/IM in divided doses q4-6h (maximum: 24 million units/day)
Penicillin V	Children <12 y: 25-50 mg/kg/day PO in divided doses q6-8h (maximum: 3 g/day) Children ≥12 y: 125-500 mg PO q6-8h
Antistaphylococcal penicillins	
Nafcillin	Infants and children: Mild-to-moderate infections: 50-100 mg/kg/day IV/IM in divided doses q6h Severe infections: 100-200 mg/kg/day IV in divided doses q4-6h (maximum: 12 g/day)
Oxacillin	Mild-to-moderate infections: 100-150 mg/kg/day IV/IM in divided doses q6h (maximum: 4 g/day) Severe infections: 150-200 mg/kg/day IV in divided doses q6h (maximum: 12 g/day)
Dicloxacillin	Children <40 kg: 25-50 mg/kg/day PO in divided doses q6h Children >40 kg: 125-500 mg PO q6h (maximum: 2 g/day)

Agent	Usual Pediatric Dosage With Normal Renal Function[a]
Aminopenicillins	
Ampicillin	Infants and children: 100-400 mg/kg/day IM/IV in divided doses q6h (maximum: 12 g/day) 50-100 mg/kg/day PO in divided doses q6h (maximum: 2-4 g/day)
Amoxicillin	Infants ≤3 mo: 20-30 mg/kg/day PO in divided doses q12h Infants and children >3 mo: 20-90 mg/kg/day PO in divided doses q8-12h
Extended-spectrum penicillin	
Piperacillin (not available in the United States)	Infants and children: 200-300 mg/kg/day IV/IM in divided doses q4-6h (maximum: 24 g/day)
Penicillins plus β-lactamase inhibitors	
Ampicillin-sulbactam	Infants >1 mo: 100-300 mg (ampicillin component)/kg/day IV/IM in divided doses q6h Children ≥1 y: 100-400 mg (ampicillin component)/kg/day IV/IM in divided doses q6h (maximum: 8 g ampicillin/day)
Amoxicillin-clavulanate	Infants <3 mo: 30 mg (amoxicillin component)/kg/day PO in divided doses q12h using the 125 mg/5 mL suspension Children <40 kg: 20-40 mg (amoxicillin component)/kg/day PO in divided doses q8h, or 25-45 mg (amoxicillin component)/kg/day in divided doses q12h using either 200 mg/5 mL or 400 mg/5 mL suspension or 200- or 400-mg (amoxicillin component) chewable tablet formulation (multidrug-resistant *Streptococcus pneumoniae* otitis media: 90 mg [amoxicillin component]/kg/day in divided doses q12h; use 7:1 BID formulation or Augmentin ES-600). Children <40 kg should not receive the 250-mg film-coated tablets.
Piperacillin-tazobactam	Safety and efficacy in children <12 y has not been established. Infants and children: 200-300 mg/kg/day in divided doses q6-8h
First-generation cephalosporins	
Cefazolin	Infants and children: 25-100 mg/kg/day IV/IM in divided doses q6-8h (maximum: 6 g/day)
Cefadroxil	Infants and children: 30 mg/kg/day PO in divided doses q12h (maximum: 2 g/day)
Cephalexin	Children >1 y: 25-100 mg/kg/day PO in divided doses q6-8h (maximum: 4 g/day)
Second-generation cephalosporins	
Cefotetan	Children: 40-80 mg/kg/day IV/IM in divided doses q12h (maximum: 6 g/day)

(continued)

Agent	Usual Pediatric Dosage With Normal Renal Function[a]
Cefoxitin	Infants ≥3 mo and children: 80-160 mg/kg/day IV/IM in divided doses q4-6h (maximum: 12 g/day)
Cefuroxime	Infants ≥3 mo to children 12 y: 75-150 mg/kg/day IV/IM in divided doses q8h up to 200-240 mg/kg/day in divided doses q6-8h (maximum: 9 g/day) Children ≥13 y: 0.75-1.5 g IV/IM q8h
Cefuroxime axetil	Infants ≥3 mo to children 12 y: Suspension: 20-30 mg/kg/day PO in divided doses q12h (maximum: 1 g/day) Tablet: 125-250 mg PO q12h Children ≥13 y: 250-500 mg PO q12h
Cefprozil	Children >6 mo to 12 y: 7.5 mg/kg PO q12h or 20 mg/kg PO q24h (maximum: 1 g/day) Children >12 y: 250-500 mg PO q12h or 500 mg PO q24h
Cefaclor	Infants >1 mo and children: 20-40 mg/kg/day PO in divided doses q8-12h (maximum: 1 g/day)
Third-generation cephalosporins	
Cefotaxime	Children 1 mo to 12 y: <50 kg: 75-100 mg/kg/day up to 150-300 mg/kg/day in divided doses q6-8h Children >12 y: 1-2 g IV q6-8h
Ceftazidime	Children 1 mo to 12 y: 100-150 mg/kg/day IV/IM q8h (maximum: 6 g/day) Children >12 y: 1-2 g IV/IM q8-12h
Ceftriaxone	Infants and children: 50-100 mg/kg/day IV/IM in divided doses q12-24h (maximum: 4 g/day)
Cefdinir	Children 6 mo to 12 y: 14 mg/kg/day PO in divided doses q12-24h (maximum: 600 mg/day) Children >12 y: 300 mg PO q12h or 600 mg PO q24h
Cefpodoxime	Children 2 mo to 12 y: 10 mg/kg/day PO in divided dose q12h (maximum: 200 mg/dose and 400 mg/day) Children >12 y: 100-400 mg PO q12h
Cefixime	Infants and children: 8 mg/kg/day PO in divided doses q12-24h (maximum: 400 mg/day)
Fourth-generation cephalosporin	
Cefepime	Children 2 mo to 16 y, ≤40 kg in weight: 50 mg/kg IV/IM q8-12h
Fifth-generation cephalosporin	

Ceftaroline	Children 2 mo to 2 y, 8 mg/kg IV q8h
	Children >2–18 y:
	  ≤33 kg: 12 mg/kg IV q8h
	  >33 kg: 400 mg IV q8h or 600 mg IV q12h

Carbapenems	

Agent	Usual Pediatric Dosage With Normal Renal Function[a]
Imipenem/cilastatin	Infants 4 wk to 3 mo: 100 mg/kg/day IV in divided doses q6h Infants ≥3 mo and children: 60-100 mg/kg/day IV in divided doses q6h (maximum: 4 g/day)
Meropenem	Children >3 mo (<50 kg): 10-40 mg/kg/day IV q8h (maximum: 1-2 g q8h) Children >50 kg: 1-2 g IV q8h
Ertapenem	Children 3 mo to 12 y: 30 mg/kg/day IV/IM in divided doses q12h (maximum: 1 g/day)
Monobactam	
Aztreonam	Children >1 mo: 30 mg/kg/dose IV/IM q6-8h up to 50 mg/kg/dose IV q6-8h (maximum: 120 mg/kg/day or 8 g/day)
Glycopeptide	
Vancomycin	Infants >1 mo and children: 40-60 mg/kg/day IV in divided doses q6-8h (maximum: 2 g/day)
Polymyxins	
Colistin (colistimethate)	2.5-5 mg/kg/day IV/IM in 2-4 divided doses
Polymyxin B	Infants, children: 12,000-15,000 units/kg IV q12h
Rifamycins	
Rifabutin	Children ≥6 y: 300 mg PO q24h
Rifampin	Tuberculosis therapy: infants and children: 10-20 mg/kg PO/IV q24h (maximum: 600 mg PO q24h)
Rifaximin	Children ≥12 y: 200 mg PO q8h
Aminoglycosides	(Doses should be adjusted based on body weight and on peak and trough concentrations.)
Streptomycin	20-30 mg/kg/day IM in divided doses q12h Tuberculosis therapy: 20-40 mg/kg IM q24h (maximum: 1 g/day)
Gentamicin	Children <5 y: 7.5 mg/kg/day IV/IM in divided doses q8h Children ≥5 y: 6-7.5 mg/kg/day IV/IM q8h Once-daily dosing: 5 mg/kg IV/IM q24h
Tobramycin	Infants and children: 6-7.5 mg/kg/day IV/IM q6-8h
Amikacin	Infants and children: 15-22.5 mg/kg/day IV/IM in divided doses q8h
Macrolides	
Erythromycin	Infants and children: base, estolate, and stearate preparations: 30-50 mg/kg/day PO in divided doses q6-8h (maximum: 2 g/day) Ethylsuccinate preparation: 30-50 mg/kg/day PO in divided doses q6-8h (maximum: 3.2 g/day) Lactobionate preparation: 15-50 mg/kg/day IV in divided doses q6h (maximum: 4 g/day)

(continued)

APPENDIX 2 — Dosing of Antibacterial Agents in Children

Agent	Usual Pediatric Dosage With Normal Renal Function[a]
Azithromycin	Children ≥6 mo: Respiratory tract infections: 10 mg/kg PO on day 1 (maximum: 500 mg/day), followed by 5 mg/kg PO q24h on days 2-5 (maximum: 250 mg/day) Otitis media: 30 mg/kg PO as a single dose (maximum: 1,500 mg) 3-d regimen: 10 mg/kg PO q24h for 3 d (maximum: 500 mg/day) 5-d regimen: 10 mg/kg PO on day 1 (maximum: 500 mg), followed by 5 mg/kg PO q24h on days 2-5 (maximum: 250 mg/day)
Clarithromycin	Infants and children: 15 mg/kg/day PO in divided doses q12h
Tetracyclines	
Tetracycline	Children >8 y: 25-50 mg/kg/day PO in divided doses q6-12h (maximum: 3 g/day)
Doxycycline	Children ≥8 y: 2.2-4.4 mg/kg/day PO/IV in divided doses q12-24h (maximum: 200 mg/day)
Minocycline	Children >8 y: 4 mg/kg PO first dose followed by 4 mg/kg/day PO in divided doses q12h
Clindamycin	Infants and children: 8-20 mg/kg/day PO as hydrochloride; 8-25 mg/kg/day PO as palmitate in divided doses q6-8h Children >1 mo: 20-40 mg/kg/day IV/IM in divided doses q6-8h
Oxazolidinones	
Linezolid	Infants and children: 30 mg/kg/day PO/IV in divided doses q8h
Tedizolid	Children >12 y: 200 mg/kg IV/PO q24h
Nitrofurantoin	Children >1 m (Furadantin, Macrodantin): 5-7 mg/kg/day PO in divided doses q6h (maximum: 400 mg/day) Children >12 y (Macrobid): 100 mg PO q12h
Trimethoprim-sulfamethoxazole	Children >2 mo: Mild-to-moderate infections: 6-10 mg (trimethoprim component)/kg/day PO/IV in divided doses q12h up to 15-20 mg (trimethoprim component)/kg/day PO/IV in divided doses q6-8h
Quinolones	Quinolones are not approved for use in children <16 y.
Metronidazole	Infants and children: 30-50 mg/kg/day PO/IV in divided doses q6-8h (maximum: 4 g/day)
Antimycobacterial agents	(Doses are those recommended for once-daily regimens.)
Isoniazid	Infants and children: 10-15 mg/kg PO/IM q24h (maximum: 300 mg/day)

APPENDIX 2 — Dosing of Antibacterial Agents in Children

Agent	Usual Pediatric Dosage With Normal Renal Function[a]
Rifampin	Tuberculosis therapy: infants and children: 10-20 mg/kg/day PO/IV q24h
Pyrazinamide	Infants and children: 15-30 mg/kg/day PO q24h (maximum: 2 g/day)
Ethambutol	Infants and children: 15-25 mg/kg/day PO q24h (maximum: 2.5 g/day) (Use cautiously in children <13 y.)

[a]Note: These dosing recommendations do not apply to neonates.
Adapted from Gilbert DN, Moellering RC Jr, Eliopoulos GM, et al. *The Sanford Guide to Antimicrobial Therapy, 2011*. 41st ed. Antimicrobial Therapy, Inc.; 2011; UpToDate. Drug Information. In: Connor RF, ed. Wolters Kluwer. Accessed June 1, 2017 and December 29, 2023. http://www.uptodate.com; Thomson M. *Micromedex Healthcare Series*. Thomson Micromedex; 2006. Accessed September 1, 2006. http://www.micromedex.com; *Clinical Pharmacology*. Gold Standard, Inc.; 2006. Accessed September 1, 2006. http://www.clinicalpharmacology.com; https://www.clinicalkey.com/pharmacology/login; and American Society of Health-System Pharmacists. *AHFS Drug Information 2011*. American Society of Health-System Pharmacists; 2011.

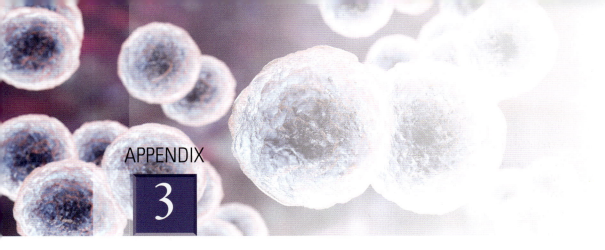

APPENDIX 3

Dosing of Antibacterial Agents in Adults With Renal Insufficiency

Agent	Creatinine Clearance (CrCl) (mL/min)	Typical Dose[a,b,c]
Natural penicillins		
Penicillin G	>50 10-50 <10	2-4 million units IV q4h 2-4 million units IV q6h 1-2 million units IV q6h
Penicillin V	>10 <10	500 mg PO q6h 500 mg PO q8h
Antistaphylococcal penicillins		
Nafcillin	Not renally dosed	2 g IV q4h
Oxacillin	<10	Adjustment to the lower range of the usual dosage
Dicloxacillin	Not renally dosed	500 mg PO q6h
Aminopenicillins		
Ampicillin	>50 10-50 <10	2 g IV q6h 2 g IV q6-12h 2 g IV q12h
Amoxicillin	>30 10-30 <10	500 mg PO q8h 500 mg PO q12h 500 mg PO q24h

APPENDIX 3 — Dosing of Antibacterial Agents in Adults With Renal Insufficiency

Agent	Creatinine Clearance (CrCl) (mL/min)	Typical Dose[a,b,c]
Extended-spectrum penicillin		
Piperacillin (not available in the United States)	>40 20-40 <20	4 g IV q8h 3-4 g IV q8h 3-4 g IV q12h
Penicillins plus β-lactamase inhibitors		
Ampicillin-sulbactam	>30 15-30 <15	2 g (ampicillin component) IV q6h 2 g IV q12h 2 g IV q24h
Amoxicillin-clavulanate	>30 10-30 <10	500 mg (amoxicillin component) PO q8h 500 mg (amoxicillin component) PO q12h (875 mg tablet should not be used with CrCl <30.) 500 mg (amoxicillin component) PO q24h
Amoxicillin-clavulanate extended release	>30 <30	2 g PO q12h Do not use
Piperacillin-tazobactam	>40 20-40 <20	3.375 g (piperacillin component) IV q6h or 4.5 g IV q6h 2.25 g IV q6h or 3.375 g IV q6h 2.25 g IV q8h or 2.25 g IV q6h
First-generation cephalosporins		
Cefazolin	>55 35-54 11-34 <10	1 g IV q6-8h 1 g IV q8h 1 g IV q12h 1 g IV q24h
Cefadroxil	>25 10-25 <10	500 mg PO q12h 500 mg PO q24h 500 mg PO q36h
Cephalexin	>40 10-40 <10	500 mg PO q6h 250 mg PO q8h 250 mg PO q12h
Second-generation cephalosporins		
Cefotetan	>30 10-30 <10	1-2 g IV q12h 1-2 g IV q24h or 1 g IV q12h 1-2 g IV q48h or 500 mg IV q12h

(continued)

Agent	Creatinine Clearance (CrCl) (mL/min)	Typical Dose[a,b,c]
Cefoxitin	>50	1-2 g IV q6h
	30-50	1-2 g IV q8-12h
	10-30	1-2 g IV q12-24h
	5-10	0.5-1 g IV q12-24h
	<5	0.5-1 g IV q24-48h
Cefuroxime	>20	750 mg IV q8h
	10-20	750 mg IV q12h
	<10	750 mg IV q24h
Cefuroxime axetil	Not renally dosed	250 mg PO q12h
Cefprozil	>30	500 mg PO q12h
	<30	250 mg PO q12h
Cefaclor	>10	500 mg PO q8h
	<10	250 mg PO q8h
Third-generation cephalosporins		
Cefotaxime	>20	1-2 g IV q8h
	<20	1 g IV q8h
Ceftazidime	>50	1-2 g IV q8h
	30-50	1-2 g IV q12h
	15-30	1-2 g IV q24h
	6-15	1 g IV q24h
	<6	1 g IV q24-48h
Ceftriaxone	Not renally dosed	1 g IV q24h
Cefdinir	>30	600 mg PO q24h
	<30	300 mg PO q24h
Cefpodoxime	>30	200 mg PO q12h
	<30	200 mg PO q24h
Cefixime	>60	400 mg PO q24h
	20-60	300 mg PO q24h
	<20	200 mg PO q24h
Fourth-generation cephalosporin		
Cefepime	>60	1-2 g IV q12h
	30-60	1-2 g IV q24h
	10-30	1 g IV q24h
	<10	500 mg IV q24h
Fifth-generation cephalosporin		
Ceftaroline	>50	600 mg IV q12h
	30-50	400 mg IV q12h
Cephalosporins plus β-lactamase inhibitors		
Ceftazidime-avibactam	>50	2.5 g IV q8h
	30-50	1.25 g IV q8h
	15-30	0.94 g IV q12h
	5-15	0.94 g IV q24h
	<5	0.94 g IV q48h

APPENDIX 3 — Dosing of Antibacterial Agents in Adults With Renal Insufficiency

Agent	Creatinine Clearance (CrCl) (mL/min)	Typical Dose[a,b,c]
Ceftolozane-tazobactam	>50	1.5 g IV q8h
	30-50	750 mg IV q8h
	<30	375 mg IV q8h
Carbapenems		
Imipenem/cilastatin	>70	(All doses are imipenem component and based on weight ≥70 kg.) 500 mg IV q6h
	40-70	500 mg IV q8h
	20-40	250 mg IV q6h
	6-20	250 mg IV q12h
	<6	Do not use
Meropenem	>50	1 g IV q8h
	25-50	1 g IV q12h
	10-25	500 mg IV q12h
	<10	500 mg IV q24h
Ertapenem	>30	1 g IV q24h
	<30	500 mg IV q24h
Imipenem-relebactam	≥90	1.25 g IV q6h
	60-89	1 g IV q6h
	30-59	750 mg IV q6h
	15-29	500 mg IV q6h
	<15	do not use
Meropenem-vaborbactam	≥50	4 g IV q8h
	30-49	2 g IV q8h
	15-29	2 g IV q12h
	<15	1 g IV q12h
Monobactam		
Aztreonam	>30	2 g IV q8h
	10-30	1 g IV q8h
	<10	500 mg IV q8h
Glycopeptides		
Vancomycin	>70	1 g (15 mg/kg) IV q12h
	50-70	1 g (15 mg/kg) IV q24h
	<50	1 g (15 mg/kg) IV with interval determined by serum levels
Telavancin	>50	10 mg/kg IV q24h
	30-50	7.5 mg/kg IV q24h
	10-30	10 mg/kg IV q48h
Dalbavancin	>30	1.5 g IV single dose or 1 g IV followed by 0.5 g IV 1 wk later
	<30	1.125 g IV single dose or 750 mg IV followed by 375 mg IV 1 wk later

(continued)

APPENDIX 3 — Dosing of Antibacterial Agents in Adults With Renal Insufficiency

Agent	Creatinine Clearance (CrCl) (mL/min)	Typical Dose[a,b,c]
Oritavancin	>30	1.2 g IV single dose
	<30	not yet defined
Daptomycin	>30	4-6 mg/kg IV q24h
	<30	4-6 mg/kg IV q48h
Rifamycins		
Rifampin	Not renally dosed	600 mg PO q24h
Rifabutin	Not renally dosed	300 mg PO q24h
Rifapentine	Not renally dosed	600 mg PO q72h
Rifaximin	Not renally dosed	200 mg PO q8h
Aminoglycosides	(Doses should be adjusted based on body weight and on peak and trough concentrations.)	
Streptomycin	>80	15 mg/kg IM q24h
	50-80	7.5 mg/kg IM q24h
	10-50	7.5 mg/kg IM q24-72h
	<10	7.5 mg/kg IM q72-96h
Gentamicin	>60	Conventional dosing: 1.7 mg/kg IV q8h; once-daily dosing: 4-7 mg/kg IV q24h
	40-60	Conventional dosing: 1.7 mg/kg IV q12h; once-daily dosing: 4-7 mg/kg IV q36h
	20-40	Conventional dosing: 1.7 mg/kg IV q24h; once-daily dosing: 4-7 mg/kg IV q48h
	<20	Based on serum levels
Tobramycin	>60	Conventional dosing: 1.7 mg/kg IV q8h; once-daily dosing: 4-7 mg/kg IV q24h
	40-60	Conventional dosing: 1.7 mg/kg IV q12h; once-daily dosing: 4-7 mg/kg IV q36h
	20-40	Conventional dosing: 1.7 mg/kg IV q24h; once-daily dosing: 4-7 mg/kg IV q48h
	<20	Based on serum levels
Amikacin	>60	Conventional dosing: 15 mg/kg/day IV in divided doses q8-12h; once-daily dosing: 15 mg/kg IV q24h
	40-60	Conventional dosing: 7.5 mg/kg IV q12h; once-daily dosing: 15 mg/kg IV q36h
	20-40	Conventional dosing: 7.5 mg/kg IV q24h; once-daily dosing: 15 mg/kg IV q48h
	<20	Based on serum levels

APPENDIX 3 — Dosing of Antibacterial Agents in Adults With Renal Insufficiency

Agent	Creatinine Clearance (CrCl) (mL/min)	Typical Dose[a,b,c]
Plazomicin	≥60	15 mg/kg IV q24h
	30-60	10 mg/kg IV q24h
	15-30	10 mg/kg IV q48h
	<15	not studied
Macrolides		
Erythromycin	Not renally dosed	1 g IV q6h 500 mg PO q6h
Azithromycin	Not renally dosed	500 mg IV q24h 500 mg PO × 1 and then 250 mg PO q24h
Clarithromycin	>30	500 mg PO q12h
	<30	250 mg PO q12h or 500 mg PO q24h
Tetracyclines		
Tetracycline	>80	500 mg PO q6h
	50-80	500 mg PO q8-12h
	10-50	500 mg PO q12-24h
	<10	Do not use
Doxycycline	Not renally dosed	100 mg IV/PO q12h
Minocycline	Not renally dosed	100 mg PO q12h
Tigecycline	Not renally dosed	100 mg IV first dose, followed by 50 mg IV q12h
Eravacycline	Not renally dosed	1 mg/kg IV q12h
Omadacycline	Not renally dosed	200 mg IV as single dose or 100 mg IV q12h on day 1, followed by 100 mg IV q24h 300 mg PO q12h on day 1 or 450 mg PO q24h on days 1 and 2, followed by 300 mg PO q24h
Clindamycin	Not renally dosed	600-900 mg IV q8h 150-450 mg PO q6h
Oxazolidinones		
Linezolid	Not renally dosed	600 mg IV/PO q12h
Tedizolid	Not renally dosed	200 mg PO/IV q24h
Nitrofurantoin	>60	Furadantin, Macrodantin: 50-100 mg PO q6h
	<60	Macrobid: 100 mg q12h contraindicated
Trimethoprim-sulfamethoxazole	>30	2.5 mg/kg IV q6h 1 DS tablet PO q12h
	15-30	1.25 mg/kg IV q6h 1 SS tablet PO q12h
	<15	Not recommended

(continued)

APPENDIX 3 — Dosing of Antibacterial Agents in Adults With Renal Insufficiency

Agent	Creatinine Clearance (CrCl) (mL/min)	Typical Dose[a,b,c]
Quinolones		
Ofloxacin	>50	400 mg PO q12h
	20-50	400 mg PO q24h
	<20	200 mg PO q24h
Ciprofloxacin	>50	400 mg IV q12h
		500 mg PO q12h
	30-50	400 mg IV q12h
		250-500 mg PO q12h
	5-30	200-400 mg IV q18-24h
		250-500 mg PO q18h
	<5	200 mg IV q24h
		250 mg PO q24h
Levofloxacin	>50	500-750 mg IV/PO q24h
	20-50	250 mg IV/PO q24h or 750 mg IV/PO q48h
	10-20	250 mg IV/PO q48h or 500 mg IV/PO q48h
Moxifloxacin	Not renally dosed	400 mg IV/PO q24h
Gemifloxacin (not available in the United States)	>40	320 mg PO q24h
	<40	160 mg PO q24h
Delafloxacin	>30	300 mg IV q12h
	15-29	450 mg PO q12h
	<15	200 mg IV q12h
		450 mg PO q12h
		Not recommended
Metronidazole	>10	500 mg IV/PO q6h
	<10	250 mg IV/PO q6h
Antimycobacterial agents		
Isoniazid	Not renally dosed	300 mg PO q24h
Rifampin	Not renally dosed	600 mg PO q24h
Pyrazinamide	>30	25-35 mg/kg PO q24h
	<30	25-35 mg/kg PO three times per week
Ethambutol	>50	15-25 mg/kg PO q24h
	10-50	15-25 mg/kg PO q24-36h
	<10	15-25 mg/kg PO q48h

[a]Actual dose may vary depending on indication, severity of infection, and patient characteristics.
[b]These recommendations do not apply to individuals receiving dialysis.
[c]Loading doses may be required for some agents.
Adapted from Blumberg HM, Burman WJ, Chaisson RE, et al. American Thoracic Society/Centers for Disease Control and Prevention/Infectious Diseases Society of America: treatment of tuberculosis. *Am J Respir Crit Care Med*. 2003;167:603-662; Cunha BA. *Antibiotic Essentials.* Physicians' Press; 2004; Gilbert

APPENDIX 3 — Dosing of Antibacterial Agents in Adults With Renal Insufficiency

DN, Moellering RC Jr, Eliopoulos GM, et al. *The Sanford Guide to Antimicrobial Therapy, 2011*. 41st ed. Antimicrobial Therapy, Inc.; 2011; UpToDate. Drug Information. In: Connor RF, ed. Wolters Kluwer. Accessed June 1, 2017 and December 29, 2023. http://www.uptodate.com; Thomson M. *Micromedex Healthcare Series*. Thomson Micromedex; 2006. Accessed September 1, 2006. http://www.micromedex.com; *Clinical Pharmacology*. Gold Standard, Inc.; 2006. Accessed September 1, 2006. http://www.clinicalpharmacology.com; https://www.clinicalkey.com/pharmacology/login; and American Society of Health-System Pharmacists. *AHFS Drug Information 2011*. American Society of Health-System Pharmacists; 2011.

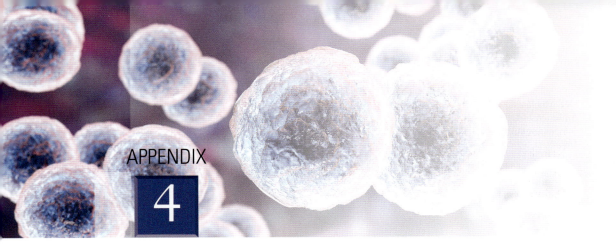

APPENDIX 4

Antibacterial Agents in Pregnancy

Antibiotics vary in their safety in pregnancy as well as in how well their use in pregnancy has been studied. As a result, the U.S. Food and Drug Administration places these agents into five categories with regard to use in pregnant women:

Category A: Adequate, well-controlled studies in pregnant women have not shown an increased risk of fetal abnormalities.

Category B: Either
1. animal studies have revealed no evidence of harm to the fetus; however, there are no adequate studies in pregnant women or
2. animal studies have shown an adverse effect, but adequate studies in pregnant women have failed to demonstrate a risk to the fetus.

Category C: Either
3. animal studies have shown an adverse effect, and there are no adequate studies in pregnant women or
4. no animal studies have been conducted, and there are no adequate studies in pregnant women.

Category D: Studies in pregnant women have demonstrated a risk to the fetus, but the benefits of therapy may outweigh the potential risk.

Category X: Studies in animals or pregnant women have demonstrated positive evidence of fetal abnormalities or risks. As a result, the use of the product is contraindicated in women who are or may become pregnant.

Agent	Pregnancy Risk Category
Natural penicillins	
Penicillin G	B
Penicillin V	B

Agent	Pregnancy Risk Category
Antistaphylococcal penicillins	
Nafcillin	B
Oxacillin	B
Dicloxacillin	B
Aminopenicillins	
Ampicillin	B
Amoxicillin	B
Extended-spectrum penicillin	
Piperacillin	B
Penicillins plus β-lactamase inhibitors	
Ampicillin-sulbactam	B
Amoxicillin-clavulanate	B
Piperacillin-tazobactam	B
First-generation cephalosporins	
Cefazolin	B
Cefadroxil	B
Cephalexin	B
Second-generation cephalosporins	
Cefotetan	B
Cefoxitin	B
Cefuroxime	B
Cefuroxime axetil	B
Cefprozil	B
Cefaclor	B
Third-generation cephalosporins	
Cefotaxime	B
Ceftazidime	B
Ceftriaxone	B
Cefdinir	B
Cefpodoxime	B
Cefixime	B
Fourth-generation cephalosporin	
Cefepime	B
Cephalosporins plus β-lactamase inhibitors	
Ceftolozane-tazobactam	B

(*continued*)

APPENDIX 4 — Antibacterial Agents in Pregnancy

Agent	Pregnancy Risk Category
Carbapenems	
Imipenem/cilastatin	C
Meropenem	B
Ertapenem	B
Monobactam	
Aztreonam	B
Glycopeptides	
Vancomycin	C
Telavancin	C
Dalbavancin	C
Oritavancin	C
Daptomycin	B
Polymyxins	
Colistin	C
Polymyxin B	C
Rifamycins	
Rifampin	C
Rifaximin	C
Rifabutin	C
Aminoglycosides	
Streptomycin	D
Gentamicin	D
Tobramycin	D
Amikacin	D
Macrolides	
Erythromycin	B
Azithromycin	B
Clarithromycin	C
Tetracyclines	
Tetracycline	D
Doxycycline	D
Minocycline	D
Tigecycline	D
Clindamycin	B

APPENDIX 4 — Antibacterial Agents in Pregnancy

Agent	Pregnancy Risk Category
Oxazolidinones	
Linezolid	C
Tedizolid	C
Nitrofurantoin	B
Trimethoprim-sulfamethoxazole	C
Quinolones	
Ofloxacin	C
Ciprofloxacin	C
Levofloxacin	C
Moxifloxacin	C
Gemifloxacin	C
Metronidazole	B
Antimycobacterial agents	
Isoniazid	C
Rifampin	C
Pyrazinamide	C
Ethambutol	B

Adapted from Bookstaver PB, Bland CM, Griffin B, et al. A review of antibiotic use in pregnancy. *Pharmacotherapy*. 2015;35:1052-1062. Gilbert DN, Moellering RC Jr, Eliopoulos GM, et al. *The Sanford Guide to Antimicrobial Therapy, 2011*. 41st ed. Antimicrobial Therapy, Inc.; 2011; Briggs GG, Freeman RK, Yaffe SJ. *Drugs in Pregnancy and Lactation*. 7th ed. Lippincott Williams & Wilkins; 2005; UpToDate. Drug Information. In: Connor RF, ed. Wolters Kluwer. Accessed June 7, 2018 and December 29, 2023. http://www.uptodate.com;

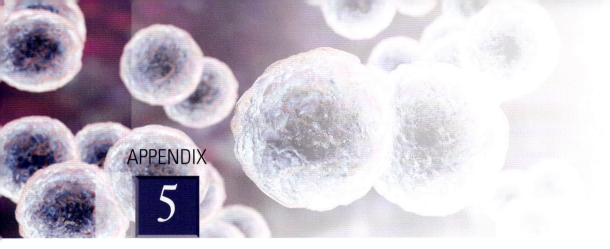

APPENDIX 5

Generic and Trade Names of Commonly Used Antibacterial Agents

Generic Name	Trade Name
amikacin	Amikin
amoxicillin	Amoxil, Polymox
amoxicillin-clavulanate	Augmentin
ampicillin	Omnipen, Polycillin, Principen
ampicillin-sulbactam	Unasyn
azithromycin	Zithromax
azithromycin ER	Zmax
aztreonam	Azactam
cefaclor	Ceclor
cefadroxil	Duricef
cefazolin	Ancef
cefdinir	Omnicef
cefepime	Maxipime
cefiderocol	Fetroja
cefixime	Suprax
cefotaxime	Claforan
cefotetan	Cefotan
cefoxitin	Mefoxin

APPENDIX 5 — Generic and Trade Names of Commonly Used Antibacterial Agents

Generic Name	Trade Name
cefpodoxime proxetil	Vantin
cefprozil	Cefzil
ceftaroline	Teflaro
ceftazidime	Fortaz, Tazicef
ceftazidime-avibactam	Avycaz
ceftriaxone	Rocephin
ceftolozane-tazobactam	Zerbaxa
cefuroxime	Kefurox, Zinacef
cefuroxime axetil	Ceftin
cephalexin	Keflex
ciprofloxacin	Cipro, Cipro XR
clarithromycin	Biaxin, Biaxin XL
clindamycin	Cleocin
clofazimine	Lamprene
colistin	Coly-Mycin M
dalbavancin	Dalvance
daptomycin	Cubicin
delafloxacin	Baxdela
dicloxacillin	Dynapen
doxycycline	Vibramycin
eravacycline	Xerava
ertapenem	Invanz
erythromycin	Ery-Tab, Eryc
erythromycin estolate	Ilosone
erythromycin ethylsuccinate	E.E.S., Ery-Ped, Pediamycin
erythromycin lactobionate	Erythrocin
erythromycin stearate	My-E
ethambutol	Myambutol
gemifloxacin	Factive
gentamicin	Garamycin
imipenem-cilastatin	Primaxin
imipenem-relebactam	Recarbrio
levofloxacin	Levaquin
linezolid	Zyvox
meropenem	Merrem

(*continued*)

APPENDIX 5 — Generic and Trade Names of Commonly Used Antibacterial Agents

Generic Name	Trade Name
meropenem-vaborbactam	Vabomere
metronidazole	Flagyl
minocycline	Minocin
moxifloxacin	Avelox
nafcillin	Nafcil, Unipen
nitrofurantoin	Furadantin, Macrobid, Macrodantin
ofloxacin	Floxin
omadacycline	Nuzyra
oritavancin	Orbactiv
oxacillin	Prostaphlin
penicillin G	Pfizerpen
penicillin V	Veetids
piperacillin	Pipracil
piperacillin-tazobactam	Zosyn
plazomicin	Zemdri
polymyxin B	—
rifabutin	Mycobutin
rifampin	Rifadin, Rimactane
rifapentine	Priftin
rifaximin	Xifaxan
tedizolid	Sivextro
telavancin	Vibativ
tigecycline	Tygacil
tobramycin	Nebcin
trimethoprim-sulfamethoxazole	Bactrim, Septra
vancomycin	Vancocin

Adapted from Gilbert DN, Moellering RC Jr, Eliopoulos GM, et al. *The Sanford Guide to Antimicrobial Therapy, 2011.* 41st ed. Antimicrobial Therapy, Inc.; 2011; UpToDate. Drug Information. In: Connor RF, ed. Wolters Kluwer. Accessed June 7, 2018 and December 29, 2023. http://www.uptodate.com;

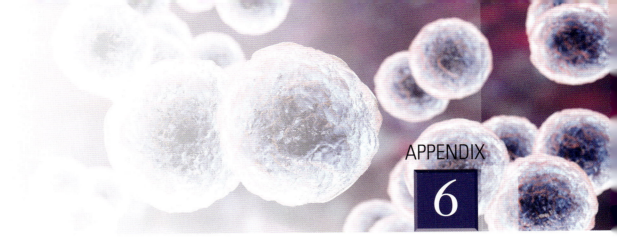

APPENDIX 6

Medical References

The information presented in this book was compiled from the following references in addition to those listed at the end of each chapter. The reader is referred to these sources for excellent overviews of clinical and microbiologic aspects of antibiotic therapy for infections caused by bacteria.

American Society of Health-System Pharmacists. *AHFS Drug Information 2023*. American Society of Health-System Pharmacists; 2023.

Bennett JE, Dolin R, Blaser MJ. *Mandell, Douglas, and Bennett's Principles and Practice of Infectious Diseases*. 9th ed. Elsevier; 2019.

Brunton LL, Knollman BC, eds. *Goodman & Gilman's: The Pharmacological Basis of Therapeutics*. 14th ed. McGraw-Hill; 2022.

Gilbert DN, Chambers HF, Saag MS, et al. *The Sanford Guide to Antimicrobial Therapy, 2023*. 53rd ed. Antimicrobial Therapy, Inc.; 2023.

Mascaretti OA. *Bacteria versus Antibacterial Agents: An Integrated Approach*. ASM Press; 2003.

UpToDate. Drug Information. In: Connor RF, ed. Wolters Kluwer. Accessed June 7, 2018 and December 29, 2023. http://www.uptodate.com;

Walsh C. *Antibiotics: Actions, Origins, Resistance*. ASM Press; 2003.

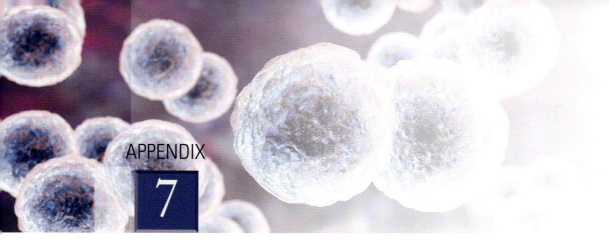

APPENDIX 7

Literary References

The quotations at the start of many of the chapters were taken from the following sources:

Ceasar J. *The Battle for Gaul*. David R. Godine; 1985.
Froissart J. *Chronicles*. Penguin Books; 1978.
Josephus F. *The Jewish War*. Penguin Books; 1986.
Musashi M. *The Book of Five Rings*. Bantam Books; 1992.
Payne-Gallwey SR. *Crossbow*. Marlboro Books, Dorset Press; 1989.
Potter KR, trans-ed. *Gesta Stephani*. Clarendon Press; 1976.
Prestwich M. *Armies and Warfare in the Middle Ages: The English Experience*. Yale University Press; 1996.
Seward D. *The Hundred Years War: The English in France, 1337–1453*. Atheneum; 1978.
Swanton M, trans-ed. *The Anglo-Saxon Chronicle*. Routledge; 1998.
Tuchman BW. *A Distant Mirror*. Ballantine Books; 1979.
Tzu S. *The Art of War*. Oxford University Press; 1971.
von Clausewitz C. *On War*. Penguin Books; 1982.
Warner P. *Sieges of the Middle Ages*. Pen & Sword; 2004.

Index

Note: Page numbers in *italics* indicate figures; t indicate tables.

A

abdominal pain
   intra-abdominal infections with, 226
   pelvic inflammatory disease with, 199
Acinetobacter baumannii, sites of infections from, 147
Acinetobacter spp.
   HAP caused by, 190, 191t
   treatment for infection with, 146–147, *147*, 147t
acquired resistance, 22
Actinomyces israelii
   aminopenicillins in treatment of, 30t
   extended-spectrum penicillins in treatment of, 30t
   natural penicillins in treatment of, 28t
acute uncomplicated cystitis
   activities of agents used to treat, *195*
   antimicrobial therapy for, 197t
   recommended empirical treatment of, 194, 197t
aerobes, 6
amikacin, 67, *67*, 67t, 68
   Acinetobacter spp. infection treatment with, 147, 147t
   Campylobacter jejuni infection treatment with, 138, 139t
   Citrobacter spp. infection treatment with, 128t, 130
   Enterobacter spp. infection treatment with, 128t, 130
   Escherichia coli infection treatment with, 127, 128t
   Klebsiella spp. infection treatment with, 127, 128t
   MAC infection treatment with, 180, 181t
   Moraxella catarrhalis infection treatment with, 145, 146t
   Morganella spp. infection treatment with, 128t, 130
   mycobacterial infections treatment with, 97
   Proteus spp. infection treatment with, 127, 128t
   Providencia spp. infection treatment with, 128t, 130
   Serratia spp. infection treatment with, 128t, 130
aminoglycosides
   Acinetobacter spp. infection treatment with, 147t
   aerobic gram-negative bacteria caused infections treatment with, *101*

amikacin, 67, *67*, 67t, 68
   antimicrobial activity of, 68t
   atypical bacteria caused infections treatment with, *101*
   Campylobacter jejuni infection treatment with, 138, 139t
   Escherichia coli infection treatment with, 127, 128t
   Francisella tularensis infection treatment with, 165t
   gentamicin, 67, 67t, 69
   Klebsiella spp. infection treatment with, 127, 128t
   Listeria monocytogenes infection treatment with, 205t
   MAC infection treatment with, 181t
   Moraxella catarrhalis infection treatment with, 145, 146t
   neomycin, 67, 67t
   plazomicin, 69
   Proteus spp. infection treatment with, 127, 128t
   Pseudomonas aeruginosa infection treatment with, 132, 134t
   Staphylococcus aureus infection treatment with, 110t
   Streptococcus agalactiae infection treatment with, 205t
   Streptococcus pyogenes penicillin-resistant infection treatment with, 117, 117t
   streptomycin, 67, 67t
   tobramycin, 67, 67t, 69
   toxicity of, 70
   Yersinia enterocolitica infection treatment with, 128t
aminopenicillins/β-lactamase inhibitor
   Borrelia burgdorferi infection treatment with, 172t
   Chlamydia spp. infection treatment with, 157t
   Haemophilus influenzae infection treatment with, 143
   Helicobacter pylori infection treatment with, 140t
   Leptospira interrogans infection treatment with, 174t
   Listeria monocytogenes infection treatment with, 205t
   meningitis treatment with, 203t
   Streptococcus agalactiae infection treatment with, 205t

aminopenicillins plus β-lactamase inhibitor
    Acinetobacter spp. infection treatment with, 146, 147t
    Haemophilus influenzae infection treatment with, 144t
    Moraxella catarrhalis infection treatment with, 146t
amoxicillin plus clarithromycin plus proton pump inhibitor
    Helicobacter pylori infection treatment with, 140t
aminopenicillins, 27t
    otitis media treatment with, 212t
aminopenicillin/β-lactamase inhibitor combinations, 27
amoxicillin, 27t, 29
amoxicillin-clavulanate, 27t, 31
    Borrelia burgdorferi infection treatment with, 172, 172t, 189t, 190
    CAP treatment with, 189t, 190
    Chlamydia spp. infection treatment with, 156, 157t
    Haemophilus influenzae infection treatment with, 143, 144t
    Helicobacter pylori infection treatment with, 139, 140t
    Leptospira interrogans infection treatment with, 173, 174t
    Moraxella catarrhalis infection treatment with, 144, 146t, 212, 212t
    otitis media treatment with, 212t, 213
AmpC, 129
ampicillin, 27t, 29, *30*
ampicillin-sulbactam, 27t, 31
    Acinetobacter spp. infection treatment with, 146, 147t
    Bacteroides spp. infection treatment with, 153, 154t
    infective endocarditis treatment with, 221, 221t
    Porphyromonas spp. infection treatment with, 153, 154t
    Prevotella spp. infection treatment with, 153, 154t
    Staphylococcus aureus infection treatment with, 110t
ampicillin/sulbactam
    CAP treatment with, 189t, 190
    enterococci infection treatment with, 119, 121t
    Escherichia coli infection treatment with, 127, 128t
    infective endocarditis treatment with, *217*, 218–219, 218t, 219t
    Klebsiella spp. infection treatment with, 127, 128t
    Leptospira interrogans infection treatment with, 173, 174t
    Listeria monocytogenes infection treatment with, 123, 123t, *204*, 205, 205t
    meningitis treatment with, 203t, 204, *204*
    Neisseria meningitidis infection treatment with, 204, *204*, 205t
    Proteus spp. infection treatment with, 127, 128t
    Streptococcus agalactiae infection treatment with, 116–117, 117t, 204, *204*, 205t
    Streptococcus pneumoniae infection treatment with, 114t
    Streptococcus pyogenes infection treatment with, 117t
    uncomplicated acute pyelonephritis treatment with, 197, 197t
anaerobes, 6
    clindamycin in treatment of, 79t
    metronidazole in treatment of, 95t
anaerobic bacteria, 18, 149
    carbapenems in treatment of, 48t
    Clostridia spp., 150–152, *150*, 151t
    glycopeptides in treatment of, 54t
    intra-abdominal infections caused by, 226, 227t
    pelvic inflammatory disease caused by, 199t
anaerobic gram-negative bacilli
    sites of infections from, 153
    treatment for infection with, 153–154, 154t
antibacterial agents
    activity of, 17
    aerobic gram-negative bacteria caused infections treatment with, 100–102, *101*
    aerobic gram-positive bacteria caused infections treatment with, 100, *101*
    anaerobic bacteria caused infections treatment with, 102, *102*
    atypical bacteria caused infections treatment with, 102–103, *103*
    categories based on mechanism of action, 17
    history of, 18
    summary, 100–103, *101*, *102*, *103*
    traffic sign representation of, 18
antibiotics
    cell envelope targeting (*See* cell envelope)
    history of, 213
    measuring susceptibility to, 14–15
    protein production blocking (*See* protein production)
antimicrobial compounds, categories based on mechanism of action, 17
antimycobacterial agents, 97
    azithromycin, 98
    clarithromycin, 98
    ethambutol, 97
    isoniazid, 98
    pyrazinamide, 98
    rifabutin, 98
    rifampin, 98
    rifapentine, 98
antipseudomonal cephalosporin, VAP treatment with, 191t, 192
antipseudomonal penicillin, VAP treatment with, 191t, 192
antistaphylococcalpenicillins, 27, 27t, 29
    antimicrobial activity of, 29t, 110t
    atypical bacteria caused infections treatment with, *101*

cellulitis treatment with, 207, 208t
infective endocarditis treatment with, *217*, 221
intravascular-related catheter infection
   treatment with, *224*, 224t
R side chain of, *29*
appendicitis, 226
atypical bacteria, 18, 155
   antibacterial agents in treatment of, 102–103, *103*
   Brucella, 162–163, *162*, 163t
   Chlamydia spp., 156–157, *156*, 157t
   Francisella tularensis, 164–165, *164*, 165t
   Legionella, 160–161, *160*, 161t
   Mycoplasma, 158–159, *158*, 158t
   Rickettsia, 166–167, *166*, 166t
azithromycin, 71, 71t, 73, 98
   Bordetella pertussis infection treatment with, 144, 145t
   Campylobacter jejuni infection treatment with, 138, 139t
   CAP treatment with, 189t, 190
   Chlamydia spp. infection treatment with, 156, 157t
   Haemophilus influenzae infection treatment with, 143, 144t
   Legionella spp. infection treatment with, 160, 161t
   MAC infection treatment with, 180, 181t
   Moraxella catarrhalis infection treatment with, 145, 146t
   Mycoplasma spp. infection treatment with, 158, 158t
   otitis media treatment with, 212t, 213
   Salmonella enterica infection treatment with, 128t, 131
   Shigella spp. infection treatment with, 128t, 131
   Staphylococcus aureus infection treatment with, 110t
   Streptococcus pneumoniae infection treatment with, 114, 114t
   Streptococcus pyogenes infection treatment with, 116, 117t
   Vibrio cholerae infection treatment with, 141, 141t
aztreonam, 51–52, *51*
   CAP treatment with, 190
   Escherichia coli infection treatment with, 127, 128t
   Klebsiella spp. infection treatment with, 127, 128t
   Proteus spp. infection treatment with, 127, 128t
   Pseudomonas aeruginosa infection treatment with, 132, 134t
   VAP treatment with, 191t, 192

B

bacilli, 4. *See also* anaerobic gram-negative bacilli; enteric gram-negative bacilli; gram-negative facultative and aerobic bacilli
bacteria. *See also* anaerobic bacteria; antibacterial agents; atypical bacteria; curved gram-negative bacteria; gram-negative bacteria; gram-positive bacteria
   cell envelope, 3–5, *4*, *5*
   DNA replication with, 1
   facultative, 7, 199t
   microaerophilic, 7
   pathogenic, 1, 6–8, *8*
   protein production, 7
   replication, 10–13, *11*, *12*, *13*
bactericidal, 14
bacteriostatic, 14
Bacteroides
   pelvic inflammatory disease with, 199
   treatment for infection with, 153–154, 154t
Bacteroides fragilis, 7, 18, 153
   carbapenems in treatment of, 48t
   clindamycin in treatment of, 79t
   intra-abdominal infections caused by, 227t
   metronidazole in treatment of, 95, 95t
   tetracycline in treatment of, 76t
Bacteroides spp.
   aminopenicillins/β-lactamase inhibitor combinations in treatment of, 31t
   extended-spectrum penicillins in treatment of, 31t
   intra-abdominal infections caused by, 227t
   penicillin plus β-lactamase inhibitor combinations in treatment of, 32t
   quinolones in treatment of, 91t
bedaquiline, multidrug-resistant (MDR) tuberculosis, 178
benzathine penicillin, 170
bezlotoxumab, 18
biliary tract infections, 226
binary fission, 10
bismuth subsalicylate, *Helicobacter pylori* infection treatment with, 139, 140t
Bordetella pertussis
   macrolides in treatment of, 72t
   sites of infections from, *145*
   treatment for infection with, 144, *145*, 145t
Borrelia burgdorferi
   macrolides in treatment of, 72t
   sites of infections from, *171*
   treatment for infection with, 171–172, *171*, 172t
Broth dilution methods, 15
Brucella abortus, 162
Brucella canis, 162
Brucella melitensis, 162
Brucella spp.
   sites of infections from, *162*
   treatment for infection with, 162–163, *162*, 163t
Brucella suis, 162

C

Campylobacter jejuni, 7
   sites of infections from, *138*
   treatment for infection with, 138, *138*, 139t, 142
CAP. *See* community-acquired pneumonia
capreomycin, mycobacterial infections treatment with, 97

carbapenems, 22
   Acinetobacter spp. infection treatment with, 147, 147t
   aerobic gram-negative bacteria caused infections treatment with, *101*
   anaerobic bacteria caused infections treatment with, *102*
   antimicrobial activity of, 110t, 48t
   atypical bacteria caused infections treatment with, *101*
   Bacteroides spp. infection treatment with, 153, 154t
   Citrobacter spp. infection treatment with, 127, 128t
   Enterobacter spp. infection treatment with, 127, 128t
   enterococci infection treatment with, 119, 121t
   ertapenem, 46, 46t, 48, 48t
   Haemophilus influenzae infection treatment with, 143, 144t
   history of, 47
   imipenem, 46, 46t
   imipenem-relebactam, 46t, 47, 48t
   intra-abdominal infection treatment with, 226, 227, 228t
   intravascular-related catheter infection treatment with, 223, *224*, 224t
   meropenem, 46, 46t
   meropenem-vaborbactam, 46t, 47–48, 48, 48–49, 48t
   Morganella spp. infection treatment with, 127, 128t
   Porphyromonas spp. infection treatment with, 153, 154t
   Prevotella spp. infection treatment with, 153, 154t
   Providencia spp. infection treatment with, 127, 128t
   Pseudomonas aeruginosa infection treatment with, 132, 134t
   Serratia spp. infection treatment with, 127, 128t
   structure of, *46*
   toxicity of, 49
   uncomplicated acute pyelonephritis treatment with, 197, 197t
   urinary tract infections treatment with, 197, 197t
   VAP treatment with, 191t, 192, *192*
cefaclor, 36t
cefadroxil, 35, 36t
cefazolin, 35, *36*, 36t
   cellulitis treatment with, 207, 208t
   Escherichia coli infection treatment with, 127, 128t
   infective endocarditis treatment with, *217*
   intravascular-related catheter infection treatment with, 223, 224t
   Klebsiella spp. infection treatment with, 127, 128t
   Proteus spp. infection treatment with, 127, 128t
   Staphylococcus aureus infection treatment with, 110t
   Streptococcus pyogenes infection treatment with, 116, 117t
cefdinir, 36t
cefdinir, otitis media treatment with, 212t, 213
cefepime, 36t, 39, *39*
   CAP treatment with, 190
   cellulitis treatment with, 209, 208t
   Citrobacter spp. infection treatment with, 128t
   Enterobacter spp. infection treatment with, 128t
   Escherichia coli infection treatment with, 127, 128t
   infective endocarditis treatment with, 217t
   intra-abdominal infection treatment with, 226, 228t
   intravascular-related catheter infection treatment with, 223, *224*, 224t
   Klebsiella spp. infection treatment with, 127, 128t
   Morganella spp. infection treatment with, 128t
   Proteus spp. infection treatment with, 127, 128t
   Providencia spp. infection treatment with, 128t
   Pseudomonas aeruginosa infection treatment with, 132, 134t
   Serratia spp. infection treatment with, 128t
   Staphylococcus aureus infection treatment with, 110t
   Streptococcus pneumoniae infection treatment with, 113–114, 114t
   urinary tract infections treatment with, 197, 197t, 197
   VAP treatment with, 191t, 192, *192*
cefiderocol, 42, *43*
cefixime, 36t
   Salmonella enterica infection treatment with, 128t, 131
   Shigella spp. infection treatment with, 128t, 131
cefotaxime, 36t, 37
   CAP treatment with, 189t, 190
   Escherichia coli infection treatment with, 128t, 205t
   Haemophilus influenzae infection treatment with, 143, 144t, 205t
   intra-abdominal infection treatment with, 226, 228t
   Klebsiella spp. infection treatment with, 128t
   meningitis treatment with, 203, 203t, 204
   Moraxella catarrhalis infection treatment with, 145, 145t
   Neisseria meningitidis infection treatment with, 136t, 205t
   PID treatment with, 200t, 201
   Proteus spp. infection treatment with, 128t
   Salmonella enterica infection treatment with, 128t
   Shigella spp. infection treatment with, 128t
   Staphylococcus aureus infection treatment with, 110t

Streptococcus pneumoniae infection treatment with, 204, 205t
cefotetan, 36, 36t, *37*
   Bacteroides spp. infection treatment with, 153, 154t
   PID treatment with, 200t, 201
   Porphyromonas spp. infection treatment with, 153, 154t
   Prevotella spp. infection treatment with, 153, 154t
cefoxitin, 36, 36t
   Bacteroides spp. infection treatment with, 153, 154t
   PID treatment with, 200t, 201
   Porphyromonas spp. infection treatment with, 153, 154t
   Prevotella spp. infection treatment with, 153, 154t
cefpodoxime proxetil, 36t
cefpodoxime, otitis media treatment with, 212t, 213
cefprozil, 36t
ceftaroline, 36t
   CAP treatment with, 189t, 190
   cellulitis treatment with, 208t, 209, *209*
   methicillin-resistant *Staphylococcus aureus* infection treatment with, 110t
ceftazidime, 36t, 37, *38*
   CAP treatment with, 190
   intra-abdominal infection treatment with, 226, 228t
   intravascular-related catheter infection treatment with, 223, *224*, 224t
   Pseudomonas aeruginosa infection treatment with, 132, 134t
   VAP treatment with, 191t, 192, *192*
ceftazidime-avibactam, 36t, 41
   Escherichia coli infection treatment with, 127, 128t
   Klebsiella spp. infection treatment with, 127, 128t
   Proteus spp. infection treatment with, 127, 128t
ceftolozane-tazobactam, 36t, 41
   Pseudomonas aeruginosa infection treatment with, 132, 134t
ceftriaxone, 36t, 37
   Borrelia burgdorferi infection treatment with, 172, 172t
   CAP treatment with, 189t, 190
   Escherichia coli infection treatment with, 127, 128t, 205t
   Haemophilus influenzae infection treatment with, 143, 144t, 205t
   infective endocarditis treatment with, 216–219, *217*, 217–219t, 221, 221t
   intra-abdominal infection treatment with, 226, 228t
   Klebsiella spp. infection treatment with, 127, 128t
   Leptospira interrogans infection treatment with, 173, 174t
   meningitis treatment with, 203t, 204, 204
   Moraxella catarrhalis infection treatment with, 145, 146t
   Neisseria gonorrhoeae infection treatment with, 136, 137t
   Neisseria meningitidis infection treatment with, 136, 136t, 205t
   PID treatment with, 200t, 201
   Proteus spp. infection treatment with, 127, 128t
   Salmonella enterica infection treatment with, 128t, 131
   Shigella spp. infection treatment with, 128t, 131
   Staphylococcus aureus infection treatment with, 110t
   Streptococcus pneumoniae infection treatment with, 205, 205t, 113–114, 114t
   Treponema pallidum infection treatment with, 170, 170t
   uncomplicated acute pyelonephritis treatment with, 197, 197t
cefuroxime, 36, 36t
   Borrelia burgdorferi infection treatment with, 172, 172t
   CAP treatment with, 189t, 190
   Haemophilus influenzae infection treatment with, 143, 144t
   intra-abdominal infection treatment with, 226, 228t
   Moraxella catarrhalis infection treatment with, 145, 146t
   otitis media treatment with, 212t, 213
   Staphylococcus aureus infection treatment with, 110t
   Streptococcus pneumoniae infection treatment with, 113–114, 114t
cefuroxime axetil, 36t
cell envelope, 3–5, *5*
   antibiotics that target, 21
      β-lactam antibiotics, 22–52, *22–25*, 22t, *27–30*, 27t, 28t, 30t, 32t, *34*, 34t, *36*, 37t, *38–40*, 39–41t, *42*, *46*, 46t, 48t, *51*, 51t
      carbapenems, 22, 46–49, *46*, 46t, 48t
      cephalosporins, 22, 34–44, *34*, 34t, *36*, 37t, *38–40*, 39–41t, *42*
      daptomycin, 58–59, *58*, 58t
      glycopeptides, 53–57, *53*, 53t, 54t, *55*
      lipoglycopeptides, 53–57, *53*, 53t
      monobactams, 22, 51–52, *51*, 51t
      penicillins, 22, 27–33, *27–30*, 27t, 28t, 30t, 32t
      polymyxins, 60–61, *60*, 60t, 61t
   defined, 3
   structure of, *4*
cellulitis
   activities of agents used to treat, *209*
   bacterial causes of, 207, 208t
   MRSA risk with, 207–210
   treatment of, 207–210, 208t

cephalexin, 36t
cephalexin, cellulitis treatment with, 208, 208t
cephalosporin plus β-lactamase inhibitors
   aerobic gram-negative bacteria caused infections treatment with, *101*
   Pseudomonas aeruginosa infection treatment with, 132, 134t
cephalosporins, 22, 34–44
   aerobic gram-negative bacteria caused infections treatment with, *101*
   anaerobic bacteria caused infections treatment with, *102*
   antipseudomonal, VAP treatment with, 191t, 192
   atypical bacteria caused infections treatment with, *102*
   Bacteroides spp. infection treatment with, 153, 154t
   β-lactamase inhibitor combinations, 34t, 41, 41t, *42*
   Borrelia burgdorferi infection treatment with, 172t
   cellulitis treatment with, 207, 208t, *209*
   Citrobacter spp. infection treatment with, 128t
   Enterobacter spp. infection treatment with, 128t
   Escherichia coli infection treatment with, 127, 128t, 204, 205t
   fifth-generation, 34t, 40–41, *40*, 40t
   first-generation, 34t, 35, *36*
   fourth-generation, 34t, 39, *39*, 39t
   Haemophilus influenzae infection treatment with, 204, 205t, 143, 144t
   history of, 44
   siderophore, 42–43, *43*, *42*
   intra-abdominal infection treatment with, 226, 227, 228t
   intravascular-related catheter infection treatment with, 223, 224t
   Klebsiella spp. infection treatment with, 127, 128t
   Leptospira interrogans infection treatment with, 174t
   meningitis treatment with, 203, 203t, 204, *204*
   methicillin-resistant *Staphylococcus aureus* infection treatment with, 110t
   Moraxella catarrhalis infection treatment with, 145, 146t
   Morganella spp. infection treatment with, 128t
   Neisseria gonorrhoeae infection treatment with, 136
   Neisseria meningitidis infection treatment with, 204, 205t, 136, 137t
   otitis media treatment with, 212t, 213
   PID treatment with, 200t, 201
   Porphyromonas spp. infection treatment with, 153, 154t
   Prevotella spp. infection treatment with, 153, 154t
   Proteus spp. infection treatment with, 127, 128t
   Providencia spp. infection treatment with, 128t
   Pseudomonas aeruginosa infection treatment with, 132, 134t
   Salmonella enterica infection treatment with, 128t, 131
   second-generation, 34t, 36, *37*, 37t
   Serratia spp. infection treatment with, 128t
   Shigella spp. infection treatment with, 128t, 131
   six Ps for, 35
   Streptococcus pneumoniae infection treatment with, 204, *204*, 205t, 113–114, 114t
   Streptococcus pyogenes infection treatment with, 116–117, 117t
   structure of, *34*
   third-generation, 34t, 37–38, *38*, 38t
   toxicity with, 43
   Treponema pallidum infection treatment with, 170t
   uncomplicated acute pyelonephritis treatment with, 197, 197t
   urinary tract infections treatment with, 197t
chills
   infective endocarditis with, 215
   intra-abdominal infections with, 226
   pelvic inflammatory disease with, 199
Chlamydia pneumoniae, 156–157, 157t
   CAP caused by, 188, 188t
Chlamydia psittaci, 156
Chlamydia spp., 18
   macrolides in treatment of, 72t
   quinolones in treatment of, 91t
   sites of infections from, *156*
   treatment for infection with, 156–157, *156*, 157t
Chlamydia trachomatis, 156–157
   pelvic inflammatory disease caused by, 199t
ciprofloxacin, 91–92
   Bordetella pertussis infection treatment with, 144, 145t
   Brucella spp. infection treatment with, 162, 163t
   Campylobacter jejuni infection treatment with, 138, 139t
   Citrobacter spp. infection treatment with, 128t, 130
   Enterobacter spp. infection treatment with, 128t, 130
   Escherichia coli infection treatment with, 127, 128t
   Francisella tularensis infection treatment with, 165, 165t
   Haemophilus influenzae infection treatment with, 143, 144t
   infective endocarditis treatment with, *217*, 221, 221t
   intra-abdominal infection treatment with, 226, 228t
   Klebsiella spp. infection treatment with, 127, 128t
   Legionella spp. infection treatment with, 160, 161t

Moraxella catarrhalis infection treatment with, 145, 146t
Morganella spp. infection treatment with, 128t, 130
Neisseria meningitidis infection treatment with, 137, 136t
Proteus spp. infection treatment with, 127, 128t
Providencia spp. infection treatment with, 128t, 130
Pseudomonas aeruginosa infection treatment with, 132, 134t
R1 side chain of, *92*
Rickettsia spp. infection treatment with, 166t, 167
Salmonella enterica infection treatment with, 128t, 131
Serratia spp. infection treatment with, 128t, 130
Shigella spp. infection treatment with, 128t, 131
Staphylococcus aureus infection treatment with, 110t
uncomplicated acute pyelonephritis treatment with, 197, 197t
urinary tract infections treatment with, 197, 197t
VAP treatment with, 192, 192t
Vibrio cholerae infection treatment with, 141, 141t
Yersinia enterocolitica infection treatment with, 128t
Citrobacter, 127–130, 128t
clarithromycin, 71, 71t, 72, 98
Bordetella pertussis infection treatment with, 144, 145t
Campylobacter jejuni infection treatment with, 138, 139t
CAP treatment with, 189t, 190
Helicobacter pylori infection treatment with, 139, 140t
Legionella spp. infection treatment with, 160, 161t
MAC infection treatment with, 180, 181t
Moraxella catarrhalis infection treatment with, 145, 146t
Mycobacterium leprae infection treatment with, 183, 182t
otitis media treatment with, 212t, 213
clavulanate
Haemophilus influenzae infection treatment with, 143, 144t
Moraxella catarrhalis infection treatment with, 145, 146t
clindamycin
anaerobic bacteria caused infections treatment with, *102*
antimicrobial activity of, 79t
atypical bacteria caused infections treatment with, *102*
Bacteroides spp. infection treatment with, 153, 154t
cellulitis treatment with, 208, 208t, *209*
Chlamydia spp. infection treatment with, 156
Clostridia spp. infection treatment with, 151
otitis media treatment with, 212t, 213
Porphyromonas spp. infection treatment with, 153, 154t
Prevotella spp. infection treatment with, 153, 154t
Staphylococcus aureus infection treatment with, 110t
Streptococcus pneumoniae infection treatment with, 114t, 114
Streptococcus pyogenes infection treatment with, 116, 117t
structure of, *78*
toxicity of, 78–79
utility of, 78
clofazimine
mycobacterial infections treatment with, 97
Mycobacterium leprae infection treatment with, 182, 182t
Clostridia spp.
aminopenicillins in treatment of, 30t
extended-spectrum penicillins in treatment of, 31t
natural penicillins in treatment of, 28t
penicillin plus β-lactamase inhibitor combinations in treatment of, 32t, 32t
quinolones in treatment of, 91t
sites of infections from, *150*
treatment for infection with, 150–152, *150*, 151t
Clostridioides difficile, 150, *150*
Clostridium botulinum, 150, *150*
Clostridium difficile, 7
Clostridium perfringens, *150*, 151
Clostridium spp., 18
cephalosporins in treatment of, 40t
clindamycin in treatment of, 79t
daptomycin in treatment of, 58t
glycopeptides in treatment of, 54t
intra-abdominal infections caused by, 227t
metronidazole in treatment of, 95, 95t
Clostridium tetani, 150–152, *150*
Coagulase-negative staphylococci, 108
infective endocarditis caused by, 216t
intravascular-related catheter infections caused by, 223, 224t, 224t
cocci, 4
coccobacilli, 4
colistin, 60–61, *60*, 60t
Acinetobacter spp. infection treatment with, 147t
VAP treatment with, 192, 192t
community-acquired pneumonia (CAP)
activities of agents used to treat, *188*
antimicrobial therapy for, 189t
atypical, 187–190
bacterial causes of, 187, 188t
optimal empiric therapy for, *188*, 188, 189t
typical, 187–188

curved gram-negative bacteria
  Campylobacter jejuni, 138, *138*, 139t, 142
  Helicobacter pylori, 138–140, *139*, 140t, 142
  Vibrio cholerae, 141, *141*, 141t
cycloserine, mycobacterial infections treatment with, 97
cystitis, acute, 194, *195*, 197, 197t, 82
cytoplasmic membrane, 3, *4*

D

dalbavancin, 53, 53t, 55–56
  cellulitis treatment with, 208, 208t
  methicillin-resistant *Staphylococcus aureus* infection treatment with, 110t
dapsone, 85–89, 85t, *87*
  antimicrobial activity of, 87t
  mycobacterial infections treatment with, 97
  Mycobacterium leprae infection treatment with, 182, 182t
  structure of, *87*
  toxicity of, 88
daptomycin
  anaerobic bacteria caused infections treatment with, *102*
  antimicrobial activity of, 58t
  atypical bacteria caused infections treatment with, *102*
  cellulitis treatment with, 208, 208t, *209*
  infective endocarditis treatment with, *217*, 220t, 221, *221*
  methicillin-resistant *Staphylococcus aureus* infection treatment with, 110t
  structure of, *58*
  toxicity of, 58
  VRE infection treatment with, 119, 121t
dATP. *See* deoxyadenosine triphosphate
dCTP. *See* deoxycytidine triphosphate
definitive therapy, 105–106
  by anaerobic bacteria, 149–154, *150*, 151t
  by anaerobic gram-negative bacilli, 153–154, 154t
  by atypical bacteria, 155–167, *156*, 157t, *158*, 158t, *160*, 161t, *162*, 163t, *164*, 165t, *166*, 166t
  by gram-negative bacteria, 125–148, *126*, 128t, *132*, *133*, 134t, *136*, 136t, *138*, *139*, 139–141t, *141*, *143*, 144–147t, *145–147*
  by gram-positive bacteria, 107–124, *108*, *109*, 110t, *113*, 114t, *116*, 117t, *120*, *120*, 121t, *123*
delafloxacin, 90, 90t, 92, *92*
  cellulitis treatment with, *209*
  methicillin-resistant *Staphylococcus aureus* infection treatment with, 110, 110t
delamanid
  multidrug-resistant (MDR) tuberculosis, 178
deoxyadenosine triphosphate (dATP), 11
deoxycytidine triphosphate (dCTP), 11
deoxyguanosine triphosphate (dGTP), 11
deoxynucleotides synthesis, 11

deoxythymidine triphosphate (dTTP), 11
dGTP. *See* deoxyguanosine triphosphate
dicloxacillin, 27t, 29
  cellulitis treatment with, 208, 208t
diverticulitis, 226
DNA
  antibiotics that target, 84
    metronidazole, 95–96, *95*, 95t
    quinolones, 90–94, *90*, 90t, 91t, *92*
    sulfa drugs, 85–89, 85t, *86*, *87*, 87t
  supercoiling of double helical structure of, *12*
DNA polymerase, 11
DNA replication, bacteria with, 1
DNA synthetic enzymes, 11–12, *12*, *13*
doxycycline plus *gentamicin*
  Brucella spp. infection treatment with, 163t
doxycycline plus rifampin
  Brucella spp. infection treatment with, 163t
doxycycline plus *streptomycin*
  Brucella spp. infection treatment with, 163t
doxycycline
  antimicrobial activity of, 75t
  Bordetella pertussis infection treatment with, 144, 145t
  Borrelia burgdorferi infection treatment with, 172, 172t
  Brucella spp. infection treatment with, 162
  Campylobacter jejuni infection treatment with, 138, 139t
  CAP treatment with, 189t, 190
  cellulitis treatment with, 208, 208t
  Chlamydia spp. infection treatment with, 156, 157t
  Francisella tularensis infection treatment with, 165, 165t
  Haemophilus influenzae infection treatment with, 143, 144t
  Leptospira interrogans infection treatment with, 173, 174t
  Moraxella catarrhalis infection treatment with, 145, 146t
  Mycoplasma spp. infection treatment with, 158, 158t
  PID treatment with, 200t, 201
  Rickettsia spp. infection treatment with, 166, 166t
  Staphylococcus aureus infection treatment with, 110t
  Streptococcus pneumoniae infection treatment with, 114t, 114
  Treponema pallidum infection treatment with, 170, 170t
  Vibrio cholerae infection treatment with, 141, 141t
  Yersinia enterocolitica infection treatment with, 128t, 131
dTTP. *See* deoxythymidine triphosphate
dyspareunia, pelvic inflammatory disease with, 199
dyspnea, infective endocarditis with, 215

E

early latent syphilis, 169
efflux pumps, 24
empiric therapy, 105, 185–186
   cellulitis, 207–210, 208t, *209*
   infective endocarditis, 215–221, 216t, *217*, 217t, 218t, 220t, 221t, 221t
   intra-abdominal infections, 226–228, *227*, 227t, 228t
   intravascular-related catheter infections, 223–225, *224*, 224t
   meningitis, 202–206, 203t, *204*, 205t
   otitis media, 211–214, 211t, *212*, 212t
   pelvic inflammatory disease, 199–201, 199t, *200*, 200t
   pneumonia, 187–193, *188*, 189t, 189t, 191–192t, 191t, *192*
   urinary tract infections, 194–198, *195*, 195t, *196*, 197t
enteric gram-negative bacilli
   intravascular-related catheter infections caused by, 224t
Enterobacter, 127–130, 128t
Enterobacterales, 131, 18
   aminoglycosides in treatment of, 68t
   aminopenicillins in treatment of, 30t
   carbapenems in treatment of, 48t
   cephalosporin plus β-lactamase inhibitor combinations in treatment of, 41t
   cephalosporins in treatment of, 39t, 40t
   Citrobacter, 127–130, 128t
   Enterobacter, 127–130, 128t
   Escherichia coli, 127–128, 128t
   extended-spectrum penicillins in treatment of, 31t
   HAP caused by, 127–128, 190, 191t
   Klebsiella spp., 128t
   monobactams in treatment of, 51t
   Morganella spp., 127–130, 128t
   nitrofurantoin in treatment of, 82t
   penicillin plus β-lactamase inhibitor combinations in treatment of, 32t
   polymyxins in treatment of, 61t, 127–128
   Proteus spp., 128t
   Providencia, 127–130, 128t
   quinolones in treatment of, 91t
   Salmonella enterica, 128t, 130–131
   Serratia, 127–130, 128t
   Shigella spp., 128t
   siderophore cephalosporins in treatment of, 42
   sites of infections from, *126*
   tetracycline in treatment of, 76t
   trimethoprim-sulfamethoxazole in treatment of, 87t
   UTI caused by, 130–131, 194, 195t
   Yersinia enterocolitica, 128t
enterococci, 18
   aminoglycosides in treatment of, 68t
   aminopenicillins in treatment of, 30t
   extended-spectrum penicillins in treatment of, 31t
   carbapenems in treatment of, 48t
   daptomycin in treatment of, 58t, 31t
   glycopeptides in treatment of, 54t
   infective endocarditis caused by, 215, 216t, 218–219, 219t
   linezolid in treatment of, 80t
   natural penicillins in treatment of, 28t
   nitrofurantoin in treatment of, 82t
   penicillin plus β-lactamase inhibitor combinations in treatment of, 32t, 32t
   sites of infections from, *120*
   tetracycline in treatment of, 76t
   treatment of infections caused by, 119–122, *120*, *120*, 121t
   UTI caused by, 194, 195t
Enterococcus faecalis, 119–121, 227t
Enterococcus faecium, 119–121, 227t
epidemic typhus, 166
eravacycline, 74–76, 74t
ertapenem, 46, 46t, 48, 48t
   Bacteroides spp. infection treatment with, 153, 154t
   Citrobacter spp. infection treatment with, 127, 128t
   Enterobacter spp. infection treatment with, 127, 128t
   Escherichia coli infection treatment with, 127, 127, 127
   Haemophilus influenzae infection treatment with, 143, 144t
   Klebsiella spp. infection treatment with, 127, 128t, 127, 128t
   Morganella spp. infection treatment with, 127
   Porphyromonas spp. infection treatment with, 153, 154t
   Prevotella spp. infection treatment with, 153, 154t
   Proteus spp. infection treatment with, 127, 128t, 127, 128t
   Providencia spp. infection treatment with, 127
   Serratia spp. infection treatment with, 127, 128t
   uncomplicated acute pyelonephritis treatment with, 197, 197t
erythromycin, 71, 71t, 72
   Bordetella pertussis infection treatment with, 145t
   structure of, *71*
   Vibrio cholerae infection treatment with, 141, 141t
ESBLs. *See* extended-spectrum b-lactamases
Escherichia coli, 127–128, 128t, 7
   cefotaxime in treatment of, 205t
   ceftriaxone in treatment of, 205t
   cephalosporins in treatment of, 205t, 204, 36t, 38–40t
   cephalosporins plus β-lactamase inhibitor combinations in treatment of, 41t
   intra-abdominal infections caused by, 227t
   meningitis caused by, 202, *204*
   pelvic inflammatory disease with, 199
   siderophore cephalosporins in treatment of, 42
   UTI caused by, 194, 195t

Etests, 14
ethambutol, 98
    MAC infection treatment with, 180, 181t
    Mycobacterium tuberculosis infection treatment with, 177, 178t
ethionamide, mycobacterial infections treatment with, 97
extended-spectrum penicillins, 27, 27t, 30–31, 30–31, 31t
    aerobic gram-negative bacteria caused infections treatment with, *101*
    anaerobic bacteria caused infections treatment with, *102*
    antimicrobial activity of, 31t
    atypical bacteria caused infections treatment with, *102*
    Bacteroides spp. infection treatment with, 154t
    Moraxella catarrhalis infection treatment with, 145, 146t
    Porphyromonas spp. infection treatment with, 154t
    Prevotella spp. infection treatment with, 154t
    Pseudomonas aeruginosa infection treatment with, 132, 134t
    R side chain of, *30*
extended-spectrum penicillin/β-lactamase inhibitor combinations, 27
extended-spectrum β-lactamases (ESBLs), 127, 130

F

facultative bacteria, 7, 199t
fever
    infective endocarditis with, 215
    intra-abdominal infections with, 226
    Mediterranean spotted, 166
    pelvic inflammatory disease with, 199
    Rocky Mountain spotted, 166
fidaxomicin
    Clostridia spp. infection treatment with, 151
50S subunit, 8, *8*
Fleming, Alexander, 22, 26
Florey, Howard, 213
fluoroquinolone, VAP treatment with, 192
fosfomycin, acute uncomplicated cystitis treatment with, 197t
Francisella tularensis
    sites of infections from, *164*
    treatment for infection with, 164–165, *164*, 165t
Fulton, John F., 213

G

Gardnerella vaginalis, pelvic inflammatory disease with, 200
gemifloxacin, 90, 90t, 92
gentamicin, 67, 67t, 69
    Brucella spp. infection treatment with, 162
    Campylobacter jejuni infection treatment with, 138, 139t
    Citrobacter spp. infection treatment with, 128t, 130
    Enterobacter spp. infection treatment with, 128t, 130
    enterococci infection treatment with, 121, 121t
    Escherichia coli infection treatment with, 127, 128t
    Francisella tularensis infection treatment with, 165, 165t
    infective endocarditis treatment with, 216–221, 217t, 218t, 219t, 220t
    Klebsiella spp. infection treatment with, 127, 128t
    Listeria monocytogenes infection treatment with, 124, 205, 205t
    Moraxella catarrhalis infection treatment with, 145, 146t
    Morganella spp. infection treatment with, 128t, 130
    Proteus spp. infection treatment with, 127, 128t
    Providencia spp. infection treatment with, 128t, 130
    Serratia spp. infection treatment with, 128t, 130
    Staphylococcus aureus infection treatment with, 110t
    Streptococcus agalactiae infection treatment with, 117, 117t, 204, 205t
    Streptococcus pyogenes penicillin-resistant infection treatment with, 117, 117t
    Yersinia enterocolitica infection treatment with, 128t, 131
glycine bridge (GGG), *5*
glycopeptides, 53–57
    antimicrobial activity of, 54t
    atypical bacteria caused infections treatment with, *101*
    cellulitis treatment with, 208t, *209*
    intravascular-related catheter infection treatment with, 224t
    meningitis treatment with, 203t
    methicillin-resistant *Staphylococcus aureus* infection treatment with, 110t
    Streptococcus pneumoniae infection treatment with, 205t
    Streptococcus pyogenes penicillin-resistant infection treatment with, 117, 117t
    structure of, *53*
    toxicity of, 56
    vancomycin, *53*, 53–55, 53t, 54t, *55*
    VAP treatment with, 191t
gram-negative bacteria, 3, *4*, 18, 125
    curved, 138–142, *138*, *139*, 139t, 140t, *141*, 141t
    Enterobacterales, 126–131, *126*, 128t
    Neisseria spp., *136*, 136–137, 136t
    other, 143–148, *143*, 144t, *145*, 145t, *146*, 146t, *147*, 147t
    Pseudomonas aeruginosa, 132–135, *132*, *133*, 134t
gram-negative facultative and aerobic bacilli, 226, 227t
gram-positive aerobic cocci, 226, 227t
gram-positive bacteria, 3, *4*, 18, 107–124
    enterococci, 119–122, *120*, 121t
    pneumococci, 113–115, *113*, 114t
    staphylococci, 108–112, *108*, *109*, 110t
    streptococci, other, 116–117, *116*, 117t
gram staining, 3
Grossman, Charles, 213

Index

H

HACEK organism
  acronym defined for, 216
  infective endocarditis caused by, 216, 216t, 221, 221t
Haemophilus influenzae, 18
  aminoglycosides in treatment of, 68t
  aminopenicillins in treatment of, 30t
  CAP caused by, 187, 188t
  carbapenems in treatment of, 48t
  cefotaxime in treatment of, 205t
  ceftriaxone in treatment of, 205t
  cephalosporins in treatment of, 39t, 40t, 204, 205t
  cephalosporins plus β-lactamase inhibitor combinations in treatment of, 41t
  extended-spectrum penicillins in treatment of, 31t
  macrolides in treatment of, 72t
  meningitis caused by, 202, *204*, 205t
  monobactams in treatment of, 51t
  natural penicillins in treatment of, 28t
  otitis media caused by, 211, 211t
  pelvic inflammatory disease with, 200
  penicillin plus β-lactamase inhibitor combinations in treatment of, 32t
  polymyxins in treatment of, 61t
  quinolones in treatment of, 91t
  rifamycins in treatment of, 65t
  sites of infections from, *143*
  tetracycline in treatment of, 76t
  treatment for infection with, 143–144, *143*, 144t
  trimethoprim-sulfamethoxazole in treatment of, 87t
HAP. *See* hospital-acquired pneumonia
Helicobacter pylori
  metronidazole in treatment of, 95
  sites of infections from, *139*
  treatment for infection with, 138–140, *139*, 140t, 142
hospital-acquired pneumonia (HAP)
  activities of agents used to treat, *192*
  bacterial causes of, 190, 191t
  empiric therapy for, 190–193, 191t
  risk factors for, 191, 191t–192t
  ventilator-associated pneumonia as, 190–193, 191t, *192*

I

imipenem, 46, 46t, 47, 48t
  Acinetobacter spp. infection treatment with, 147, 147t
  Bacteroides spp. infection treatment with, 153, 154t
  CAP treatment with, 190
  cellulitis treatment with, 208t, 209
  Citrobacter spp. infection treatment with, 127, 128t
  Enterobacter spp. infection treatment with, 127, 128t
  enterococci infection treatment with, 119, 121t
  Escherichia coli infection treatment with, 127, 128t
  Haemophilus influenzae infection treatment with, 143, 144t
  intra-abdominal infection treatment with, 226, 228t
  intravascular-related catheter infection treatment with, 223, 224t
  Klebsiella spp. infection treatment with, 127, 128t
  Morganella spp. infection treatment with, 127, 128t
  Porphyromonas spp. infection treatment with, 153, 154t
  Prevotella spp. infection treatment with, 153, 154t
  Proteus spp. infection treatment with, 127, 128t
  Providencia spp. infection treatment with, 127, 128t
  Pseudomonas aeruginosa infection treatment with, 132, 134t
  Serratia spp. infection treatment with, 127, 128t
  Staphylococcus aureus infection treatment with, 110t
  uncomplicated acute pyelonephritis treatment with, 197, 197t
  urinary tract infections treatment with, 197, 197t
  VAP treatment with, 191t, 192
imipenem-relebactam, 46t, 48–49
  Escherichia coli infection treatment with, 127
  Klebsiella spp. infection treatment with, 127
  Proteus spp. infection treatment with, 127
immune system, bacteria eradication ineffectiveness of, 15
infective endocarditis
  activities of agents used to treat, *217*
  bacterial causes of, 215–221, 216t
  coagulase-negative staphylococci caused, 216t
  empiric antimicrobial regimens examples for, 217t
  enterococci caused, 215, 216t, 218–219, 219t
  etiology of, 215
  HACEK organism caused, 216t, 221, 221t
  physical examination findings for, 215
  staphylococci caused, 220t, 221
  treatment of, 215–222, *217*, 217t, 218t, 219t, 220t, 221t
  viridans group streptococci caused, 215, 216t, 217–218, 218t
intra-abdominal infections
  abdominal imaging studies for, 226
  activities of agents used to treat, *227*
  bacterial causes of, 226, 227t
  laboratory examination for, 226
  presentations of patients with, 226
  syndromes of, 226
  treatment for, 226–228, 228t
intravascular-related catheter infections
  activities of agents used to treat, *224*
  bacterial causes of, 223, 224t
  diagnosis of, 223
  treatment of, 223–225, 224t

intrinsic resistance, 22
isoniazid, 98
  Mycobacterium tuberculosis infection treatment with, 177, 178t
isoniazid plus rifampin
  Mycobacterium tuberculosis infection treatment with, 178
isoniazid plus rifapentine
  Mycobacterium tuberculosis infection treatment with, 178

J
Janeway lesions, infective endocarditis with, 215

K
Kirby-Bauer method, 14
Klebsiella pneumoniae
  cephalosporins in treatment of, 36t, 38t, 39t, 40t
  cephalosporins plus β-lactamase inhibitor combinations in treatment of, 41t
  siderophore cephalosporins in treatment of, 42
Klebsiella pneumoniae carbapenemases (KPCs), 127, 130
Klebsiella spp., 127–128, 128t
  intra-abdominal infections caused by, 227t
  UTI caused by, 194, 195t

L
β-lactam antibiotics, 127, 130
  CAP treatment with, 189t, 190
  carbapenems, 22, 46, 46–49, 46t, 48t
  cephalosporins, 22, 34–44, *34*, 36t, *37*, *38*, 38t, *39*, 39t, *40*, 40t, 41t, *42*, *43*
  history of, 26
  list of, 22t
  mechanism of action of, *23*
  monobactams, 22, *51*, 51–52, 51t
  PBPs inhibition by, 22–24, *24*
  penicillins, 22, 27, *27*–33, 27t, *28*, 28t, *29*, *30*, 30t, 31t, 32t
  resistance to, 22–23
  six Ps of, 23–25, *25*
  structure of, 22
β-lactamase inhibitor
  aerobic gram-negative bacteria caused infections treatment with, *101*
  atypical bacteria caused infections treatment with, *102*
  uncomplicated acute pyelonephritis treatment with, 197, 197t
β-lactam/β-lactamase inhibitor combinations
  Bacteroides spp. infection treatment with, 153, 154t
  Porphyromonas spp. infection treatment with, 153, 154t
  Prevotella spp. infection treatment with, 153, 154t
  Staphylococcus aureus infection treatment with, 110t
β-lactam ring, 22, *22*
late latent syphilis, 169
latent syphilis, 169
Legionella pneumophila, 18, 72t, 155, 160
Legionella spp.
  CAP caused by, 188, 188t
  quinolones in treatment of, 91t
  sites of infections from, *160*
  treatment for infection with, 160–161, *160*, 161t
leprosy, 182–183
Leptospira interrogans
  sites of infections from, *173*
  treatment for infection with, 173–174, *173*, 174t
Leptospira spp., natural penicillins in treatment of, 28t
leptospirosis, 168, 173–174
levofloxacin, 90, 90t, 92
  Bordetella pertussis infection treatment with, 144, 145t
  Brucella spp. infection treatment with, 162, 163t
  Campylobacter jejuni infection treatment with, 138, 139t
  CAP treatment with, 189t, 190
  Chlamydia spp. infection treatment with, 157t
  Citrobacter spp. infection treatment with, 128t, 130
  Enterobacter spp. infection treatment with, 128t, 130
  Escherichia coli infection treatment with, 127, 128t
  Haemophilus influenzae infection treatment with, 143, 144t
  intra-abdominal infection treatment with, 226, 228t
  Klebsiella spp. infection treatment with, 127, 128t
  Legionella spp. infection treatment with, 160, 161t
  Moraxella catarrhalis infection treatment with, 145, 146t
  Morganella spp. infection treatment with, 128t, 130
  multidrug-resistant (MDR) tuberculosis, 178
  Mycobacterium leprae infection treatment with, 182t
  Mycoplasma spp. infection treatment with, 158, 158t
  Proteus spp. infection treatment with, 127, 128t
  Providencia spp. infection treatment with, 128t, 130
  Pseudomonas aeruginosa infection treatment with, 132, 134t
  Salmonella enterica infection treatment with, 128t, 131
  Serratia spp. infection treatment with, 128t, 130
  Shigella spp. infection treatment with, 128t, 131
  Staphylococcus aureus infection treatment with, 110t
  uncomplicated acute pyelonephritis treatment with, 197, 197t
  urinary tract infections treatment with, 197, 197t
  VAP treatment with, 192, 192t
lincosamide antibiotics
  clindamycin as, 78
  history of, 79
linezolid, 80–81
  antimicrobial activity of, 80t
  CAP treatment with, 189t, 190
  cellulitis treatment with, 208t, 209

methicillin-resistant *Staphylococcus aureus* infection treatment with, 110t
multidrug-resistant (MDR) tuberculosis, 178
structure of, *80*
VAP treatment with, 191t, 192
lipoglycopeptides, 53–57
   dalbavancin, 53, 53t, 55–56
   oritavancin, 53, 53t, 56
   structure of, *53*
   telavancin, 53, 53t, 56
   toxicity of, 56
lipopolysaccharide (LPS), 3
Listeria monocytogenes, 18, 107
   aminoglycoside in treatment of, 205t
   aminopenicillins in treatment of, 205t
   ampicillin, 205, 205t
   carbapenems in treatment of, 48t, 203, 205t
   gentamicin, 205, 205t
   meningitis caused by, *204*
   natural penicillins in treatment of, 28t, *204*
   penicillin, 205t
   penicillin G, 30t, 68t, *204*, 205, 205t
   penicillin plus β-lactamase inhibitor combinations in treatment of, 32t
   sites of infections from, *123*
   tetracycline in treatment of, 76t
   treatment of infections caused by, 123–124, *123*
   trimethoprim-sulfamethoxazole in treatment of, 87t
LPS. *See* lipopolysaccharide
Lyme disease, 171–172

M

MAC. *See Mycobacterium avium* complex
macrolides
   aerobic gram-negative bacteria caused infections treatment with, *101*
   antimicrobial activity of, 72t
   atypical bacteria caused infections treatment with, *103*
   azithromycin, 71, 71t, 73
   Bordetella pertussis infection treatment with, 144
   Campylobacter jejuni infection treatment with, 138, 139t
   CAP treatment with, 189t, 190
   cellulitis treatment with, *209*
   Chlamydia spp. infection treatment with, 156
   clarithromycin, 71, 71t, 72
   erythromycin, 71, *71*, 71t, 72
   Haemophilus influenzae infection treatment with, 144t, 145t
   Helicobacter pylori infection treatment with, 140t
   Legionella spp. infection treatment with, 160, 161t
   MAC infection treatment with, 181t
   macrocyclic lactone ring with, 71
   Moraxella catarrhalis infection treatment with, 145, 146t
   Mycobacterium leprae infection treatment with, 182t
   otitis media treatment with, 212t, 213
   resistance with, 71
   Salmonella enterica infection treatment with, 128t
   Shigella spp. infection treatment with, 128t
   Staphylococcus aureus infection treatment with, 110t
   toxicity of, 73
   Vibrio cholerae infection treatment with, 141, 141t
MBC. *See* minimum bactericidal concentration
Mediterranean spotted fever, 166
meningitis
   activities of agents used to treat, *204*
   bacterial causes of, 202, 205t
   empiric antimicrobial therapy for, 202–206, 203t, *204*, 205t
   pathogenesis of, 203, *204*, 205t
meropenem, 46, 46t, 47–48
   Acinetobacter spp. infection treatment with, 147, 147t
   Bacteroides spp. infection treatment with, 153, 154t
   CAP treatment with, 190
   cellulitis treatment with, 208t, 209
   Citrobacter spp. infection treatment with, 127, 128t
   Enterobacter spp. infection treatment with, 127, 128t
   enterococci infection treatment with, 119, 121t
   Escherichia coli infection treatment with, 127, 128t
   Haemophilus influenzae infection treatment with, 143, 144t
   intra-abdominal infection treatment with, 226, 228t
   intravascular-related catheter infection treatment with, 223, 224t
   Klebsiella spp. infection treatment with, 127, 128t
   Morganella spp. infection treatment with, 127, 128t
   Porphyromonas spp. infection treatment with, 153, 154t
   Prevotella spp. infection treatment with, 153, 154t
   Proteus spp. infection treatment with, 127, 128t
   Providencia spp. infection treatment with, 127, 128t
   Pseudomonas aeruginosa infection treatment with, 132, 134t
   Serratia spp. infection treatment with, 127, 128t
   Staphylococcus aureus infection treatment with, 110t
   uncomplicated acute pyelonephritis treatment with, 197, 197t
   urinary tract infections treatment with, 197, 197t
   VAP treatment with, 191t, 192

meropenem-vaborbactam, 46t, 48
   Escherichia coli infection treatment with, 127, 128t
   Klebsiella spp. infection treatment with, 127, 128t
   Proteus spp. infection treatment with, 127, 128t
messenger RNA (mRNA), 7, 63
methicillin-resistant S. aureus (MRSA), 221
methicillin-resistant *Staphylococcus aureus* (MRSA), 29
methicillin-resistant *Staphylococcus epidermidis* (MRSE), 29
   ceftaroline in treatment of, 110t
   cellulitis with risk of, 207–210, 208t
   cephalosporins in treatment of, 110t
   dalbavancin in treatment of, 110t
   daptomycin in treatment of, 110t
   delafloxacin in treatment of, 110t
   glycopeptides in treatment of, 110t
   linezolid in treatment of, 110t
   mechanisms for, *109*
   omadacycline in treatment of, 110t
   oritavancin in treatment of, 110t
   oxazolidinones in treatment of, 110t
   quinolones in treatment of, 110t
   tedizolid in treatment of, 110t
   telavancin in treatment of, 110t
   vancomycin in treatment of, 110t
metronidazole
   anaerobic bacteria caused infections treatment with, *102*
   antimicrobial activity of, 95t
   Bacteroides spp. infection treatment with, 153, 154t
   Clostridia spp. infection treatment with, 150, 151t
   Helicobacter pylori infection treatment with, 139
   history of, *96*
   intra-abdominal infection treatment with, 226, 227, 228t
   PID treatment with, 200t, 201
   Porphyromonas spp. infection treatment with, 153, 154t
   Prevotella spp. infection treatment with, 153, 154t
   resistance to, 95
   structure of, *95*
   toxicity of, 96
metronidazole plus clarithromycin plus proton pump inhibitor, *Helicobacter pylori* infection treatment with, 140t
MIC. *See* minimum inhibitory concentration
microaerophilic bacteria, 7
minimum bactericidal concentration (MBC), 14
minimum inhibitory concentration (MIC), 14–15
minocycline
   Mycobacterium leprae infection treatment with, 182t, 183

   Staphylococcus aureus infection treatment with, 110t
monobactams, 22, 51–52
   aerobic gram-negative bacteria caused infections treatment with, *101*
   antimicrobial activity of, 51t
   Pseudomonas aeruginosa infection treatment with, 132, 134t
   structure of, *51*
   toxicity of, 52
   VAP treatment with, 191t, 192
Morganella spp., 127–130, 128t
moxifloxacin, 90, 90t, 92
   Bacteroides spp. infection treatment with, 153, 154t
   Bordetella pertussis infection treatment with, 144, 145t
   Brucella spp. infection treatment with, 162, 163t
   CAP treatment with, 189t, 190
   Chlamydia spp. infection treatment with, 157t
   Citrobacter spp. infection treatment with, 128t, 130
   Enterobacter spp. infection treatment with, 128t, 130
   Escherichia coli infection treatment with, 127, 128t
   Haemophilus influenzae infection treatment with, 143, 144t
   Klebsiella spp. infection treatment with, 127, 128t
   Legionella spp. infection treatment with, 160, 161t
   Moraxella catarrhalis infection treatment with, 145, 146t
   Morganella spp. infection treatment with, 128t, 130
   multidrug-resistant (MDR) tuberculosis, 178
   Mycobacterium leprae infection treatment with, 182t
   Mycoplasma spp. infection treatment with, 158, 158t
   Porphyromonas spp. infection treatment with, 153, 154t
   Prevotella spp. infection treatment with, 153, 154t
   Proteus spp. infection treatment with, 127, 128t
   Providencia spp. infection treatment with, 128t, 130
   Serratia spp. infection treatment with, 128t, 130
   Staphylococcus aureus infection treatment with, 110t
mRNA. *See* messenger RNA
MRSA. *See* methicillin-resistant *Staphylococcus aureus*
MRSE. *See* methicillin-resistant *Staphylococcus epidermidis*
multidrug-resistant (MDR) tuberculosis, 178
murine typhus, 166

mycobacteria, 175–183
  Mycobacterium avium complex, 180–181, *180*, 181t
  Mycobacterium leprae, 182–183, *182*, 182t
  Mycobacterium tuberculosis, 177–179, *177*, 178t
Mycobacterium avium, 97
Mycobacterium avium complex (MAC), 176
  aminoglycosides in treatment of, 68t, 181t
  macrolides in treatment of, 181t
  quinolones in treatment of, 91t
  rifamycins in treatment of, 65t, 180–181, *180*
  treatment for infection with, 72t, 181t
Mycobacterium leprae, 97
  dapsone in treatment of, 87, 87t
  macrolides in treatment of, 72t
  quinolones in treatment of, 91t
  rifamycins in treatment of, 65t
  treatment for infection with, *182*, 182–183, 182t
Mycobacterium tuberculosis, 7, 97, 176
  aminoglycosides in treatment of, 68t
  quinolones in treatment of, 91t
  rifamycins in treatment of, 65t
  treatment for infection with, 177–179, *177*, 178t
Mycoplasma pneumoniae, 158
  CAP caused by, 188, 188t
  quinolones in treatment of, 91t
Mycoplasma spp., 18
  macrolides in treatment of, 158
  sites of infections from, *158*
  tetracycline in treatment of, 158
  treatment for infection with, 72t, 76t, 158, 158t, *158*

N

N-acetylglucosamine (NAGA), 5, *23*
N-acetylmuramic acid (NAMA), 5, *23*
nafcillin, 27t, 29, *29*, 109
  cellulitis treatment with, 207, 208t
  infective endocarditis treatment with, 219, 220t, 221
  intravascular-related catheter infection treatment with, 223, 224t
NAGA. *See N*-acetylglucosamine
NAMA. *See N*-acetylmuramic acid
natural penicillins, 27–28, 27t
  ampicillin in treatment of, 204, *204*
  antimicrobial activity of, 28t
  cephalosporin in treatment of, 204
  extended-spectrum penicillins in treatment of, 31t
  Leptospira interrogans infection treatment with, 174t
  meningitis caused by, *204*
  natural penicillins in treatment of, 28t
  penicillin G in treatment of, *204*, 205t
  R side chain of, *28*
  treatment for infection with, *136*, 136–137, 136t
Neisseria gonorrhoeae, pelvic inflammatory disease caused by, 199t

Neisseria meningitidis
  aminopenicillins in treatment of, 30t
  extended-spectrum penicillins in treatment of, 31t
  doxycycline in treatment of, 75t
  meningitis caused by, 202t, 203, *204*
  rifamycins in treatment of, 65t
  tetracycline in treatment of, 75t
  treatment for infection with, 136t
Neisseria spp., 18
  carbapenems in treatment of, 48t
  cephalosporins in treatment of, 39t, 40t
  cephalosporins plus β-lactamase inhibitor combinations in treatment of, 41t
  macrolides in treatment of, 72t
  monobactams in treatment of, 51t
  penicillin plus β-lactamase inhibitor combinations in treatment of, 32t
  quinolones in treatment of, 91t
  sites of infections from, *136*
  tetracycline in treatment of, 76t
  treatment for infection with, *136*, 136–137, 136t
neomycin, 67, 67t
night sweats, infective endocarditis with, 215
nitrofurantoin
  acute cystitis treatment with, 82
  acute uncomplicated cystitis treatment with, 194, 197t
  antimicrobial activity of, 82t
  structure of, *82*
  toxicity of, 82

O

ofloxacin, 90, 90t, 92
omadacycline, 74–76, 74t
  cellulitis treatment with, 208t, 209
  methicillin-resistant *Staphylococcus aureus* infection treatment with, 110t, 112t
Orientia tsutsugamushi, 166
oritavancin, 53, 53t, 56
  cellulitis treatment with, 208, 208t
  methicillin-resistant *Staphylococcus aureus* infection treatment with, 110t
Osler nodes, infective endocarditis with, 215
otitis media
  activities of agents used to treat, *212*
  bacterial causes of, 211, 211t
  children with, 211–212
  pathogenesis of, 211
  treatment of, *212*, 212–213, 212t
outer membrane, 3, *4*
oxacillin, 27t, 29, 109
  cellulitis treatment with, 207, 208t
  infective endocarditis treatment with, 219, 220t, 221
  intravascular-related catheter infection treatment with, 223, 224t

oxazolidinone
    CAP treatment with, 189t
oxazolidinones
    atypical bacteria caused infections treatment with, 101
    cellulitis treatment with, 208, 208t, 209
    linezolid, 80, 80–81, 80t
    methicillin-resistant *Staphylococcus aureus* infection treatment with, 110t
    tedizolid, 80–81
    toxicity of, 81
    VAP treatment with, 191t
    VRE infection treatment with, 119, 121t

P

P-aminosalicylic acid, mycobacterial infections treatment with, 97
pathogenic bacteria, 1
PBPs. *See* penicillin-binding proteins
pelvic inflammatory disease (PID)
    abdominal pain with, 199
    activities of agents used to treat, 200
    antimicrobial therapy for, 200t
    bacterial causes of, 199, 199t
    bleeding with, 199
    chills with, 199
    dyspareunia with, 199
    empiric treatment of, 200–201, 200t
    fever with, 199
    laboratory examination for, 199
    pathogenesis of, 199–200, 199t, 200
    vaginal discharge with, 199
penetration, 23, 25
    cephalosporins with, 35
    penicillins with, 28
penicillin, 27–33, 108
    adverse reactions to, 32
    aminopenicillins, 27, 27t, 29–30, 30
    aminopenicillin/β-lactamase inhibitor combinations, 27, 30t
    anaerobic bacteria caused infections treatment with, 102
    antistaphylococcal penicillins, 27, 27t, 29, 29, 29t
    atypical bacteria caused infections treatment with, 102
    Clostridia spp. infection treatment with, 150, 151t
    core of, 22
    extended-spectrum penicillins, 27, 27t, 30–31, 30, 31t
    list of, 27t
    Listeria monocytogenes infection treatment with, 205t
    natural penicillins, 27–28, 27t, 28, 28t
    Neisseria meningitidis infection treatment with, 136, 136t
    penicillin plus β-lactamase inhibitor combinations, 32t
    penicillin/β-lactamase inhibitor combinations, 31–32
    resistance to, 28
    six Ps for, 28
    Streptococcus agalactiae infection treatment with, 116, 117t, 205t
    Streptococcus pneumoniae infection treatment with, 114, 114t
    Streptococcus pyogenes infection treatment with, 117, 117t
    structure of, 27
    toxicity with, 32
    Treponema pallidum infection treatment with, 169, 170t
penicillin G, 27, 27t
    Clostridia spp. infection treatment with, 151t
    enterococci infection treatment with, 119, 121t
    infective endocarditis treatment with, 217–218, 218t, 219t
    Leptospira interrogans infection treatment with, 173, 174t
    Listeria monocytogenes infection treatment with, 204, 205, 205t
    Neisseria meningitidis infection treatment with, 204
    Streptococcus agalactiae infection treatment with, 207t
    Streptococcus pneumoniae infection treatment with, 114t
    Treponema pallidum infection treatment with, 170t
penicillin plus clindamycin
    Clostridia spp. infection treatment with, 151
penicillin/β-lactamase inhibitor combinations, 31–32, 32t
    intra-abdominal infection treatment with, 226, 227, 228t
penicillin-binding proteins (PBPs), 4, 5, 109
    cephalosporins with, 35
    penicillins with, 28
    Streptococcus pneumoniae producing, 211
    β-lactam antibiotics in inhibition of, 22–24, 24
penicillins plus β-lactamase inhibitors, 27t
    aerobic gram-negative bacteria caused infections treatment with, 101
    anaerobic bacteria caused infections treatment with, 102
    atypical bacteria caused infections treatment with, 102
    intravascular-related catheter infection treatment with, 223, 224, 224t
    otitis media treatment with, 212t
penicillin V, 27, 27t
Penicillium, 22
peptidoglycan, 24, 25
    cephalosporins with, 35
    cross-linking of, 4
    penicillins with, 28
    structure of, 5
Peptostreptococcus spp., pelvic inflammatory disease with, 199

periplasm, 3
periplasmic space, 3, *4*
peritonitis, 226
PID. *See* pelvic inflammatory disease
piperacillin, 27t, 30, *30*
   Bacteroides spp. infection treatment with, 153, 154t
   enterococci infection treatment with, 119, 121t
   Moraxella catarrhalis infection treatment with, 145, 146t
   Porphyromonas spp. infection treatment with, 153, 154t
   Prevotella spp. infection treatment with, 153, 154t
   Pseudomonas aeruginosa infection treatment with, 132, 134t
piperacillin-tazobactam, 27t, 31
   Bacteroides spp. infection treatment with, 153, 154t
   CAP treatment with, 190
   Escherichia coli infection treatment with, 127, 128t
   intra-abdominal infection treatment with, 226, 228t
   intravascular-related catheter infection treatment with, 223, 224t
   Klebsiella spp. infection treatment with, 127, 128t
   Porphyromonas spp. infection treatment with, 153, 154t
   Prevotella spp. infection treatment with, 153, 154t
   Proteus spp. infection treatment with, 127, 128t
   Staphylococcus aureus infection treatment with, 110t
   uncomplicated acute pyelonephritis treatment with, 197, 197t
   urinary tract infections treatment with, 197, 197t
   VAP treatment with, 191, 191t, *192*
plazomicin, 67, 67t, 69
   Citrobacter spp. infection treatment with, 128t, 130
   Enterobacter spp. infection treatment with, 128t, 130
   Escherichia coli infection treatment with, 127, 128t
   Klebsiella spp. infection treatment with, 127, 128t
   Morganella spp. infection treatment with, 128t, 130
   Proteus spp. infection treatment with, 127, 128t
   Providencia spp. infection treatment with, 128t, 130
   Serratia spp. infection treatment with, 128t, 130
pneumococci, 113–115, *113*, 114t
pneumonia
   community-acquired, 187–190, *188*, 188t, 189t
   hospital-acquired, 190–193, 191–192t, 191t, *192*
polymyxins, *60*, 60–61, 60t, 61t, 192, *192*, 192t
   Acinetobacter spp. infection treatment with, 147, 147t
   aerobic gram-negative bacteria caused infections treatment with, *101*
polymyxin B, 60t, 192, 192t
polymyxin E, 60t
porins, 4, 23–24, *25*
   cephalosporins with, 35
   penicillins with, 28
Porphyromonas spp. treatment for infection with, 153–154, 154t
pretomanid, multidrug-resistant (MDR) tuberculosis, 178
Prevotella spp., treatment for infection with, 153–154, 154t
probenecid, PID treatment with, 200t
protein production
   antibiotics that block, 63
      aminoglycosides, *67*, 67–70, 67t, 68t
      clindamycin, 78–79, *78*, 79t
      doxycycline, 75t
      macrolides, *71*, 71–73, 71t, 72t
      nitrofurantoin, *82*, 82–83, 82t
      oxazolidinones, *80*, 80–81, 80t
      rifamycins, *64*, 64t, 64–66
      tetracyclines, *74*, 74–77, 74t, 75t
   bacteria, 1, 6–8, *7*, *8*
   raw materials in, 6–7, *7*
   transcription in, 7–8
   translation in, 8, *8*
Proteus mirabilis
   cephalosporins in treatment of, 36t, 37t
Proteus spp., 127–128, 128t
   cephalosporins in treatment of, 39t, 40t
   cephalosporins plus β-lactamase inhibitor combinations in treatment of, 41t
   siderophore cephalosporins in treatment of, 42
proton motive force, 7
Providencia spp., 127–130, 128t
Pseudomonas aeruginosa, 18
   carbapenems in treatment of, 48t
   cephalosporins in treatment of, 39t
   cephalosporins plus β-lactamase inhibitor combinations in treatment of, 41t
   HAP caused by, 190, 191t
   intra-abdominal infection treatment with, 226
   intra-abdominal infections caused by, 227t
   intravascular-related catheter infections caused by, 224t
   monobactams in treatment of, 51t
   penicillin plus β-lactamase inhibitor combinations in treatment of, 32t
   polymyxins in treatment of, 61t
   quinolones in treatment of, 91t
   resistance mechanisms of, *133*
   siderophore cephalosporins in treatment of, 42
   sites of infections from, *132*
   treatment for infection with, 132–135, *132*, *133*, 134t
   UTI caused by, 194, 195t

pumps, 24, *25*
    cephalosporins with, 35
    penicillins with, 28
pyelonephritis, uncomplicated acute, 194
    activities of agents used to treat, *196*
    antimicrobial therapy for, 197, 197t
pyrazinamide, 98
    Mycobacterium tuberculosis infection treatment with, 177, 178t

Q

quinolones
    aerobic gram-negative bacteria caused infections treatment with, *101*
    antimicrobial activity of, 91t
    atypical bacteria caused infections treatment with, *103*
    Bacteroides spp. infection treatment with, 153, 154t
    Bordetella pertussis infection treatment with, 144, 145t
    Brucella spp. infection treatment with, 162, 163t
    Campylobacter jejuni infection treatment with, 138, 139t
    CAP treatment with, 189t, 190
    Chlamydia spp. infection treatment with, 157t
    ciprofloxacin, 91–92
    Citrobacter spp. infection treatment with, 128t, 130
    delafloxacin, 90, 90t, 92, *92*
    Enterobacter spp. infection treatment with, 128t, 130
    Escherichia coli infection treatment with, 128t
    gemifloxacin, 92, *92*
    Haemophilus influenzae infection treatment with, 143, 144t
    Klebsiella spp. infection treatment with, 128t
    Legionella spp. infection treatment with, 160, 161t
    levofloxacin, 92
    methicillin-resistant *Staphylococcus aureus* infection treatment with, 110t
    Moraxella catarrhalis infection treatment with, 145, 146t
    Morganella spp. infection treatment with, 128t, 130
    moxifloxacin, 92, *92*
    mycobacterial infections treatment with, 97
    Mycobacterium leprae infection treatment with, 182t
    Mycoplasma spp. infection treatment with, 158, 158t
    ofloxacin, 92
    Porphyromonas spp. infection treatment with, 153, 154t
    Prevotella spp. infection treatment with, 153, 154t
    Proteus spp. infection treatment with, 128t
    Providencia spp. infection treatment with, 128t, 130
    Pseudomonas aeruginosa infection treatment with, 132, 134t
    Rickettsia spp. infection treatment with, 166t
    Salmonella enterica infection treatment with, 128t, 130
    Serratia spp. infection treatment with, 128t, 130
    Shigella spp. infection treatment with, 128t, 130
    Staphylococcus aureus infection treatment with, 110t
    toxicity of, 93–94
    uncomplicated acute pyelonephritis treatment with, 197, 197t
    urinary tract infections treatment with, 197, 197t
    Vibrio cholerae infection treatment with, 141, 141t
    Yersinia enterocolitica infection treatment with, 128t

R

raxibacumab, 18
replication
    antibiotics that target, 84
        metronidazole, *95*, 95–96, 95t
        quinolones, 90–94, 90t, *91*, 91t, *92*
        sulfa drugs, 85–89, 85t, *86*, *87*, 87t
    bacteria, 10–13, *11*, *12*, *13*
    bacterial chromosome, *13*
    binary fission with, 10
    deoxynucleotides synthesis with, 11
    DNA synthetic enzymes with, 11–12, *12*, *13*
    supercoiling of double helical structure of DNA in, *12*
resistance to antibiotics
    acquired, 22
    intrinsic, 22
    macrolides with, 71
    metronidazole with, 95
    penicillins with, 28
    Pseudomonas aeruginosa with, *133*
    Staphylococcus aureus with, *109*
    β-lactam antibiotics with, 22–23
ribosomal RNA (rRNA), 8
ribosomes, 8
Rickettsia akari, 166
Rickettsia conorii, 166
Rickettsia prowazekii, 166, 167
Rickettsia rickettsii, 166
Rickettsia spp.
    macrolides in treatment of, 72t
    sites of infections from, *166*
    treatment for infection with, 166, 166–167, 166t
Rickettsia typhi, 166
rickettsialpox, 166
rifabutin, 64, 64t, 65, 98
    MAC infection treatment with, 180
    Mycobacterium tuberculosis infection treatment with, 177

rifampin, 64, *64*, 64t, 65, 98
  Acinetobacter spp. infection treatment with, 147, 147t
  Brucella spp. infection treatment with, 162
  Haemophilus influenzae infection treatment with, 144, 144t
  infective endocarditis treatment with, 216, 217t, 220t, 221
  Mycobacterium leprae infection treatment with, 182, 182t
  Mycobacterium tuberculosis infection treatment with, 177–178, 178t
  Neisseria meningitidis infection treatment with, 136t, 137
  Staphylococcus aureus infection treatment with, 110t

rifamycins
  Acinetobacter spp. infection treatment with, 147t
  antimicrobial activity of, 65t
  atypical bacteria caused infections treatment with, *101*
  Haemophilus influenzae infection treatment with, 144t
  history of, 66
  Neisseria meningitidis infection treatment with, 136t
  rifabutin, 64, 64t
  rifampin, 64, *64*, 64t
  rifapentine, 64, 64t, 65
  rifaximin, 64, 64t, 65
  Staphylococcus aureus infection treatment with, 110t
  toxicity of, 65

rifapentine, 64, 64t, 65, 98
rifaximin, 64, 64t, 65
RNA polymerase, 7–8
Rocky Mountain spotted fever, 166
Roth spots, infective endocarditis with, 215
rRNA. *See* ribosomal RNA

S

S. *See* Svedberg units
Salmonella enterica, 128t, 130–131
scrub typhus, 166
Serratia, 127–130, 128t
70S bacterial ribosome, 8, *8*
Shigella spp., 128t, 130–131
spirochetes, 4, 168
  Borrelia burgdorferi, 171–172, *171*, 172t
  Leptospira interrogans, 173–174, *173*, 174t
  Treponema pallidum, 169–170, *169*, 170t
splenic abscesses, 226
splinter hemorrhages
  infective endocarditis with, 215
staphylococci, 108–112, *109*, 110t
  aminoglycosides in treatment of, 68t
  coagulase-negative, 224t
  daptomycin in treatment of, 58t
  infective endocarditis caused by, 221
  linezolid in treatment of, 80t
  rifamycins in treatment of, 65t
  sites of, *108*
  tetracycline in treatment of, 76t
  trimethoprim-sulfamethoxazole in treatment of, 87t

Staphylococcus aureus, 7, 18, 107–112
  aminoglycosides in treatment of, 110t
  ampicillin-sulbactam in treatment of, 110t
  antimicrobial agents for treatment of infections caused by, 110t
  antistaphylococcalpenicillins in treatment of, 110t
  azithromycin in treatment of, 110t
  CAP caused by, 48t, 187
  carbapenems in treatment of, 110t
  cefazolin in treatment of, 110t
  cefepime in treatment of, 110t
  cefotaxime in treatment of, 110t
  ceftriaxone in treatment of, 110t
  cefuroxime in treatment of, 110t
  cellulitis caused by, 207, 208t
  cephalosporins in treatment of, 36t, 38t, 39t, 79t
  ciprofloxacin in treatment of, 110t
  clindamycin in treatment of, 110t
  doxycycline in treatment of, 110t
  gentamicin in treatment of, 110t
  glycopeptides in treatment of, 54t
  HAP caused by, 190, 191t
  imipenem in treatment of, 110t
  intra-abdominal infection treatment with, 226
  intravascular-related catheter infections caused by, 72t, 223, 224t
  β-lactamase inhibitor combinations in treatment of, 110t
  levofloxacin in treatment of, 110t
  macrolides in treatment of, 110t
  mechanisms of antibiotics resistance by, *109*
  meropenem in treatment of, 110t
  minocycline in treatment of, 110t
  moxifloxacin in treatment of, 110t
  penicillin plus β-lactamase inhibitor combinations in treatment of, 32t, 91t
  piperacillin-tazobactam in treatment of, 110t
  quinolones in treatment of, 110t
  rifampin in treatment of, 110t
  rifamycins in treatment of, 110t
  sulfa drugs in treatment of, 110t
  tetracyclines in treatment of, 110t
  trimethoprim-sulfamethoxazole in treatment of, 29t, 110t

Staphylococcus aureus, infective endocarditis caused by, 215–216, 216t, 219, 220t, 221
Staphylococcus epidermidis, 108, 223
  antistaphylococcalpenicillins in treatment of, 29t
  glycopeptides in treatment of, 54t

Staphylococcus saprophyticus, 108
   nitrofurantoin in treatment of, 82t
   UTI caused by, 194, 195t
streptococci
   aminoglycosides in treatment of, 68t
   cellulitis caused by, 207, 208t
   clindamycin in treatment of, 79t
   quinolones in treatment of, 91t
   sites of infections from, *116*
   tetracycline in treatment of, 76t
   treatment of infections caused by, 116–117, 117t
Streptococcus agalactiae
   aminoglycosides in treatment of, 205t
   aminopenicillins/β-lactamase inhibitor, 205t
   ampicillin/sulbactam in treatment of, 116–117, 117t, 204, *204*, 205t
   penicillin G in treatment of, 207t
   penicillin/β-lactamase inhibitor combinations, 116, 117t, 205t
Streptococcus mitis, 216
Streptococcus mutans, 216
Streptococcus pneumoniae, 18, 105, 107
   aminopenicillins in treatment of, 30t
   ampicillin in treatment of infection from, 113
   azithromycin in treatment of infection from, 114t
   CAP caused by, 187, 188t
   carbapenems in treatment of, 48t
   cefepime in treatment of infection from, 113–114, 114t
   cefotaxime in treatment of infection from, 203, 205t
   ceftriaxone in treatment of infection from, 113–114, 114t
   cefuroxime in treatment of infection from, 113–114, 114t
   cephalosporins in treatment of, 39t, 40t
   cephalosporins in treatment of infection from, 113–114, 114t
   cephalosporins plus β-lactamase inhibitor combinations in treatment of, 41t, 79t
   clindamycin in treatment of infection from, 114t
   daptomycin in treatment of, 54t, 58t
   doxycycline in treatment of infection from, 114t
   extended-spectrum penicillins in treatment of, 31t
   glycopeptides in treatment of, 205t
   linezolid in treatment of, 80t
   macrolides in treatment of, 72t, 202, 203t
   meningitis caused by, 36t, 38t, 204, *204*
   natural penicillins in treatment of, 28t
   otitis media caused by, 211, 211t
   penicillin-binding proteins produced by, 211
   penicillin G in treatment of infection from, 113
   penicillin in treatment of infection from, 113–114, 114t
   penicillin plus β-lactamase inhibitor combinations in treatment of, 32t
   quinolones in treatment of, 76t, 87, 91t, 92, 116–117, *116*, 117t
   sites of infections from, *113*
   sulfa drugs in treatment of infection from, 114t
   tetracyclines in treatment of infection from, 114t
   treatment of infections caused by, 113–115, 114t
   trimethoprim-sulfamethoxazole in treatment of infection from, 114, 114t
   vancomycin in treatment of, 203, *204*, 205t
Streptococcus pyogenes
   aminopenicillins in treatment of, 30t
   clindamycin in treatment of, 79t
   extended-spectrum penicillins in treatment of, 31t
   linezolid in treatment of, 80t
   macrolides in treatment of, 72t
   tetracycline in treatment of, 76t
Streptococcus sanguinis, 216
Streptococcus spp., intra-abdominal infections caused by, 227t
streptomycin, 67
   Brucella spp. infection treatment with, 162
   Francisella tularensis infection treatment with, 165, 165t
   mycobacterial infections treatment with, 97
sulbactam
   Acinetobacter spp. infection treatment with, 146
   Haemophilus influenzae infection treatment with, 143, 144t
   Moraxella catarrhalis infection treatment with, 145, 146t
sulfa drugs
   aerobic gram-negative bacteria caused infections treatment with, *101*
   antimicrobial activity of, 87t
   atypical bacteria caused infections treatment with, *101*
   Bordetella pertussis infection treatment with, 145t
   Brucella spp. infection treatment with, 163t
   cellulitis treatment with, 208t
   Citrobacter spp. infection treatment with, 128t
   dapsone, 85–89, 85t, *87*
   Enterobacter spp. infection treatment with, 128t
   Escherichia coli infection treatment with, 128t
   Haemophilus influenzae infection treatment with, 144t
   history of, 87
   Klebsiella spp. infection treatment with, 128t
   Moraxella catarrhalis infection treatment with, 146t
   Morganella spp. infection treatment with, 128t
   Proteus spp. infection treatment with, 128t
   Providencia spp. infection treatment with, 128t
   Salmonella enterica infection treatment with, 128t
   Serratia spp. infection treatment with, 128t
   Shigella spp. infection treatment with, 128t

Staphylococcus aureus infection treatment with, 110t
Streptococcus pneumoniae infection treatment with, 114, 114t
sulfisoxazole, 85, 85t
toxicity of, 88
trimethoprim-sulfamethoxazole, *85*, 85–89, 85t, 87t
Yersinia enterocolitica infection treatment with, 128t
sulfamethoxazole. *See also* trimethoprim-sulfamethoxazole
  structure of, *86*
sulfisoxazole, 85, 85t
Svedberg units (S), 8
syphilis, 169–170, *169*

T
tedizolid, 80–81
  cellulitis treatment with, 208t, *209*
  methicillin-resistant *Staphylococcus aureus* infection treatment with, 110t
telavancin, 53, 53t, 56
  cellulitis treatment with, 208, 208t
  methicillin-resistant *Staphylococcus aureus* infection treatment with, 110t
TEM-1, 129
tetracyclines
  aerobic gram-negative bacteria caused infections treatment with, *101*
  anaerobic bacteria caused infections treatment with, *102*
  antimicrobial activity of, 75t
  atypical bacteria caused infections treatment with, *103*
  Bordetella pertussis infection treatment with, 144, 145t
  Borrelia burgdorferi infection treatment with, 172t
  Campylobacter jejuni infection treatment with, 138, 139t
  CAP treatment with, 189t
  cellulitis treatment with, 208t, *209*
  Chlamydia spp. infection treatment with, 156, 157t
  doxycycline, 74
  eravacycline, 74–76, 74t
  Francisella tularensis infection treatment with, 165, 165t
  Haemophilus influenzae infection treatment with, 143, 143t
  Helicobacter pylori infection treatment with, 139, 140t
  Legionella spp. infection treatment with, 160, 161t
  Leptospira interrogans infection treatment with, 174t
  minocycline, 74, 74t
  Moraxella catarrhalis infection treatment with, 145, 146t
  Mycobacterium leprae infection treatment with, 182t
  Mycoplasma spp. infection treatment with, 158, 158t
  omadacycline, 74–76, 74t
  Rickettsia spp. infection treatment with, 166t, 167
  Staphylococcus aureus infection treatment with, 110t
  Streptococcus pneumoniae infection treatment with, 114, 114t
  structure of, *74*
  toxicity of, 76
  Treponema pallidum infection treatment with, 170, 170t
  Vibrio cholerae infection treatment with, 141, 141t
  Yersinia enterocolitica infection treatment with, 128t
tetracyclines plus aminoglycosides
  Brucella spp. infection treatment with, 163t
tetracyclines plus rifamycins
  Brucella spp. infection treatment with, 163t
tetrahydrofolate (THF), 85, 88
  bacterial synthesis of, 11, *11*
30S subunit, 8, *8*
tigecycline, 74, 74t, 75–76
  Acinetobacter spp. infection treatment with, 147, 147t
  Bacteroides spp. infection treatment with, 153, 154t
  Porphyromonas spp. infection treatment with, 153, 154t
  Prevotella spp. infection treatment with, 153, 154t
  structure of, *75*
  VRE infection treatment with, 121t
tobramycin, 67, 67t, 69
  Campylobacter jejuni infection treatment with, 138, 139t
  Citrobacter spp. infection treatment with, 128t, 130
  Enterobacter spp. infection treatment with, 128t, 130
  Escherichia coli infection treatment with, 127, 128t
  Klebsiella spp. infection treatment with, 127, 128t
  Moraxella catarrhalis infection treatment with, 145, 146t
  Morganella spp. infection treatment with, 128t, 130
  Proteus spp. infection treatment with, 127, 128t
  Providencia spp. infection treatment with, 128t, 130
  Pseudomonas aeruginosa infection treatment with, 132, 134t
  Serratia spp. infection treatment with, 128t, 130

transcription, 7–8
transfer RNA (tRNA), 8
translation, 8, *8*
Treponema pallidum
    macrolides in treatment of, 72t
    natural penicillins in treatment of, 28t
    sites of infections from, *169*
    treatment for infection with, 169–170, *169*, 170t
trimethoprim-sulfamethoxazole, 85–89, 85t
    acute uncomplicated cystitis treatment with, 194, 197t
    antimicrobial activity of, 87t
    Bordetella pertussis infection treatment with, 145t
    Brucella spp. infection treatment with, 162, 163t
    cellulitis treatment with, 208, 208t, *209*
    Citrobacter spp. infection treatment with, 128t, 130
    Enterobacter spp. infection treatment with, 128t, 130
    Escherichia coli infection treatment with, 127, 128t
    Haemophilus influenzae infection treatment with, 143, 144t
    inhibition of tetrahydrofolate synthesis by, *85*
    Klebsiella spp. infection treatment with, 127, 128t
    Moraxella catarrhalis infection treatment with, 145, 146t
    Morganella spp. infection treatment with, 128t, 130
    Proteus spp. infection treatment with, 127, 128t
    Providencia spp. infection treatment with, 128t, 130
    Salmonella enterica infection treatment with, 128t, 131
    Serratia spp. infection treatment with, 128t, 130
    Shigella spp. infection treatment with, 128t, 131
    Staphylococcus aureus infection treatment with, 112t
    Streptococcus pneumoniae infection treatment with, 114, 114t
    toxicity of, 88
    Yersinia enterocolitica infection treatment with, 128t
tRNA. *See* transfer RNA

U

uncomplicated acute pyelonephritis, 194
    activities of agents used to treat, *196*
    antimicrobial therapy for, 197, 197t
urinary tract infection (UTI)
    activities of agents used to treat
        complicated infections, *196*
        uncomplicated acute cystitis, *195*
        uncomplicated acute pyelonephritis, *196*
    antimicrobial therapy for, 197t
    bacterial causes of, 194, 195t
    complicated, 194, 195t, *196*, 197
    treatment of, 194–198, 197t
    uncomplicated, 194–197, *195*, 195t, *196*

V

vaginal discharge, pelvic inflammatory disease with, 199
vancomycin, 53, 53–55, 53t, 54t, *55*, 226
    anaerobic bacteria caused infections treatment with, *102*
    CAP treatment with, 189t
    cellulitis treatment with, 208t, 209
    Clostridia spp. infection treatment with, 151
    history of, 53
    infective endocarditis treatment with, 216, *217*, 217t, 218–221, 219t, 221t
    intravascular-related catheter infection treatment with, 223, *224*, 224t
    meningitis treatment with, 203t, *204*
    methicillin-resistant *Staphylococcus aureus* infection treatment with, 110t
    Streptococcus pneumoniae infection treatment with, 204, *204*, 205t
    VAP treatment with, 191t
Vancomycin-resistant enterococci (VRE), 119, 121t
Vibrio cholerae, infection treatment with, 141, 141t
Viridans streptococci
    aminopenicillins in treatment of, 30t
    cephalosporins in treatment of, 36t
    extended-spectrum penicillins in treatment of, 31t
    penicillin plus β-lactamase inhibitor combinations, 32t
ventilator-associated pneumonia (VAP)
    activities of agents used to treat, *192*
    bacterial causes of, 190, 191t
    defined, 190
    empiric therapy for, 191–193, 191–192t
    risk factors for, 191, 191–192t
viridans group streptococci
    aminopenicillins in treatment of, 30t
    carbapenems in treatment of, 48t
    cephalosporins in treatment of, 36t, 38t, 39t, 40t
    cephalosporins plus β-lactamase inhibitor combinations in treatment of, 41t
    clindamycin in treatment of, 79t
    daptomycin in treatment of, 58t
    extended-spectrum penicillins in treatment of, 31t
    glycopeptides in treatment of, 54t
    infective endocarditis caused by, 215, 216t, 217–218, 218t
    linezolid in treatment of, 80t
    macrolides in treatment of, 72t
    natural penicillins in treatment of, 28t
    penicillin plus β-lactamase inhibitor combinations in treatment of, 32t
    quinolones in treatment of, 91t
    tetracycline in treatment of, 76t
VRE. *See* Vancomycin-resistant enterococci

Y

Yersinia enterocolitica, 128t